Butterworths International Medical Reviews

*Ophthalmology 1*

# Disorders of the Vitreous, Retina and Choroid

Butterworths International Medical Reviews

*Ophthalmology*



*Next Volume in the Series*

Cataract Surgery

Butterworths
International
Medical
Reviews

# *Ophthalmology 1*

# Disorders of the Vitreous, Retina and Choroid

*Edited by*
**Jack J. Kanski,** FRCS
Consultant Surgeon
Prince Charles Eye Unit
King Edward VII Hospital
Windsor
Berkshire, UK

*and*

**Peter H. Morse,** MD, FACS
Professor of Ophthalmology
University of Chicago
Chicago
Illinois, USA

**Butterworths**
London Boston Durban
Singapore Sydney Toronto Wellington

First published 1983



**British Library Cataloguing in Publication Data**

Ophthalmology. – 1 – (Butterworths international medical reviews. Ophthalmology ISSN 0260-0145; 1)
1. Ophthalmology – Serials.
617′.7′005 RE1

ISBN 0-407-02340-2

Photoset by Butterworths Litho Preparation Department
Printed and bound in England by Robert Hartnoll Ltd., Bodmin, Cornwall

# Preface

This volume on disorders of the vitreous, retina and choroid initiates a series intended to keep the ophthalmologist up to date with recent advances as well as to stimulate thought on problems yet to be solved. We commence with the frequently overlooked evaluation of visual functions with a codified methodical approach. Other chapters on disorders of the retinal pigmented epithelium are of contemporary interest as the importance of the retinal pigmented epithelium in visual function is much more complex than hitherto imagined. Metabolic diseases and enzymatic deficiencies are also burgeoning in number and assume a critical importance, not only in research but also in clinical management.

We have included a condensation of the important points in scleral buckling operations for retinal separation, as well as the more difficult surgical techniques involved with the management of the giant retinal breaks, particularly with inverted flaps.

An enormous and rapidly expanding field was opened with the introduction of vitrectomy. The instruments used have many applications to the anterior segment as well as the posterior segment. The latter also involves removal of epiretinal membranes and also permits management of severe proliferative diabetic retinopathy, which was previously untreatable. The instrumentation for this type of surgery is quite important and therefore we have included a chapter discussing the development of these instruments.

Retinal vascular disease, its evaluation and treatment, such as the most commonly seen diabetes mellitus and retinal vein occlusion, is treated with photocoagulation which is eminently successful if applied at the appropriate stages of development of the disease.

Subretinal neovascular membranes associated with numerous ocular and systemic diseases are also discussed with respect to the natural history, modalities of treatment and in particular emphasizing the choice of laser wavelength, which is assuming increasing importance.

The topic of human chorioretinal biopsy either for diagnosis or resection of malignant tumours is a dramatic subject which we also felt should be discussed.

Finally, the advances in management of choroidal malignant melanoma and retinoblastoma are presented, as these are subjects in which there have been numerous recent revisions in thinking.

The authors in the current volume were selected as those actively involved in the investigation and treatment of the various diseases discussed. The scope of this book is not encyclopedic but rather addresses the various subjects which all ophthalmic surgeons encounter. Subsequent volumes will concentrate on different topics or further abbreviated advances in those already covered.

We feel that this is an exciting international co-operative venture comparing and digesting views from each side of the Atlantic, incorporating published and spoken communications in various subjects from the world at large.

It is hoped that all ophthalmologists reading these volumes will feel free to communicate their criticisms, reflections on the subject matter, and desires with respect to further coverage.

Jack Kanski
Peter Morse

# List of Contributors

*Rolf K. Blach*, MD, FRCS
Consultant Surgeon, Moorfields Eye Hospital, London, UK

*Janet V. Burch*, MD
Clinical Associate, Department of Ophthalmology and the Eye Research Laboratories, University of Chicago, Chicago, Illinois, USA

*Devron H. Char*, MD
Director, Ocular Oncology Unit and Associate Professor, Department of Ophthalmology and the Francis I. Proctor Foundation, University of California, San Francisco, California, USA

*Iain H. Chisholm*, MA, FRCS, DO
Southampton Eye Hospital;
Moorfields Eye Hospital, London, UK

*Robert J. Cooling*, FRCS
Senior Lecturer in Clinical Ophthalmology, Institute of Ophthalmology and Honorary Consultant Surgeon, Moorfields Eye Hospital, London, UK

*Jay L. Federman*, MD
Attending Surgeon; Professor of Ophthalmology, Thomas Jefferson Medical College, Pennsylvania, and Director of Research, Wills Eye Hospital, Philadelphia, Pennsylvania, USA

*Alistair Fielder*, FRCS
Reader in Ophthalmology, University of Leicester, and Honorary Consultant Ophthalmologist, Leicester Royal Infirmary, Leicester, UK

*List of contributors*

*H. MacKenzie Freeman*, MD
Associate Clinical Professor of Ophthalmology, Harvard Medical School; Vice-President, Eye Research Institute of Retina Foundation and Associate Surgeon in Ophthalmology, Massachusetts Eye and Ear Infirmary, Boston, Massachusetts, USA

*Rodney H. B. Grey*, MA, FRCS
Consultant Ophthalmic Surgeon, Bristol Eye Hospital and Clinical Teacher in Ophthalmology, University of Bristol, Bristol, UK

*A. M. Peter Hamilton*, FRCS
Honorary Consultant Surgeon, Moorfields Eye Hospital and Consultant Ophthalmologist, The Middlesex Hospital, London, UK

*Jack J. Kanski*, FRCS
Consultant Surgeon, Prince Charles Eye Unit, King Edward VII Hospital, Windsor, Berkshire, UK

*Marvin F. Kraushar*, MD, FACS, FICS
Clinical Associate Professor of Ophthalmology, The Mount Sinai Medical School, New York, and Chief, Retina Service, Department of Ophthalmology, Beth Israel Medical Center, New York, Retina Service, The Eye Institute, Saint Barnabas Medical Centre, Livingstone, New Jersery, USA

*David McLeod*, BSc, FRCS
Consultant Surgeon, Moorfields Eye Hospital, London and Recognized Teacher, University of London, London, UK

*Peter H. Morse*, MD, FACS
Chief, Retina Service, Department of Ophthalmology and Eye Research Laboratories, University of Chicago, Pritzker School of Medicine, Chicago, Illinois, USA

*Miriam E. Ridley*, MD, FRCS(C)
Lecturer, Department of Ophthalmology, University of Toronto, Retina-Vitreous Surgeon, Toronto General Hospital, Toronto, Ontario, Canada

*Charles L. Schepens*, MD
President and Founder, Eye Research Institute of Retina Foundation, Boston, Massachusetts; Clinical Professor, Department of Ophthalmology, Harvard Medical School and Senior Consulting Surgeon, Massachusetts Eye and Ear Infirmary, Boston, Massachusetts, USA

*Jeffrey L. Shakin*, MD
Assistant Attending Surgeon, Manhattan Eye, Ear and Throat Hospital, New York, USA

*John S. Shilling*, FRCS
Consultant Ophthalmic Surgeon, St. Thomas' Hospital, London, UK

*M. Madison Slusher*, MD, FACS
Attending Surgeon, Forsyth Memorial Hospital, Winston-Salem, North Carolina, USA

*David Taylor*, MRCP, FRCS
Consultant Ophthalmologist, Hospital for Sick Children, Great Ormond Street, and The National Hospital for Nervous Diseases, London; Honorary Senior Lecturer, University of London, UK

*Rodger Whitelocke*, PhD, FRCS
Consultant Ophthalmic Surgeon, St. Bartholomew's Hospital, London and Recognized Teacher in Ophthalmology, University of London, UK

# Contents

# 1
# Evaluation of retinal disease

Marvin F. Kraushar

When evaluating patients with posterior segment disease it is important for the clinician to have a well-planned sequence and to follow the same routine for each patient while making appropriate modifications as indicated by the results of each previous test. The initial examination should be simple, inexpensive, reliable and non-invasive.

## OFFICE EVALUATION

### History

Patients with posterior segment disorders typically present with visual loss or visual field defects, or entoptic phenomena such as photopsia and floaters. However, since the posterior segment can be visualized in eyes with clear media, a history is slightly less important to the ophthalmologist than to an internist.

### Ophthalmoscopy

Careful ophthalmoscopy is unquestionably the most useful means of evaluating posterior segment lesions. Unfortunately, it is frequently done without the compulsive attention to detail that is required.

Binocular indirect ophthalmoscopy (Kraushar, 1974) should be the first step in the examination. However, no matter how the examiner manipulates the condensing lens, the patient's eye, and his own head, to obtain additional information, the examination is incomplete without seleral indentation (Kraushar, 1979). This maneuver is indispensable in the evaluation of retinal detachment involving the ora serrata, cysts of the pars plana, and small peripheral retinal breaks in aphakic eyes. By using this dynamic examination technique, many lesions can be seen in profile and their true nature more clearly appreciated.

Binocular indirect ophthalmoscopy allows the examiner to perform ophthalmodynamometry without the help of an assistant. This is much more difficult to perform with the direct ophthalmoscope or with the slit-lamp and fundus contact lens because movements of the eye during compression usually cause the observer to lose the view of the optic disc and its vessels (*Figure 1.1*).

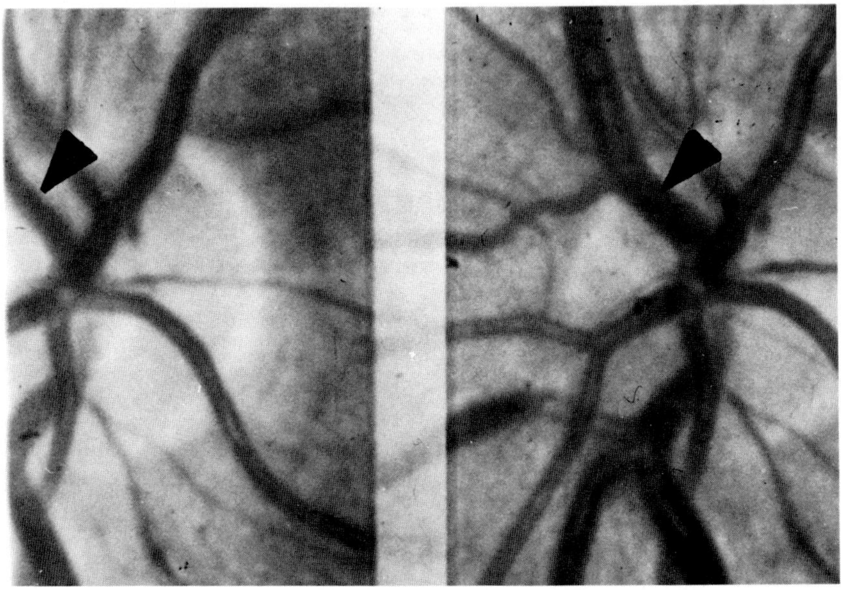

*Figure 1.1* Venous pulsation on the optic disc produced at diastole as visualized during ophthalmodynamometry

Direct ophthalmoscopy is useful for observing fine details of lesions previously detected with the indirect ophthalmoscope. It is not a suitable method for detecting large lesions since the diameter of the field is only slightly larger than that of the optic disc in an emmetropic eye. It is often helpful to examine highly myopic eyes through the patient's spectacles in order to avoid the greatly reduced field of view of the fundus caused by magnification.

## Slit-lamp biomicroscopy

If greater magnification is required the fundus should be examined using a slit-lamp and fundus contact lens. This is far superior to a Hruby lens and if a special contact lens holder with an built-on indentation tip is used, scleral depression can be performed simultaneously. The new fish-eye (Rodenstock) contact lens gives the same inverted view as the indirect ophthalmoscope but with a larger field. This lens is particularly useful for panretinal photocoagulation, laser treatment of tumors and photocoagulation of peripheral retinal lesions.

If doubt still remains as to the presence or absence of posterior segment disease, the macula and optic nerve can be evaluated more thoroughly with several other modalities readily availably in the office (Kraushar and Margolis, 1981).

## Monochromatic light

Ophthalmoscopy with monochromatic light makes subtle lesions easier to recognize than with standard illumination. Because shorter wavelengths of light (blue end of the spectrum) do not penetrate the retina well, they are most useful for examination of the inner retinal layers. Longer wavelengths (red end of the spectrum) penetrate the retina most deeply and are appropriate for examining the retinal pigmented epithelium and choroid. The best single wavelength for examining the retina is the green (red-free). Red-free filters are available in most ophthalmoscopes and slit-lamps. Red-free ophthalmoscopy is particularly useful in the detection of retinal nerve fiber bundle defects due to optic nerve disease. It is also excellent for visualization of the fundus through mild nuclear cataracts and vitreous hemorrhage. Lesions on the retinal surface such as wrinkling of the internal limiting membrane and foveal cysts are more readily seen with the aid of a red-free filter, and outlines of serous detachments of the sensory retina more sharply delineated.

## Color vision testing

Color vision tests can be used to screen and quantify congenital defects, and also to follow the clinical course of acquired lesions. Ishihara plates and the American Optical Hardy–Rand–Rittler plates primarily detect red–green defects. The Farnsworth–Munsell D-15 and D-10 hue tests are excellent for testing or quantifying both red–green and blue–yellow defects. The Nagel anomaloscope gives a more precise diagnosis of red–green color blindness and can detect female carriers.

Optic nerve lesions typically affect color vision very early. Thus, color desaturation in the absence of an obvious fundus lesion is very suggestive of optic nerve disease. However, defects in color vision due to macular disease are not often noted until the lesion is relatively advanced and easily detected ophthalmoscopically. Therefore, color vision testing is more helpful in detecting early optic nerve disease than in macular disease.

## Amsler grid

The Amsler grid is an easy and rapid screening test for macular and paramacular lesions. Using this test lesions can often be discovered before there is any discernible fundus abnormality. This test is particularly useful for detecting disorders that distort the orientation of the photoreceptors, such as serous or hemorrhagic detachment of the sensory retina, and preretinal macular fibrosis. Two of the most valuable uses of the Amsler grid are to detect recurrences of macular lesions in presumed ocular histoplasmosis and to detect early leakage from subretinal neovascular membranes in the fellow eyes of patients with disciform macular degeneration. The natural course of macular lesions can be followed by having the patient draw on the chart what he sees for comparison at a later date.

## Photostress test

The macular photostress test is a gross version of the dark adaptation test. It is a simple and reliable test by which one can detect the earliest stages of macular disease.

The test is based on the fact that when visual pigment is bleached by a light stimulus a temporary state of retinal insensitivity is produced which the patient perceives as a scotoma. The recovery of retinal sensitivity is dependent on the resynthesis of visual pigment by the photoreceptors. This requires healthy photoreceptors which must also be in apposition with the retinal pigmented epithelium. The ability of the photoreceptors to resynthesize visual pigment will therefore be adversely affected by degenerative diseases as well as disorders in which the photoreceptors are separated from the retinal pigmented epithelium.

When performing this test, the best corrected visual acuity is determined and then the patient fixates for 10 sec on a pocket flashlight held approximately 25 mm from the eye. The patient is then timed until he can read three letters on the pretest acuity line. The test is performed on both eyes separately and the results compared. A photostress recovery time (PSRT) greater than 50 sec is considered abnormal. Patients with early macular disease may require several minutes to recover their pretest visual acuity, whereas in patients with optic nerve disease the PSRT is within normal limits. By using this test it is also possible to detect the earliest stages of central serous choroidopathy, senile maculopathy and retinal drug toxicity. In addition, the test can be used to quantify progression or recovery in many of these diseases.

## Flying corpuscle test

The flying corpuscles (blue field entoptic) pheomenon consists of seeing one's own white blood cells travelling through the perifoveal capillaries. Perception of the 'flying corpuscles' is dependent upon intact photoreceptors and patent macular capillaries.

The physiological basis for the test is the fact that blue light is absorbed by the hemoglobin in the red blood cells but not by the white blood cells. The blue light that is not absorbed stimulates the photoreceptors. The white corpuscles are perceived as slightly elongated moving spots.

When performing this test a blue field entoptoscope is held close to the patient's eye, in alignment with the pupillary axis, and the patient is asked to describe what he sees.

A normal response is when the patient sees at least 15 corpuscles moving in a pulsatile manner in the entire visual field apart from the central area of fixation which corresponds to the capillary-free zone. In an abnormal response the patient reports that portions of the field are without corpuscles or when only a few corpuscles are seen. A low corpuscular speed and a uniform rather than pulsatile movement of the corpuscles is also abnormal.

This test is particularly well-suited in the detection of early macular disorders, retinal vascular disease and glaucoma. It is also extremely useful, and more accurate than color perception and two-point discrimination tests, in assessing potential visual function in eyes with opaque media. In these cases the intensity of the blue light has to be increased. A normal response indicates a visual capacity of at least 20/40.

### Contrast sensitivity gratings

Visual perception of complex images depends on the ability to detect differences in brightness between borders of adjacent contours. A measure of this visual function is called contrast sensitivity. Spatial frequency is a measure of spacing between contrasting borders of adjacent objects. The visual contrast sensitivity threshold can be clinically tested by changing the contrast (degree of whiteness-to-blackness) until the stripes vanish at each spatial frequency. By testing various combinations of spatial frequency and contrast a much broader range of visual function can be evaluated than by performing a simple Snellen visual acuity test.

Until recently, contrast sensitivity testing could be performed only in the laboratory using a bar pattern generated on an oscilloscope. Now this test can be performed in the office by utilizing a booklet of contrast sensitivity plates. Reduction of contrast sensitivity has been reported in very early diabetic retinopathy, glaucoma and neuro-ophthalmological diseases. Cystoid macular edema with normal vision is also associated with loss of contrast sensitivity.

If after the above tests have been performed and there is still doubt as to the presence or absence of posterior segment disease, or as to the exact nature of whatever disease may be present, it may be necessary to perform other more sophisticated tests.

## SPECIAL INVESTIGATIONS

### Fluorescein angiography

Retinal fluorescein angiography is one of the most important advances in the field of ophthalmology in recent decades. It has provided the ophthalmologist with insight into the pathophysiology of many disease states and it is an invaluable teaching aid for demonstrating disease processes.

Retinal fluorescein angiography, however, should not be thought of as primarily a diagnostic modality because most fundus lesions can be accurately diagnosed without resorting to this invasive test. Occasionally, however, a diagnosis cannot be made by any other means and it is appropriate to do a fluorescein study. In clinical practice the primary use of fluorescein angiography is to identify diseases requiring laser photocoagulation. The test is also extremely useful in locating the area to be treated and also assessing the efficacy of treatment.

## Hypofluorescence

Hypofluorescence may be due either to a vascular filling defect or blocking of fluorescence. In vascular filling defects fluorescence is absent because the obstructed vessel is unable to carry dye to its normal location. This may be due to branch or central obstruction of retinal arterioles or veins, or capillary non-perfusion. Hypofluorescence due to blockage of normal fluorescence is caused by a pathological process between the fluorescein dye and the camera. This occurs by retinal edema, blood exudate or other fluid, as well as excessive pigment in the retina or choroid.

The normal macula is hypofluorescent and appears black on the angiogram. This is because of the avascularity of the foveal zone, the greater concentration of pigment granules in the retinal pigmented epithelium at the macula, and the presence of xanthophyll pigment at the macula.

## Hyperfluorescence

Hyperfluorescence may be due to a window defect (Keno and Green, 1978) in the retinal pigmented epithelium which allows increased transmission of background choroidal fluorescence. Window defects in eyes with drusen or toxic maculopathies appear early because the dye reaches the choroid before it reaches the central retinal artery (*Figure 1.2*). No change in size is noted in the hyperfluorescent area with the passage of time (*Figure 1.3*).

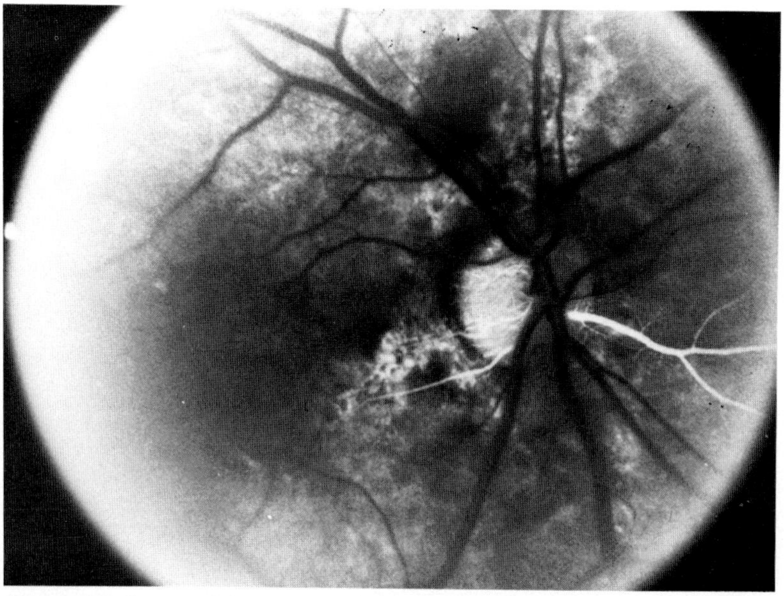

*Figure 1.2* Prearterial stage of retinal fluorescein angiography. Two cilioretinal arterioles have filled and there is early choroidal fluorescence

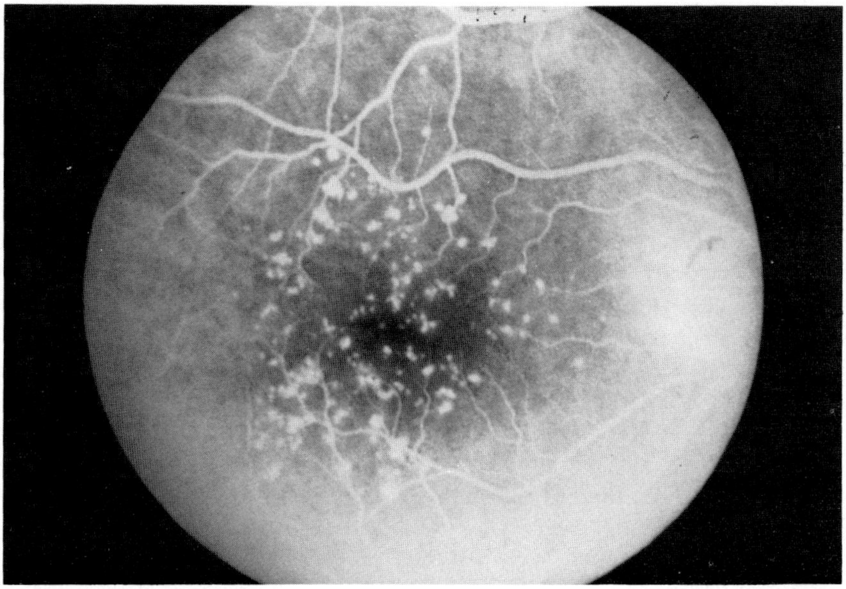

*Figure 1.3* Late-stage angiogram showing transmitted fluorescence from defects in the retinal pigmented epithelium from drusen. The hyperfluorescent defects are sharply outlined, of constant size and do not become confluent

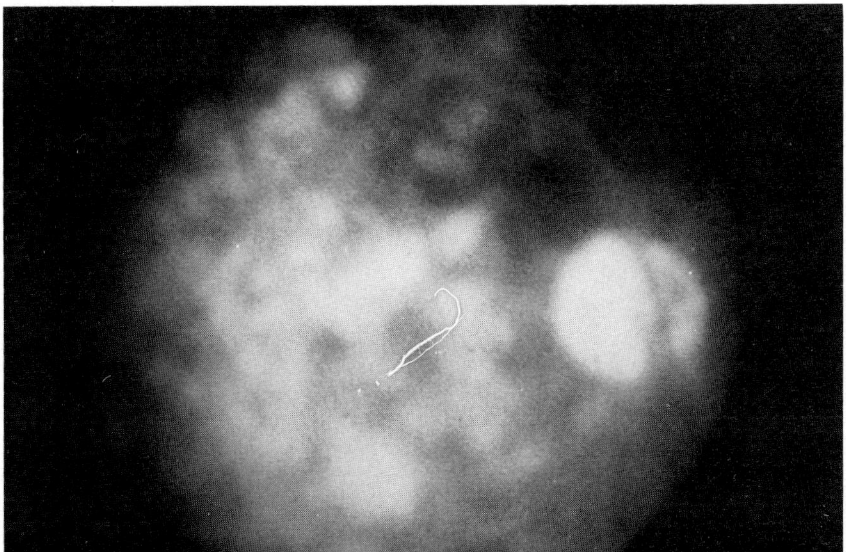

*Figure 1.4* Late stage angiogram showing leakage from microaneurysms. The areas of hyperfluorescence have enlarged, have indistinct borders and are becoming confluent (compare with *Figure 1.3*)

Hyperfluorescence may also be caused by vascular abnormalities such as microaneurysms (*Figure 1.4*), collaterals, and new vessels as in proliferative diabetic retinopathy or choroidal neovascularization. Abnormal vessels will fluoresce early and the hyperfluorescent area will expand with the passage of time and will have indistinct borders. Leaks generally appear in the late stages of an angiogram and can be divided into the subcategories of pooling and tissue staining. Pooling may be either preretinal (intravitreal), intraretinal in the outer plexiform layer, or subretinal under the sensory retina or under the retinal pigmented epithelium. When leaking from optic disc neovascularization occurs into the vitreous it will expand continuously with indistinct borders since it is not in a confined space. When pooling is intraretinal as in cystoid macular edema it usually occurs in multiple discrete foci which expand with the passage of time and tend to become confluent. Pooling under the sensory retina as in central serous choroidopathy has an initial patchy distribution with sharp borders since it is confined to a definite anatomical space. As time progresses it will become more homogenous and more intense. Pooling under the retinal pigmented epithelium is generally homogeneous from the onset because it is in a confined space wherein the first drop of dye is sufficient to fill the entire area. As time progresses this area will fluoresce more intensely but will not expand. Tissue staining is a late phenomenon wherein the dye is bound to collagen in normal or pathologic ocular tissues. This includes structures such as the lamina cribosa, optic-nerve drusen, choroidal ruptures, and fibrotic disciform scars.

To alleviate expense and inconvenience to the patient it may on occasion be appropriate to perform fluorescein angioscopy in the office using a cobalt blue filter. Oral fluorescein may be administered to children, patients with inaccessible veins and those with a history of mild reaction to dye by the intravenous route. A dose of 1 g/50 kg of body weight is given and photography is done at 30 and 60 min. The detail will not be as fine as when fluorescein is administered intravenously. Foci of leakage can be identified but cannot be localized sharply enough for accurate laser treatment. The main clinical indication for oral fluorescein is the confirmation of leaks such as cystoid macular edema, or papilledema. In such instances the diagnosis can be confirmed with a high degree of confidence.

Fundus photography should be performed on all patients with choroidal nevi or suspected malignant melanomas. This is the only accurate method of determining a change in the appearance of the smallest lesions with the passage of time. Also the discovery of so-called 'double circulation' caused by visualization of the tumor vessel may be helpful in diagnosis.

## Electroretinography

### Standard electroretinogram

The electroretinogram (ERG) waveform consists of the summation of electrical activity from different layers of the retina in response to a light stimulus. In the normal healthy eye the electroretinogram response takes place in less than a quarter of a second. The α-wave has negative polarity and originates from the rods and cones. The β-wave has positive polarity and originates from the Müller cells. By altering the intensity of light as well as by using colored filters and single flashes it is possible to selectively stimulate either the rod or cone system. Rod function is tested in a scotopic, dark-adapted state, and the cones are tested in a light-adapted, photopic state. Because the electroretinogram is a mass retinal response, disease processes must involve a large portion of the retina before the electroretinogram is affected.

### Focal electroretinogram

The focal electroretinogram is a test which can be restricted to one area of the macula. This requires computed summation of the electrical response which is minimal since only a small area of the retina is stimulated. At present this is such a complex procedure that few centers are capable of the sophistication required.

### Early receptor potential

The early receptor potential occurs almost simultaneously with the flash of the electroretinogram and at least 1 ms before the onset of the α-wave. Although it has been applied with some success to studies of widespread retinal degenerations, it is not currently considered to be a useful diagnostic modality.

## Electro-oculography

The electro-oculogram (EOG) records alterations in corneo-retinal standing potential. Like the electroretinogram it is a mass retinal response. The standing potential of the eye requires a healthy choriocapillaris, intact retinal pigmented epithelium intracellular junctions, and a healthy retinal pigmented epithelium–photoreceptor complex. The measurements are made in both the light-adapted and dark-adapted states and their ratio is expressed as a fraction. The origins of the light-induced voltage changes are not clear. There are certain eye diseases with inexplicable electro-oculogram findings. For example, a reduced electro-oculogram has been noted in patients with vitelliform macular dystrophy, occasionally in fundus flavimaculatus, and malignant melanoma, despite the fact that there is no clinical evidence of widespread disease of the retinal pigmented epithelium in any of these disorders.

## Dark adaptometry

Dark adaptometry is useful in evaluating patients with night blindness. The result is a two-part response which can be recorded from the peripheral or central retina. This is essentially a qualitative and not a quantitative test.

## Fundus reflectometry

Fundus reflectometry compares the reflectivity of the dark-adapted fundus with the change in reflectivity after the eye is exposed to an intense bleaching by light. This can be done in the peripheral retina to assess the density of the rod pigment, or at the fovea to assess the cone pigment. This test provides valuable data regarding photoregeneration of retinal pigment, particularly in patients with night blindness.

## Visually evoked cortical potential

The visually evoked cortical potential (VECP) (VEP) (VER – visual evoked response) is a summation of the electrical signals generated by the occipital cortex in response to light stimulation of the retina. It can assess the integrity of the visual pathway from the macula to the visual cortex. Because the response of the visually evoked potential is so small, a computer is required to produce an interpretable waveform. The primary use of the visually evoked potential is to assess macular function or to detect optic nerve disease. In the presence of opacities in the ocular media a bright light is required to stimulate the retina. A more effective pattern-reversal stimulus such as an alternating checkerboard may be used in the patient with clear media. A normal visually evoked potential response suggests normal macular, optic nerve and visual pathway function. Compressive lesions of the optic pathway alter the appearance of the waveform, whereas demyelinating diseases alter the impulse conduction time of the visually evoked potential through the visual pathway. This is also an excellent test for ruling out malingering or hysteria.

## Ultrasonography

Ultrasonography may be helpful in differentiating lesions which are visible ophthalmoscopically. Deep drusen of the optic nerve and calcification within a retinoblastoma may be detected at reduced sound levels. Tumors may usually be differentiated from hemorrhage by ultrasonography (*Figure 1.5*). This modality is often helpful in detecting an increase in tumor size which may necessitate theraputic intervention, or a decrease in tumor size as a response to therapy.

Radioisotope studies may be extremely useful in the diagnosis of intraocular tumors. These findings, when combined with ultrasonography, fluorescein angiography and ophthalmoscopy often help to confirm the diagnosis.

## EVALUATION OF EYES WITH OPAQUE MEDIA

An attempt should be made to evaluate the posterior segment in all patients with opaque media. In such cases it is essential to rule out the presence of retinal disease which may preclude a useful visual result after anterior segment surgery. A patient with an immature cataract may have a suspicious-appearing macula which cannot be adequately evaluated by objective means such as ophthalmoscopy or slit-lamp and contact lens examination.

In the presence of advanced macular degeneration there will be a reduction of the direct pupillary response to light (Marcus Gunn reaction) (Newsome, Milton and Gass, 1981). As has been mentioned earlier, the flying corpuscles test is helpful in evaluating macular function in eyes with a moderately opaque media. Laser interferometry (Green and Cohen, 1971) may be useful in patients with immature cataract. A grating of alternating parallel light and dark bars is projected on to the macula through the least dense portion of the cataract. The visual acuity of the patient can be assessed by determining the narrowest width of alternating light and dark bars that can be perceived.

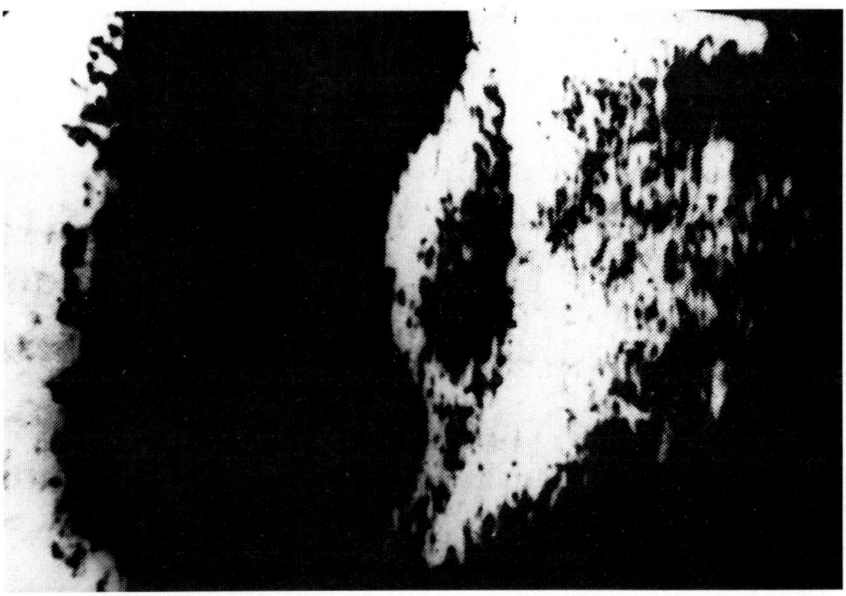

*Figure 1.5* B-mode ultrasonogram showing typical changes of a tumor. There is a sharp anterior border echo, hollowing of the internal portion of the lesion and shadowing of the orbital fat echo. This lesion was histologically proven to be a malignant choroidal melanoma

When the media are too opaque to permit the use of subjective tests, A and B mode ultrasonography can be helpful in ruling out vitreous hemorrhage, tumor, and retinal detachment. Fundus lesions which are elevated at least 1 mm may be identified with ultrasonography. Ultrasonography may define the location, thickness, shape, distribution and surface configuration of intraocular lesions. In patients with extremely dense vitreous hemorrhage a bright-flash electroretinogram (Fuller, Knighton and Machemer, 1975) can determine whether the retina is sufficiently viable to consider complicated surgery in eyes with severe diabetic retinopathy or excessive trauma. X-ray studies may be used to establish the presence and location of intraocular calcium and foreign bodies. Computerized tomography (CT) is even more valuable with respect to precise localization.

## References

Fuller, D. G., Knighton, R. W. and Machemer, R. (1975) Bright-flash electroretinography for the evaluation of eyes with opaque vitreous. *American Journal of Ophthalmology*, **80,** 214–223

Green, D. G. and Cohen, M. M. (1971) Laser interferometry in the evaluation of potential macular function in the presence of opacities in the ocular media. *Transactions of the American Academy of Ophthalmology and Otolaryngology*, **75,** 629–637

Keno, D. D. and Green, W. R. (1978) Retinal pigment epithelial window defect. *Archives of Ophthalmology*, **96,** 854–856

Kraushar, M. F. (1974) Simplified binocular indirect opthalmoscopy as a routine office procedure. *Annals of Ophthalmology*, **6,** 475–485

Kraushar, M. F. (1979) Learning scleral depression with binocular indirect ophthalmoscopy. *American Journal of Ophthalmology*, **87,** 97–99

Kraushar, M. F. and Margolis, S. (1981) Why can't my patient see 20/20?: simplifed evaluation of macular function. *Perspectives in Ophthalmology*, **4,** 289–296

Newsome, D. A., Milton, R. C. and Gass, J. D. M. (1981) Afferent pupillary defect in macular degeneration. *American Journal of Ophthalmology*, **92,** 396–402

# 2
# Laser treatment of macular disease: is the choice of wavelength important?

Charles L. Schepens

## INTRODUCTION

Macular photocoagulation of subretinal new vessels requires the use of a laser because it is the only known light source capable of causing retinal burns nearly as small as 50 μ. Xenon arc photocoagulation does not generate an energy density sufficient to obtain burns this small. Practically, lasers that are available for fundus photocoagulation operate with either argon or krypton. Each laser source produces a number of discrete wave bands in the visible spectrum, some of which are powerful enough to be easily used in photocoagulation (*Table 2.1*).

*Table 2.1* Laser wavelengths (in nm) usable in photocoagulation

| *Source* | *Blue** | *Green* | *Yellow* | *Red** |
|---|---|---|---|---|
| Argon | 476.5<br>488.0<br>496.5 | 514.5 | None | None |
| Krypton | None | 530.9 | 568.2 | 647.1<br>676.4 |

* The main wavelength in blue is 488.0 nm, and in red 647.1 nm

This chapter is divided into two parts – physical properties of light that are important in laser photocoagulation, and clinical considerations.

## PHYSICAL PROPERTIES OF LIGHT

Photocoagulation near or in the macula must destroy abnormal tissue but disturb neighboring structures only minimally. Since the effect of a strong beam of light on eye tissue varies according to its wavelength, it is important to determine the most efficient wavelength for use in the macular area. In this respect three properties of light are relevant: scattering, absorption by pigment and phototoxicity.

## Scattering of light

Scattering occurs when a light beam hits particles whose refractive index is different from that of the interstitial medium. Clinicians see this phenomenon when they examine the transparent ocular media with the slit-lamp; it is called the Tyndall effect. The scattered light is deviated away from the light beam and thus represents a loss in the beam intensity. Light scattering depends on the size and separation of the scattering particles. If the particles and their spacing are smaller than a light wavelength, scattering varies inversely with the fifth power of the wavelength ($S = 1/\lambda^5$). This is the type of scattering that occurs in a normal cornea (Feuk, 1970, 1971; Feuk and McQueen, 1971), and there are indications that it follows the same law in the other transparent media. This type of scattering is maximal with the blue light of argon; it is 23% less with the green light of argon, 35% less with the green light of krypton, 53% less with the yellow light of krypton, and 76% less with the red light of krypton. Thus, to obtain the delivery of equal energies per unit of area at the pigmented epithelium, one requires about twice as much blue light as yellow light delivered to the cornea, and about four times as much blue light as red light. In addition, it must be remembered that the intensity of scattering increases with the patient's age, particularly as a result of normal lens changes.

## Light absorption by pigment

Three types of pigment in the eye can absorb enough light to cause a burn: melanin, hemoglobin and xanthophyll. Light absorption in the photopigments of the visual receptors contributes little to a fundus burn.

Melanin is present in the retinal pigmented epithelium and the choroid. Because the latter is much thicker than the former, more heat can be developed by light absorption in the choroid than in the pigmented epithelium. The short wavelengths

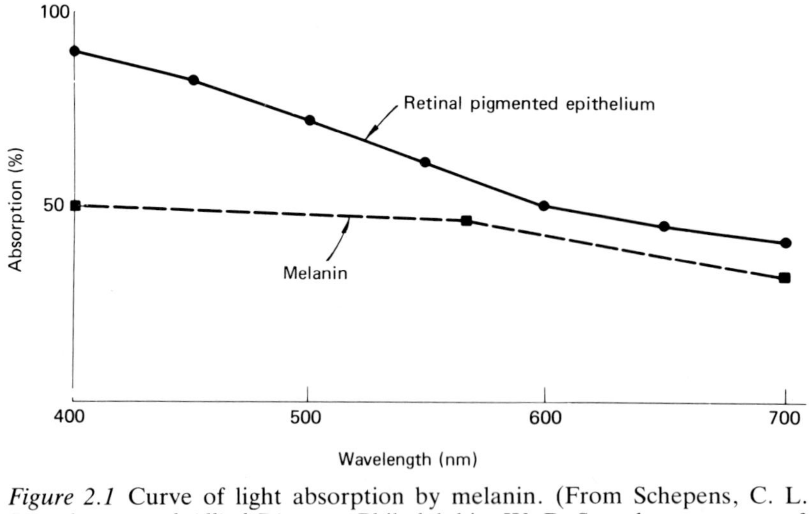


*Figure 2.1* Curve of light absorption by melanin. (From Schepens, C. L. (1983) *Retinal Detachment and Allied Diseases*, Philadelphia: W. B. Saunders, courtesy of the Publishers)

are absorbed better by the melanin than are the longer wavelengths, but the difference is not very marked (*Figure 2.1*). What is more important to consider is the variable density of pigmentation in the pigmented epithelium and choroid. Absorption of visible light in a darkly pigmented fundus is about twice that in a pale fundus (Geeraets *et al.*, 1962).

Hemoglobin does not absorb red wavelengths (Van Assendelft, 1970). It absorbs argon blue and green well, but its most avid absorption is in the krypton green and yellow (*Figure 2.2*).

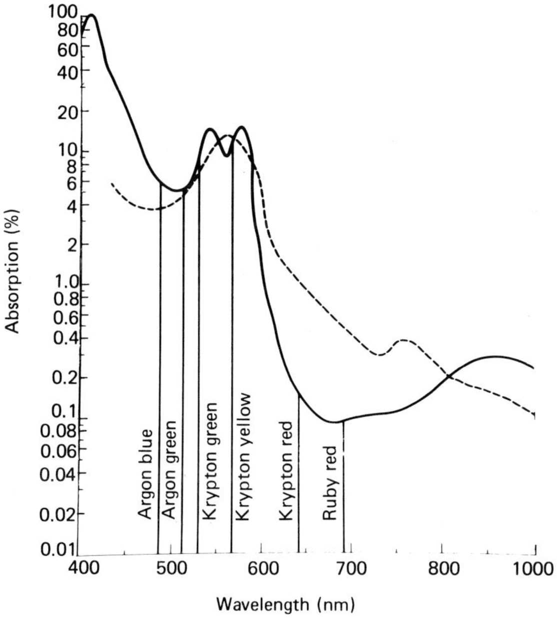


*Figure 2.2* Curves of light absorption by hemoglobin. Solid line, absorption by oxyhemoglobin; dashed line, absorption by reduced hemoglobin. Absorption scale is logarithmic. (From Schepens, C. L. (1983) *Retinal Detachment and Allied Diseases*, Philadelphia: W. B. Saunders, courtesy of the Publishers)

Xanthophyll is the yellow pigment that is present in the inner layers of the macula (*Figure 2.3*). A similar pigment also appears in the lens of subjects over 40 years of age. Xanthophyll absorbs the blue light of argon about eight times more avidly than its green component (Wald, 1945). Absorption of longer wavelengths by xanthophyll is negligible (*Figure 2.4*).

The above data indicate that before reaching the fundus a light beam is weakened by scattering in the transparent media and, in older patients, by absorption due to xanthophyll in the lens (Boettner and Wolter, 1962). Thus, light transmission to the fundus is much poorer for blue light than for longer wavelengths. For instance, in young patients 60% of the krypton red light is transmitted to the fundus, but only 48% of the argon blue (Delori, 1981). Transmission of argon blue light to the fundus is almost five times less in old than in young patients, whereas for krypton red it is only 1.5 times less (*Table 2.2*).

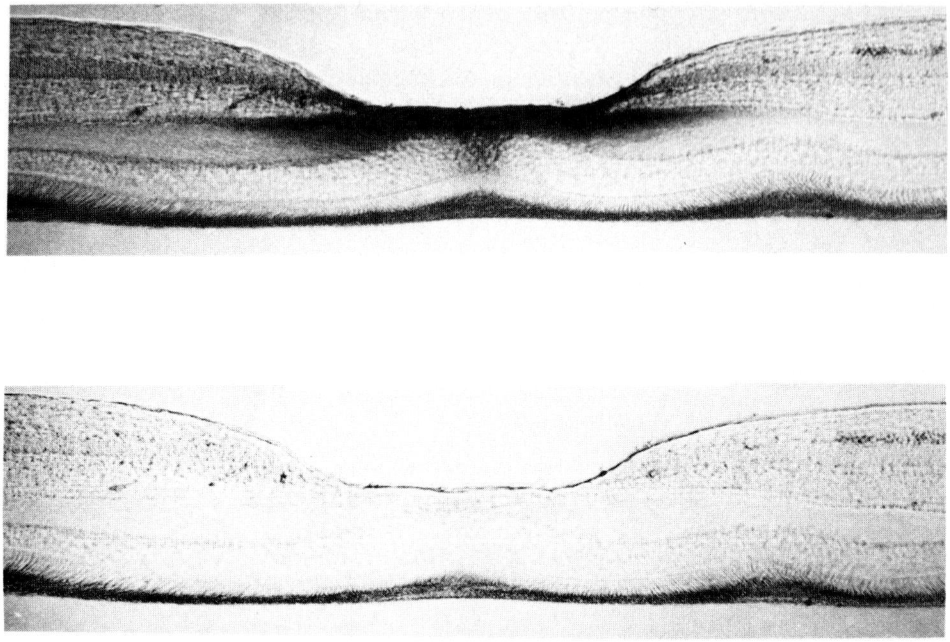

*Figure 2.3* Cross-section of macular area. *Above*, viewed in blue light; dark zone in inner retinal layers indicates location of xanthophyll. *Below*, macular area viewed with yellow light is transparent (courtesy of D. M. Snodderly)

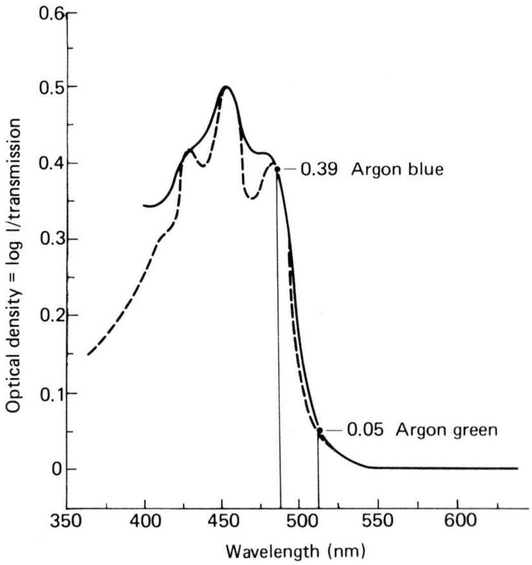


*Figure 2.4* Curves of light absorption by xanthophyll. Solid line, absorption by macular xanthophyll; dashed line, absorption by crystalline xanthophyll. Absorption of argon blue light is about eight times that of argon green (logarithmic scale). (From Schepens, C. L. (1983) *Retinal Detachment and Allied Diseases*, Philadelphia: W. B. Saunders, courtesy of the Publishers)

## Phototoxicity

Phototoxicity is manifested by light damage to the visual cells that may occur in addition to or even in the absence of a burn. The lesions produced by sun-gazing or in eclipse retinitis are phototoxic rather than thermal (Ham *et al.*, 1979). The relation between wavelength and phototoxicity has been well studied (Ham, Mueller and Sliney, 1976). To produce a threshold retinal lesion, namely, one that is barely visible clinically, the amount of light needed, measured at the cornea, is 1000 times less for 441 nm, which causes a predominantly phototoxic effect, than for 1064 nm, which produces an exclusively thermal effect (Ham *et al.*, 1979).

*Table 2.2* Light transmission through ocular media

| *Source* | *Wavelength (nm)* | *Per cent transmission in young subjects* | *Decreased transmission in old compared with young subjects* |
|---|---|---|---|
| Argon | 488.0 (blue) | 48 | 4.8X |
| | 514.5 (green) | 52 | 2.6X |
| Krypton | 530.9 (green) | 55 | 2.3X |
| | 568.2 (yellow) | 58 | 1.7X |
| | 647.1 (red) | 60 | 1.5X |

The phototoxic effect increases steadily through the spectrum of the wavelengths of light, being almost absent at 1064 nm and very strong at 441 nm. At 488 nm, the effect is largely phototoxic but there is also a thermal element. For 514.5 nm and longer wavelengths, the effect is preponderantly thermal (Ham *et al.*, 1979). The mechanism of the phototoxic effect is unknown, but it is accelerated by a rise in temperature in the retina and seems to affect primarily the melanin granules (Ham *et al.*, 1980).

In a study of the macular photoreceptors, it was demonstrated that intense blue light destroys permanently the blue-sensitive cones (Sperling and Harwerth, 1972; Harwerth and Sperling, 1975). In contrast, intense green light causes only temporary damage to the green-sensitive cones. In fact, exposure of the macula to green or red light that is 20 times more intense than a cone-destroying dose of blue light fails to destroy green- or red-sensitive cones.

## CLINICAL CONSIDERATIONS

In laser treatment of the macular area, the primary goal is to arrest or improve the visual damage caused by subretinal neovascularization. It is hoped that this is accomplished by permanent closure of the new vessels, with minimal damage to macular or paramacular structures. Successful treatment should bring about improvement or at least stabilization of the visual acuity and of the size of the paracentral scotoma. A choice must be made among the five available wavelengths of argon and krypton lasers. At the short end of the spectrum is the argon blue light, and at the long end, the krypton red. In between are argon green, krypton green, and krypton yellow.

## The worst choice: blue light

The most popular machine presently used for laser treatment is a bichromatic argon laser in which about 70% of the energy is blue light and about 30% green light. The instrument is bichromatic because it does not deliver enough energy in either color to be clinically effective. The laser beam forms two foci in the fundus. If one focus happens to be on the pigmented epithelium, the other will necessarily be either in the choroid or in the retina. These are not optimal physical conditions for photocoagulation of subepithelial new vessels.

The data presented in the previous section make it clear that blue light is the worst possible wavelength for macular photocoagulation. The reasons for this lie in its scattering properties, its strong absorption by macular and lens xanthophyll, and its phototoxicity. Clinical considerations resulting from the physical properties of blue light are summarized as follows:

### Effect on cornea and lens

As a result of the strong scattering of argon blue and its absorption by crystalline and macular xanthophyll, more blue light than any other available wavelength must be delivered to the cornea to obtain an adequate burn in the fundus. This is particularly true in patients over 40 years of age. The great majority of patients with new vessels under the pigmented epithelium are in this older age group. Consequently, a statistically significant decrease of the corneal endothelial cell population may occur. Such an effect was documented in panphotocoagulation with a bichromatic (predominantly blue) laser (Pardos and Krachmer, 1981). Aging not only increases the scattering properties of the transparent media but it also causes the appearance of lens xanthophyll, which absorbs blue light avidly. Absorption of blue light by the lens xanthophyll may warm the lens enough to accelerate the development of cataract. In addition, aging often causes not only a marked increase in the scattering by the lens but also lens opacities or premature nuclear sclerosis, which render laser photocoagulation difficult with any laser wavelength but frequently impossible with blue light.

Theoretically, the intensity of a blue laser beam needed for adequate photocoagulation is 4.8 times greater in an old than in a young patient (Delori, 1981). This difference decreases gradually with increasing wavelength (*see Table 2.2*). Clinical observations in patients 65 years old and over with diabetic retinopathy confirm these facts. With the green light of an argon laser an adequate reaction was visible with 70 mw, whereas under the same conditions in the same eye, 230 mw of blue argon light was required (Pomerantzeff *et al.*, 1976).

### Effect on the retina

Once the beam reaches the retina, two burn foci tend to develop, because available blue lasers are bichromatic, and, most important, because the absorption of blue light by macular xanthophyll causes a second burn focus in the inner retinal layers (*see Figure 2.3*). The result of this phenomenon is that, when treating through macular xanthophyll, a blue beam is attentuated by 50% (Ham *et al.*, 1979). The xanthophyll-induced burn, which increases in intensity as the beam nears the fovea, has two severe disadvantages. First, it has been implicated as a potential cause of postoperative foveal denervation and intraretinal fibrosis (Marshall, Hamilton and Bird, 1974; Marshall and Bird, 1979). Second, the white retinal burns produced by argon blue light impede immediate re-treatment of subretinal vessels in the same locus. Then, for many days after treatment, these white burns hinder angiographic observation of residual or recrudescent new vessels. One is therefore obliged to wait several weeks to obtain a clear angiographic picture and be able to re-treat a previously treated area that needs it.

Another disadvantage of the use of blue light is its phototoxicity for the retina. Of all the wavelengths available for laser treatment, blue is by far the most phototoxic, especially to blue-sensitive cones. The latter are concentrated in the macular area. Experimental proof is still lacking that phototoxicity unnecessarily damages macular function when treating subretinal neovascularization near the fovea with blue light. However, until the phototoxic effects of blue light have been proven harmless in macular laser treatment, there is no excuse for using it. There is no evidence that phototoxicity can cause or even contribute to the obliteration of subepithelial new vessels. In conclusion, blue light offers many disadvantages and not a single advantage for the treatment of macular disease.

## Possible usefulness of red light

Krypton red has several advantages over blue light. It is scattered four times less during the intraocular transit. This property allows effective treatment even through a thin layer of preretinal blood. However, such a circumstance is probably less frequent in patients with treatable disciform degeneration of the macula than in those with treatable diabetic retinopathy. Since krypton red is practically not absorbed by xanthophyll, it does not produce a second burn in the inner macular layers, nor does it heat the lens of older patients. Therefore, early post-treatment fluorescein angiography and early re-treatment are possible following the use of red krypton light. Finally, it has the least photochemical effect of all the wavelengths available for laser treatment.

Red light, however, has one severe disadvantage as it is not absorbed by blood (*see Figure 2.2*). This creates several problems:

(1) Its thermal effects result solely from absorption of light by melanin in the pigmented epithelium and choroid. Because of irregularities in fundus pigmentation, the variability of the fundus burns is three times greater with krypton red than with shorter wavelengths that show significant absorption by hemoglobin (Pomerantzeff and Delori, 1968).
(2) Since the burns are due solely to absorption by melanin in the pigmented epithelium and choroid, the burns are located in the deeper layers of the fundus and affect the choroid more than do burns caused by shorter wavelengths. As a result, they are less prominent ophthalmoscopically and, clinically, their intensity is harder to evaluate. The latter factor, combined with the greater absorption variability of kryton red, is responsible for reports of the increased frequency of hemorrhage with krypton red photocoagulation. The same problem was noted years ago with ruby lasers. Such hemorrhages are often small but, when they occur near the fovea, they may have catastrophic effects on central vision.
(3) A subretinal hemorrhage caused by a laser application may keep increasing during treatment; it cannot be stopped by additional treatment with krypton red but is generally stopped promptly with a laser light of any other color.
(4) The deeper lesions of krypton red are often more painful. This can be offset by retrobulbar anesthesia, but in the combined experience of my associates and myself, repeated laser treatments at short intervals are often indicated. We think that to associate multiple re-treatments at short intervals with retrobulbar anesthesia is unacceptable because retrobulbar injection is painful and potentially dangerous.

## What is the best wavelength?

The foregoing considerations indicate that the best wavelength for the treatment of macular subretinal neovascularization must be in the middle of the spectrum. Of the three middle wavelengths now available – argon green (514.5 nm), krypton green (530.9 nm), and krypton yellow (568.2 nm) – the latter appears to be the most suitable, at least on theoretical grounds. When comparing the physical properties of these three wavelengths, the following facts become apparent:

(1) Krypton yellow is the least scattered by the transparent media.
(2) It is the best transmitted to the fundus (*see Table 2.2*).
(3) It is the most transparent to xanthophyll (*see Figures 2.3* and *2.4*).
(4) Along with krypton green, krypton yellow is best absorbed by blood (*see Figure 2.2*).

Krypton green appears preferable to argon green because its transmission through the transparent media and its absorption by blood are superior. Also, its absorption by xanthophyll is less than for argon green.

The advantage of argon green is that we already have a solid amount of experience with it; my associates and I have used it for 10 years. In a recent review of 74 consecutive patients who showed decreased visual acuity due to subretinal neovascularization in the macular area, Trempe was able to close the new vessels in 93% of the cases, stabilize or decrease the paracentral scotoma in 76%, and stabilize or improve visual acuity in 70% (Trempe *et al.*, 1982). In an earlier study, Bird (1974) reported similar though somewhat less favorable results. However, his criteria for patient selection were not identical with Trempe's and he used a bichromatic (blue/green) argon laser for treatment. The Retina Associates are currently carrying out an analogous program using krypton yellow, with encouraging results. However, the number of cases is yet too small to be statistically significant. Longer experience will tell whether krypton yellow, in our hands, is more effective than argon green.

## References

Bird, A. C. (1974) Recent advances in the treatment of senile disciform macular degeneration by photocoagulation. *British Journal of Ophthalmology*, **58,** 367–376

Boettner, E. A. and Wolter, J. R. (1962) Transmission of the ocular media. *Investigative Ophthalmology*, **1,** 776–783

Delori, F. C. (1981) Physics of photocoagulation. Optical properties of ocular tissues. In *Ninth Annual Course, Practical Aspects of Photocoagulation*, I-1 to I-6. Boston: Eye Research Institute of Retina Foundation

Feuk, T. (1970) On the transparency of the stroma in the mammalian cornea. *IEEE Transactions on Bio-Medical Engineering*, **BME–17,** 186–190

Feuk, T. (1971) The wavelength dependence of scattered light intensity in rabbit corneas. *IEEE Transactions on Bio-Medical Engineering*, **BME–18,** 92–96

Feuk, T. and McQueen, D. (1971) The angular dependence of light scattered from rabbit corneas. *Investigative Ophthalmology*, **10,** 294–299

Geeraets, W. J., Williams, R. C., Chan, G., Ham, W. T. Jr., Guerry, D. III and Schmidt, F. H. (1962) The relative absorption of thermal energy in retina and choroid. *Investigative Ophthalmology*, **1,** 340–347

Ham, W. T. Jr., Mueller, H. A., Ruffalo, J. J. Jr. and Clarke, A. M. (1979) Sensitivity of the retina to radiation damage as a function of wavelength. *Photochemistry and Photobiology*, **29,** 735–743

Ham, W. T., Mueller, H. A. and Sliney, D. H. (1976) Retinal sensitivity to damage from short wavelength light. *Nature*, **260,** 153–155

Ham, W. T. Jr., Ruffolo, J. J. Jr., Mueller, H. A. and Guerry, D. III. (1980) The nature of retinal radiation damage: dependence on wavelength, power level and exposure time. *Vision Research*, **20,** 1105–1111

Harwerth, R. S. and Sperling, H. G. (1975) Effects of intense visible radiation on the increment-threshold spectral sensitivity of the rhesus monkey eye. *Vision Research*, **15,** 1193–1204

Marshall, J. and Bird, A. C. (1979) A comparative histopathological study of argon and krypton laser irradiations of the human retina. *British Journal of Ophthalmology*, **63,** 657–668

Marshall, J., Hamilton, A. M. and Bird, A. C. (1974) Intra-retinal absorption of argon laser irradiation in human and monkey retinae. *Experientia*, **30,** 1335–1337

Pardos, G. J. and Krachmer, J. H. (1981) Photocoagulation: its effect on the corneal endothelial cell density of diabetics. *Archives of Ophthalmology*, **99,** 84–86.

Pomerantzeff, O. and Delori, F. C. (1968) Physical aspects of ruby-laser and xenon-arc photocoagulation. In *New and Controversial Aspects of Retinal Detachment*, edited by A. McPherson, 247–260. New York: Harper and Row

Pomerantzeff, O., Kaneko, H., Donovan, R. H., Schepens, C. L. and McMeel, J. W. (1976) Effect of the ocular media on the main wavelengths of argon laser emission. *Investigative Ophthalmology*, **15,** 70–77

Schepens, C. L. (1983) *Retinal Detachment and Allied Diseases*. Philadelphia: W. B. Saunders

Sperling, H. G. and Harwerth, R. S. (1972) Intense spectral light effects on spectral sensitivity. *Optica Acta*, **19,** 395–399

Trempe, C. L., Mainster, M. A., Pomerantzeff, O., Avila, M. P., Jalkh, A. E., Weiter, J. J., McMeel, J. W. and Schepens, C. L. (1982) Macular photocoagulation: optimal wavelength selection. *Ophthalmology*, **89,** 721–728

Van Assendelft, O. W. (1970) *Spectrophotometry of Haemoglobin Derivatives*. Springfield, Illinois: Charles C. Thomas

Wald, G. (1945) Human vision and the spectrum. *Science*, **101,** 653–658

# 3
# The management of diabetic maculopathy

Rodger Whitelocke, Rolf K. Blach and
A. M. Peter Hamilton

## INTRODUCTION

Diabetic maculopathy consists of background diabetic retinopathy with macular involvement. We shall consider the evolution of this complex condition which leads to a clinical and therapeutic subclassification that may be used as a guide to patient management. Techniques of photocoagulation are described.

## THE EVOLUTION OF DIABETIC MACULOPATHY

The earliest histological changes of diabetic retinopathy that have been identified consist of basement membrane thickening, pericyte (mural cell) degeneration and endothelial proliferation. These are associated with metabolic changes and give rise to haemodynamic disturbances in the retina that may result in dilated veins, microaneurysm formation and abnormal capillary permeability. It has been suggested that the integrity of the blood-retinal barrier breaks down at an early stage in diabetes, before there is ophthalmoscopic evidence of retinopathy. Some evidence for this has been derived from vitreous fluorophotometry studies (Cunha-Vaz *et al.*, 1975).

The microaneurysms, which can vary from 10–100 μ, may either thrombose or decompensate with leakage of blood constituents, giving rise to haemorrhage or oedema. Permeability changes also affect the retinal capillary network generally and, in addition, it is possible that the blood–retinal barrier at the level of the pigmented epithelium may be altered, all mechanisms giving rise to oedema and haemorrhage. Fluid accumulates within the retina, initially between the outer plexiform and nuclear layers, and later in the nerve fibre and inner plexiform layers and may eventually involve its entire thickness. There is a predilection for the accumulation of fluid at the macula. Because of its particular anatomical structure, this can take the form of microcysts in the superficial retinal layers, which may coalesce into larger cysts giving rise to cystoid macular oedema. These changes are readily visible biomicroscopically and on fluorescein angiography.

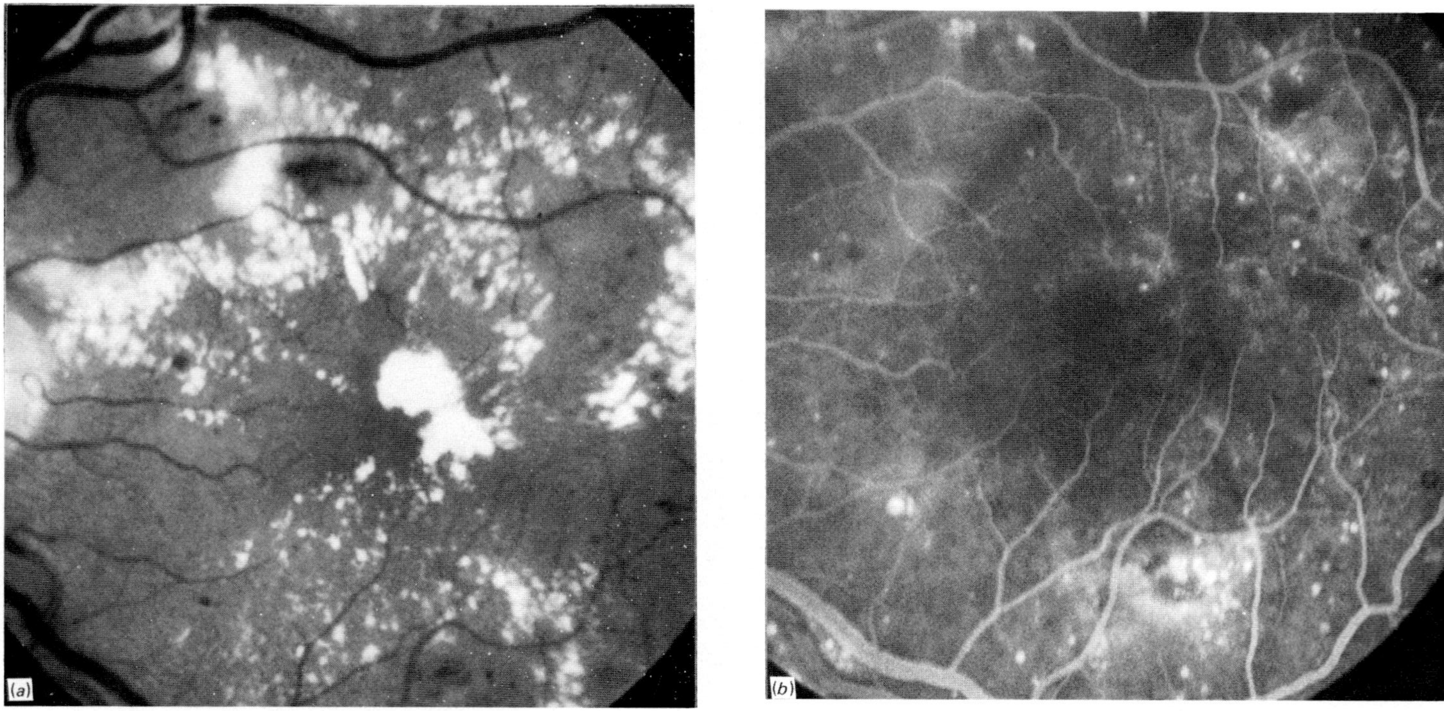


*Figure 3.1* A case of diabetic maculopathy. (*a*) and (*b*) Before treatment. Visual acuity 6/18. Photograph (*left*) of patient's left eye, showing extensive circinate exudates and a parafoveal plaque. Microaneurysms and haemorrhages are also seen. The fluorescein angiogram (*right*) reveals areas of focal leakage, but does not show exudates

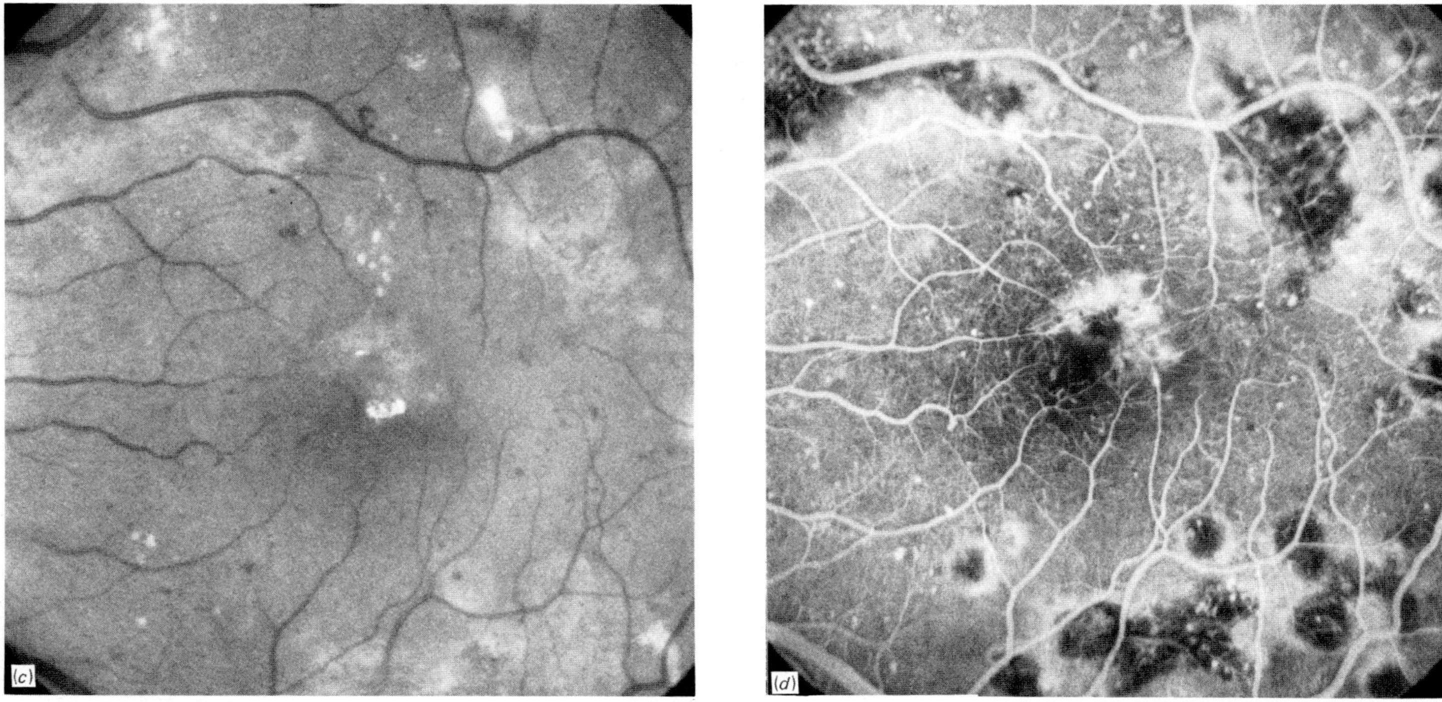


(*c*) and (*d*) 8 months after treatment. Visual acuity 6/6. Photograph (*left*) demonstrates a marked reduction in exudates. The fluorescein angiogram (*right*) reveals the areas of photocoagulation more clearly

At the margin of oedematous retina, lipid material may be deposited between the outer plexiform and nuclear layers. These exudates usually take the form of rings, or arcs of rings, centered on intraretinal microvascular abnormalities (IRMA), but may also lie in the perivascular spaces or as a plaque at the macula (*Figure 3.1*).

Many of the early vascular changes of diabetic retinopathy are subtle and difficult to detect on clinical examination, but can be easily demonstrated by fluorescein angiography, which may reveal microaneurysms and small areas of capillary non-perfusion. It is not known what determines the capillary response in any individual case. However, the influences that may determine these responses are indicated in Chapter 8.

Diabetic maculopathy therefore can evolve following focal leakage, generalized oedema or ischaemia. Depending on which of these features is dominant, three broad groups of diabetic maculopathy may be identified:

(1) focal,
(2) cystoid, and
(3) ischaemic.

The clinical management of diabetic maculopathy is based upon the recognition of these three groups.

## CLINICAL FEATURES

### Symptoms

Early diabetic retinopathy is usually asymptomatic. The patient may later complain of microscotomas which are most apparent on close rather than distance vision. Once exudates, haemorrhages or oedema have affected the fovea there is usually a reduction in visual acuity. Areas of ischaemia are not usually visible ophthalmoscopically and it is often difficult to correlate the ophthalmoscopic and angiographic appearances with the patient's objective visual acuity. With further involvement of the macula, vision may be markedly reduced although the field of vision usually remains relatively normal. Only with the possible subsequent development of proliferative retinopathy is the peripheral field and navigational vision threatened. Extensive and valuable work on other psychophysical functions has been undertaken, and may well eventually give rise to clues to the nature of diabetic retinopathy. However, for our immediate clinical purposes, visual acuity is the only retinal function that influences the management of diabetic maculopathy. Other changes in visual function have been described; these include alterations in colour vision (chiefly blue-yellow) (Birch and Hamilton, 1981). It is believed that the oscillatory potentials are affected at an early stage (Yonemura, Aoki and Tsuzuki, 1962; Simonsen, 1966). Other electrodiagnostic tests are of little clinical importance in diabetic retinopathy.

## Classification and signs of diabetic maculopathy

According to which features dominate, diabetic maculopathy may be subdivided into three groups: focal, cystoid and ischaemic. However, these groups are not mutually exclusive, and a fourth group, mixed maculopathy, is clinically useful. In order to define these groups, ophthalmoscopic, biomicroscopic and fluorescein examinations are required.

### Focal diabetic maculopathy

The features of focal diabetic maculopathy are microaneurysms, haemorrhages and usually well-defined circinate exudates. Associated with these changes may be mild oedema of the macula, or exudates or oedema threatening the macula. Fluorescein angiography demonstrates adequate macular capillary perfusion, and areas of focal leakage are seen (*Figures 3.1* and *3.2*).

### Cystoid diabetic maculopathy

The features of cystoid diabetic maculopathy are microaneurysms, haemorrhages, relatively few or no exudates in the presence of marked macular oedema, frequently with cystoid spaces which are visible biomicroscopically. Fluorescein angiography shows a marked increase in permeability of the vessels at the posterior pole, and loculated leakage is often observed (*Figure 3.3*).

### Ischaemic diabetic maculopathy

The features of ischaemic diabetic maculopathy are microaneurysms and haemorrhages with few exudates. Deep blot-like haemorrhages, often associated with retinal ischaemia, are commonly present. Macular oedema, varying from mild to cystoid, is frequently an associated finding. Fluorescein angiography reveals areas of capillary non-perfusion in the macular and paramacular areas (*Figure 3.4*).

### Mixed diabetic maculopathy

Where exudates, oedema and ischaemia are each of significant importance one may talk of mixed maculopathy.

## EPIDEMIOLOGY

The incidence of background diabetic retinopathy is largely related to the duration of the diabetes, with a significant increase in prevalence after 10 years, rising to

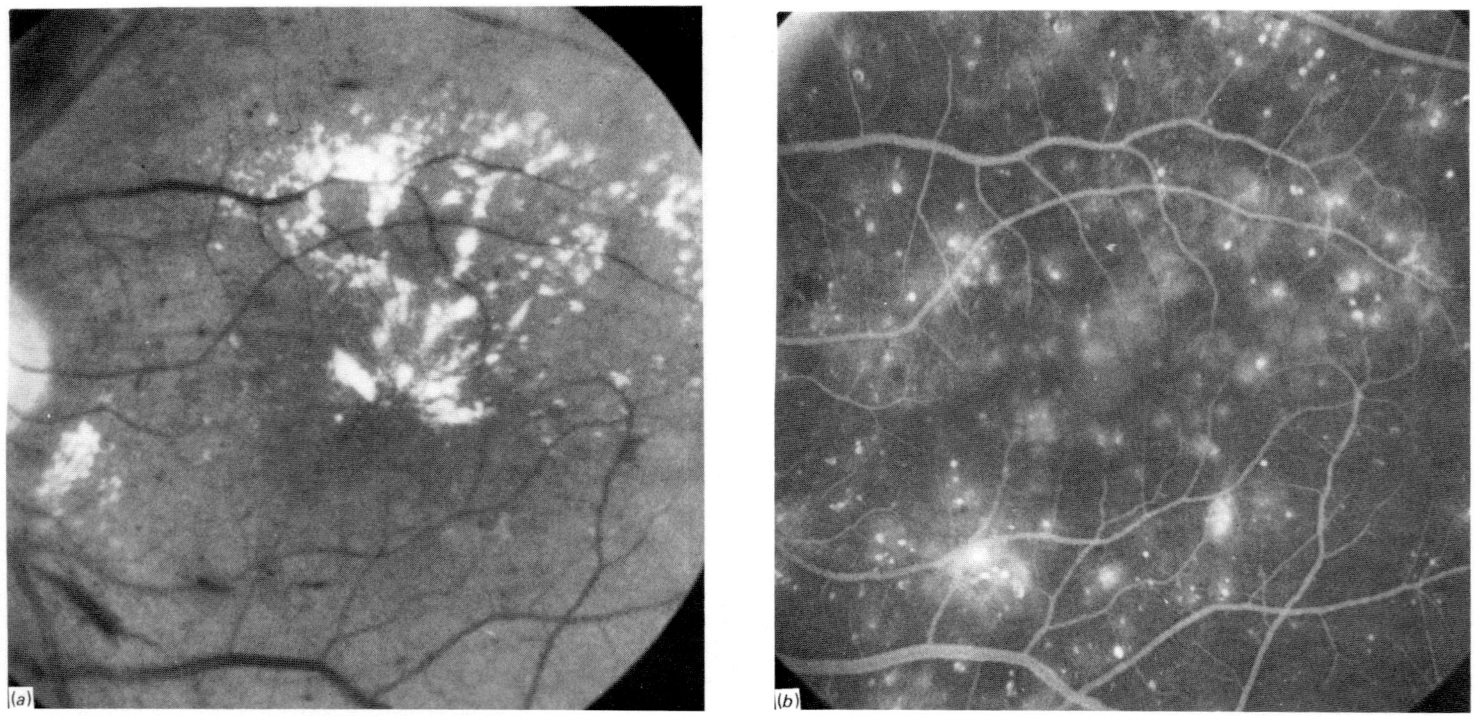


*Figure 3.2* A case of focal diabetic maculopathy. (*a*) and (*b*) Before treatment. Visual acuity 6/18. Photograph (*left*) showing exudates and fluorescein angiogram (*right*) reveals areas of leakage

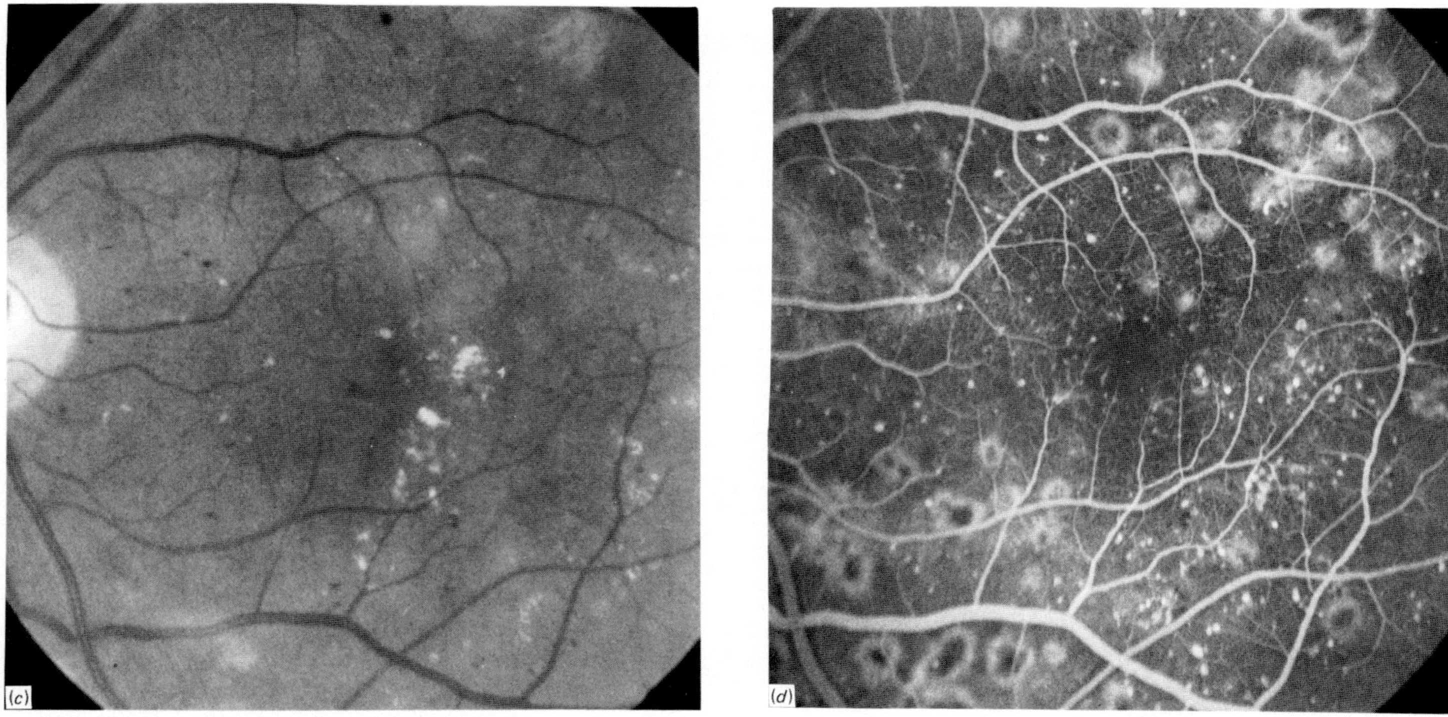

(*c*) and (*d*) After treatment. Visual acuity 6/9 which has been maintained for the past 4 years. Photograph (*left*) shows reduction in exudates and fluorescein angiogram (*right*) reveals areas of laser photocoagulation

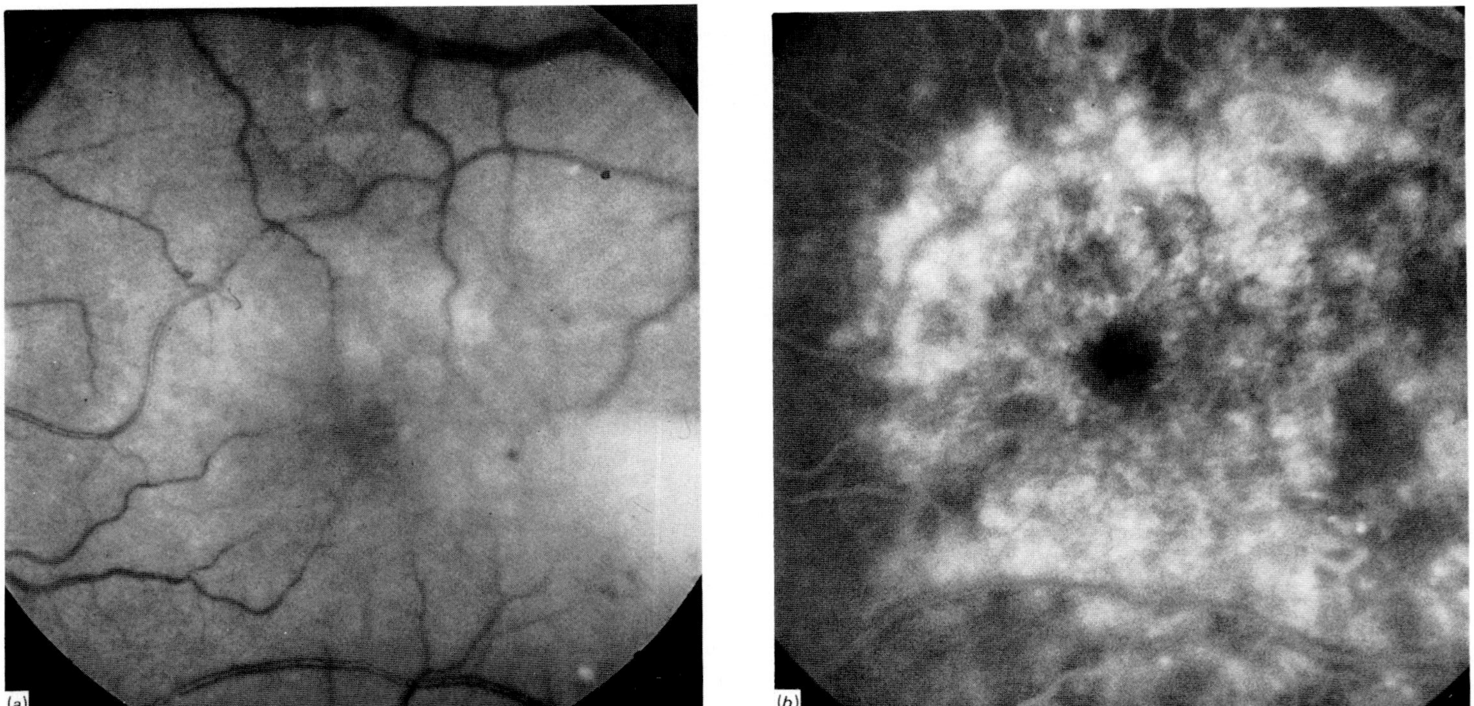

*Figure 3.3* A case of cystoid diabetic maculopathy. (*a*) and (*b*) Before treatment. Visual acuity 6/60. Photograph (*left*) showing a rather featureless retina. The fluorescein angiogram (*right*) shows extensive macular oedema

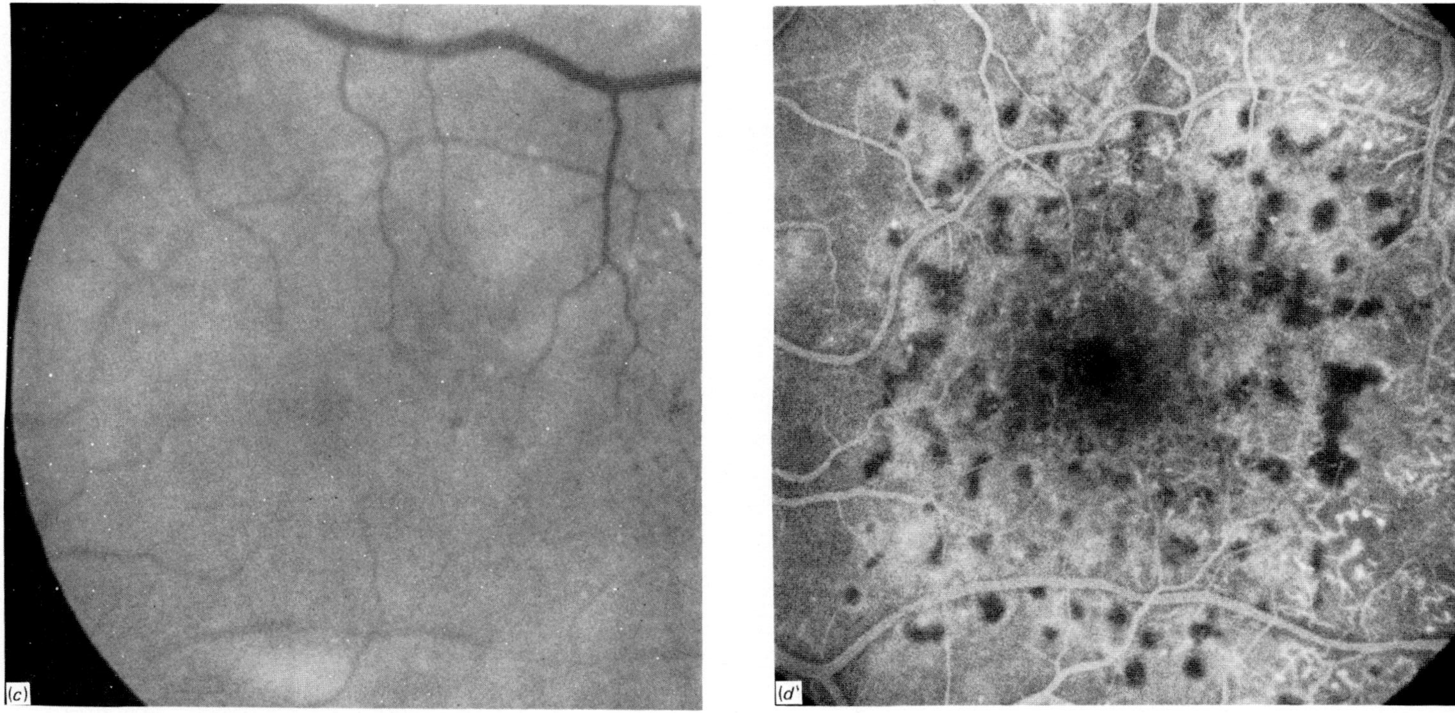

(*c*) and (*d*) After grid photocoagulation treatment. Visual acuity 6/36 which subsequently improved to 6/18 and this has been maintained for 3 years. The gentle photocoagulation scars which do not involve the fovea are not shown on direct ophthalmoscopy (*left*) but only on fluorescein angiography (*right*)

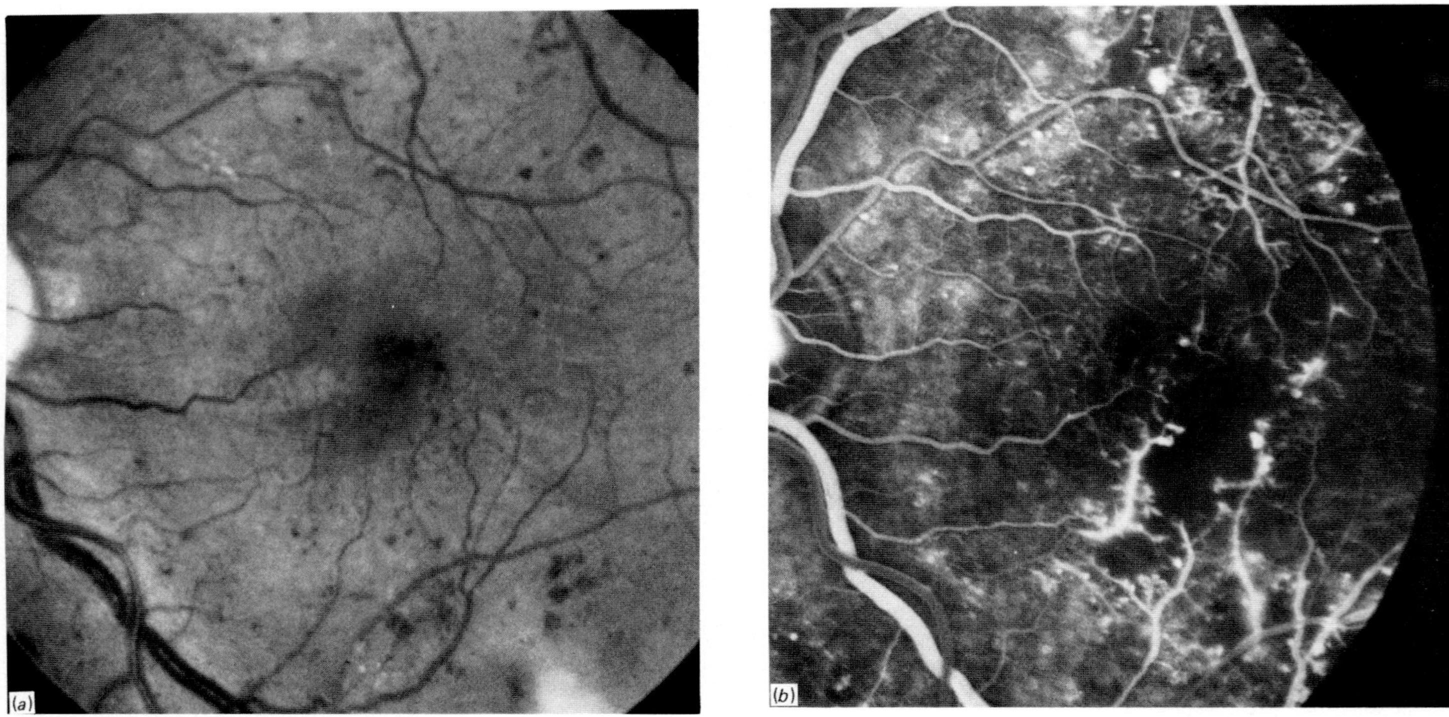


*Figure 3.4* A case of ischaemic diabetic maculopathy. Visual acuity 6/18. Photograph (*a*) showing characteristic deep 'blot' haemorrhages which are associated with ischaemia. The fluorescein angiogram (*b*) reveals areas of capillary non-perfusion. Disc new vessels developed 7 months later and these were treated with panretinal photocoagulation; 3 years later vision is 6/24

85% after 26 years (Lestradet *et al.*, 1981). Donovan (1978) found that nearly 23% of diabetics attending a diabetic clinic of a district general hospital had diabetic retinopathy, of whom 6.1% had maculopathy. Diabetic maculopathy tends to occur more frequently in type 2 (non-insulin dependent) diabetics and 75% of patients with diabetic maculopathy are diagnosed after the age of 40 years (Kohner, 1978). In a study of 100 consecutive diabetic patients with severe retinopathy who were referred to a diabetic retinopathy clinic, Bodansky *et al.* (1982) confirmed a significant association between type 2 diabetes and maculopathy. Of the 100 consecutive cases, 43% had maculopathy, or severe background retinopathy with macular involvement.

The majority of diabetic patients have the type 2 variety, and in this older age-group females predominate. Maculopathy therefore tends to affect older patients, and is more frequent than proliferative retinopathy. However, maculopathy may also occur in association with proliferative retinopathy, thereby being a feature in younger diabetics (Sigelman, 1980).

Numerically, maculopathy is a commoner cause of blindness in diabetics than proliferative retinopathy (Keen, 1972).

## MANAGEMENT

Screening for diabetic retinopathy is best undertaken by ophthalmologists, because of the complex diagnostic techniques involved and the subtlety of many of the physical signs. Indeed, both retinal oedema and retinal ischaemia require special techniques for their identification. The consequences of this precept, given the large diabetic population, poses considerable problems in relation to training and staffing.

It is of importance to identify retinopathy in its early stages, before there is irreversible damage.

### Options in the treatment of diabetic maculopathy

When considering the therapy of diabetic macular disease, consideration must be given to:

(1) Good glycaemic control
(2) Treatment of associated hypertension
(3) Commercial preparations
(4) Low visual aids
(5) Photocoagulation

#### Good glycaemic control

Good glycaemic control in the early stages of diabetes probably delays the onset and reduces the severity of diabetic retinopathy (Colwell, 1966), although it is not prevented. More recently, the beneficial effect of strict metabolic control for diabetic microangiopathy has been reported (Steno study group, 1982). However, once diabetic retinopathy has become established, good control will rarely be effective in reversing the microangiopathy. Indeed, where excellent control is introduced in an established retinopathy as in continuous subcutaneous insulin infusion, serious retinovascular decompensation may occur (Keen, personal communication). In epidemiological studies over 5 years, Jarrett and Keen (1976) showed a correlation between patients with poor glucose tolerance and the development of retinopathy. A relationship between the degree of initial glucose intolerance, the duration of diabetes and the development of retinopathy in non-insulin dependent diabetic patients has also been described (Hautecouverture *et al.*, 1973; Pettitt *et al.*, 1980).

Present methods of therapy have not been successful in preventing vascular complications in non-insulin dependent (type 2) diabetics. However, in insulin-dependent (type 1) diabetics, there is a slower rate of progression in the number of microaneurysms in patients receiving divided insulin injections when compared with patients receiving only a single daily injection (Eschwege *et al.*, 1979).

Animal experiments also indicate that every attempt should be made to restore a normal physiological cellular environment in diabetic patients, as this may minimize degenerative complications (Engerman, Bloodworth and Nelson 1977; Mauer *et al.*, 1976).

Evidence continues to accumulate that poor glycaemic control is an important factor in the aetiology of diabetic retinopathy (Tchobroutsky, 1978; Pirart, 1978).

In conclusion, good glycaemic control in the early stages of diabetes appears to be important in delaying complications. However, we feel that there is no point in introducing feelings of guilt in either the patient or his physician, if, as a result of inadequate control, serious retinopathy has developed, since by this stage the game has been lost.

## Treatment of associated hypertension

Hypertension is commonly found in diabetic patients, especially those with renal involvement. It is important to treat any associated hypertension as this has a detrimental effect on the already vulnerable retinal vasculature.

## Commercial medications

Although many claims have been made with respect to the benefit of medical therapy on diabetic maculopathy, no single drug has yet proved to have any significant effect on the visual outcome. These drugs include salicylates, calcium debosilate and clofibrate. However, clofibrate may cause a reduction in exudates (Duncan *et al.*, 1968). This is not to say that clinical trials may not eventually demonstrate valuable therapeutic agents for diabetic retinopathy.

## Low vision aids

The success of low vision aids depends on the motivation of the patient, and the special interest of the optician. The most successful group of patients tends to be young and intelligent with specific requirements. Results tend to be less satisfactory in the elderly.

Macular blindness is less disabling than the blindness resulting from proliferative diabetic retinopathy, since peripheral vision is maintained, which permits navigational vision and therefore social independence. This group of patients therefore does not require navigational aids. It should be remembered that as many patients with diabetic maculopathy may progress to proliferative diabetic retinopathy, they should be kept under regular review, so that proliferative changes may be treated at an early stage.

## Photocoagulation

The only form of therapy that has been proved by clinical trials to modify the visual outcome in diabetic retinopathy is photocoagulation (British Multicentre Study, 1975, 1979), either with the xenon arc photocoagulator or the argon laser. Other studies have shown the beneficial effect of photocoagulation in diabetic maculopathy (Patz *et al.*, 1973; Spalter, 1971). However, none of these studies differentiated among different types of maculopathy.

Subsequently, Whitelocke *et al.* (1979) showed that the different types of maculopathy offer different therapeutic problems and carry different prognoses. In this study, which was not a controlled trial, it was clearly shown that photocoagulation for focal maculopathy was an effective form of treatment. Patients with cystoid maculopathy treated by grid photocoagulation either maintained their already reduced vision or showed a modest improvement. The results of this type of treatment were not strong enough to recommend grid photocoagulation routinely. Patients with ischaemic maculae did not benefit from focal photocoagulation, however, they were at high risk of developing disc new vessels (32% over 2 years), thus raising the question of when to treat these patients.

It may well be that while the result of the British Multicentre Trial is positive, but not overwhelmingly so, is because this study includes all types of maculopathy. The good results to be expected from the treatment of focal diabetic maculopathy were compromised by the inclusion of the oedematous and ischaemic groups. In this study, eyes with an initial visual acuity of less than 6/36 did not show any significant improvement.

Eyes with focal maculopathy, with exudates threatening the fovea, but vision better than 6/12, carry the best prognosis with regard to treatment. In contrast, eyes with a visual acuity of 6/36 or below, due either to macular deposits, oedema or ischaemia, carry the worst prognosis.

The aims of treatment by photocoagulation are to maintain or improve the patient's visual acuity, and to prevent the development of proliferative retinopathy. Three types of photocoagulator are generally used: the xenon arc photocoagulator, the argon laser and the krypton laser.

All xenon arc photocoagulators use a direct ophthalmoscopic delivery system, allowing a monocular view of the retina. The exceptions are the Fankhauser slit-lamp fitting to a xenon arc photocoagulator (Fankhauser and Lotmar, 1972), and the indirect ophthalmoscope attachment to the O'Malley photocoagulator. All xenon arc photocoagulation requires retrobulbar anaesthesia, or occasionally, general anaesthesia. They have in common the feature that the larger the burn the more powerful it is. By and large, xenon arc photocoagulators are not suitable to treat the parafoveal areas.

The argon laser photocoagulators use a slit-lamp delivery system, allowing excellent magnification and stereopsis. They require only topical anaesthesia; only rarely is retrobulbar anaesthesia necessary. Very exact localization in the parafoveal area is possible, thus making the argon laser currently the most appropriate method of photocoagulation for diabetic maculopathy.

The krypton laser has been used in the treatment of diabetic maculopathy, and in our experience has no advantage over the argon laser in the management of patients with this condition.

In view of the dangers of burning the patient's fovea, meticulous technique is required. Indeed, the overall importance of photocoagulation technique, which is specific for each type of diabetic retinopathy, cannot be overestimated (Blach and Hamilton, 1978).

While many patients with a minor amount of maculopathy can be treated at a single outpatient attendance, there are those with extensive macular involvement where multiple treatment sessions are necessary. Indeed, there may be dangers of oedema following excessive treatment at a single photocoagulation session. Prior to carrying out photocoagulation, patients should be carefully assessed. Colour fundus photographs are certainly useful to document the progress of the disease, and the response to photocoagulation. Fluorescein angiograms are essential to monitor oedema and ischaemia, but are not a prerequisite for the treatment of focal maculopathy.

The pattern of the vessels will guide the observer to the foveal area. It will be remembered that the fovea is situated slightly below a horizontal line which bisects the optic disc, and is about two-and-a-half disc diameters to the temporal side. A useful guide to the indentification of the fovea is the luteal pigment using red-free (green) illumination when the luteal pigment will be darker than the adjacent macular area. However, the contrast is reduced when the macula is oedematous, and the increased sensitivity following dark adaptation usually allows the observer to overcome this difficulty. Undoubtedly, the most devastating complication of photocoagulation is a foveal burn.

## Focal diabetic maculopathy

The aim of photocoagulation in focal diabetic maculopathy is to destroy the localized vascular malformations which produce the classical lesions. A small spot size, 50–200 μ of moderate intensity and short duration (*Table 3.1*), is used to treat the centre of circinate lesions, individual microaneurysms, and other vascular malformations (*Figures 3.1, 3.2* and *3.5*).

The intensity is not assessed by the absolute power, but by the immediate blanching of the retina. Treatment is applied to all the red dots and vascular

*Table 3.1* A guide to argon laser settings in diabetic maculopathy

| | *Size* (μ) | *Number* | *Intensity* |
|---|---|---|---|
| Focal | 50–200 | As required | Moderate |
| Cystoid | 200 | Approximately 200 | Very low |
| Ischaemic | 500 | 1000 (prophylaxis)<br>2000 (therapeutic) | Low |

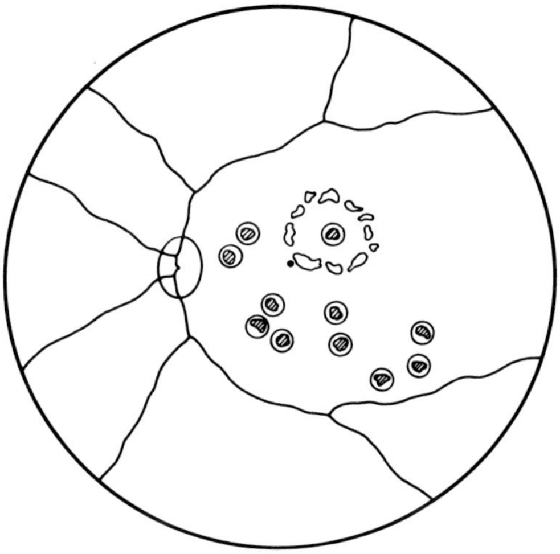

*Figure 3.5* Diagram showing technique of laser photocoagulation used to treat focal diabetic maculopathy. Individual vascular malformations and centres of circinate lesions treated focally

malformations at the posterior pole except those at the fovea, but superficial retinal haemorrhages are not treated because of damage to the nerve fibre layer. Ideally, all major leaking dots seen on the fluroescein angiogram should be treated. In practice, the red dots seen on biomicroscopy (far fewer in number) may be sufficient. Following treatment, patients are reviewed at approximately 3 months, when further lesions may be visible following absorption of oedema and exudates, and more treatment may then be given.

## Cystoid diabetic maculopathy

Patients with cystoid diabetic maculopathy present a far greater problem, and photocoagulation may be of limited benefit only. In cases where cystoid diabetic maculopathy is present without any obvious focal lesion (*see Figure 3.3*), a gentle 'grid' of photocoagulation to the macula, carefully avoiding the fovea (*Figure 3.6*), may result in a reduction in the oedema and a slight improvement in vision (Whitelocke *et al.*, 1979). The technique consists of treating the macular area with a spot size of approximately 200 μ at very low intensity and short duration, so as to produce a grid-like pattern over the macular area (*Figure 3.3*), avoiding the fovea. About 100–200 burns are applied. Because of the exceedingly low intensity used in this technique, the burns should only just be visible during the photocoagulation session, and once the initial oedema has settled, there should be little or no evidence of photocoagulation on ophthalmoscopy (*see Figure 3.3*). The lesions, at the pigment epithelial layer, are readily indentifiable on fluorescein angiography (*see Figure 3.3*). In cases where there are focal lesions, these should be treated first.

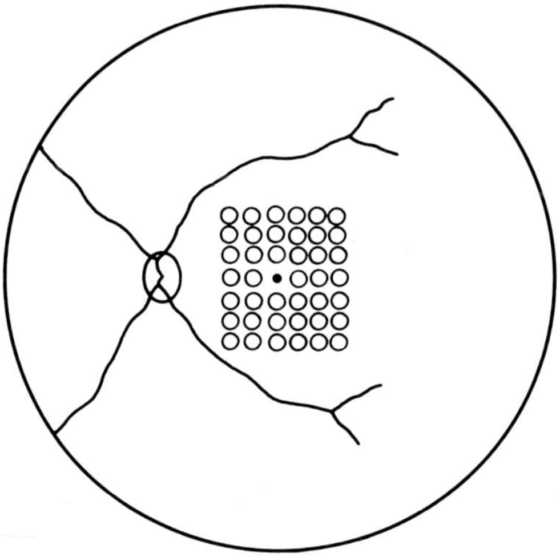

*Figure 3.6* Diagram showing technique of laser photocoagulation used to treat cystoid diabetic maculopathy. A gentle grid which avoided the fovea was applied to the macula

After an interval of about 6–12 weeks patients may be be reviewed and a decision taken whether or not to carry out more extensive treatment such as the grid photocoagulation described.

## Ischaemic diabetic maculopathy

Photocoagulation to the already ischaemic macula is not generally beneficial. However, where new vessels develop, the technique for photocoagulation as described for new vessels (in the chapter on proliferative retinopathy) should be undertaken. It will be remembered that in the case of established disc new vessels, at least 2000 burns of 500 μ in diameter should be given in the form of panretinal photocoagulation. If it is decided to give this form of treatment prophylactically to an ischaemic retina without new vessels, then about 1000 burns of 500 μ in diameter will often be sufficient.

## Mixed diabetic maculopathy

The management of mixed maculopathy by photocoagulation presents the ophthalmologist with a difficult problem, as each case is unique and the balance of the features will determine the technique of treatment. In those cases where central vision is already compromised and there is widespread ischaemia, panretinal photocoagulation may involve too great a sacrifice in peripheral vision to justify treatment.

## DISCUSSION

The first question is how early background diabetic retinopathy, the precursor of diabetic maculopathy, should be treated. Meyer-Schwickerath has for many years advocated early treatment. However, the answer to this important question can only be obtained by means of a controlled clinical trial. Such a trial is in progress at the present time in America: the Early Treatment Diabetic Retinopathy Study. We feel that background diabetic retinopathy should be treated if there is a threat to the macula.

Therefore, focal diabetic maculopathy, which is the most satisfactory of the maculopathies to treat, should be anticipated where circinate exudates threaten the fovea, and it is reasonable to treat these areas before the fovea is actually involved and vision is reduced. It is not necessary to treat all leaking spots in a focal maculopathy, but only those areas which are associated with exudates or oedema.

The place of grid photocoagulation in the treatment of oedematous diabetic maculopathy has not been established. The management of macular oedema resulting from other ophthalmological conditions such as aphakia or uveitis has not been helpful in our understanding of the management of diabetic macular oedema. The rationale of grid photocoagulation has been given some support by the studies of Tso *et al.* (1980) who suggest that the blood–retinal barrier at the level of the pigmented epithelium can be affected by this form of treatment. Other techniques of photocoagulation for this condition have proved disappointing.

It is clearly illogical to apply photocoagulation to already ischaemic maculae. However, since we know that these cases are at risk of developing neovascularization, the question of prophylactic photocoagulation needs to be faced. There is no doubt that a lesser amount of photocoagulation is required prophylactically than therapeutically, and it may well be correct to treat cases that are likely to be lost to follow-up. However, it is more satisfactory to keep these cases under observation and only treat them as soon as neovascularization develops.

For the future, the main interest lies in whether the newer methods of greatly improved diabetic control, started early in the disease, will prevent the development of diabetic maculopathy. Until the underlying mechanisms in the development of diabetic microangiopathy are more clearly understood, more precise drug therapy is unlikely to be developed. For the present, photocoagulation, empirical though it is, remains the most effective form of therapy for diabetic maculopathy.

## CONCLUSIONS

The evidence for the beneficial effects of the treatment of focal diabetic maculopathy is very strong. The treatment of ischaemic diabetic maculopathy revolves around the management of preproliferative and proliferative retinopathy. Undoubtedly the management of oedematous diabetic maculopathy remains the greatest challenge.

## References

Birch, J. and Hamilton, A. M. (1981) Xenon arc and argon laser photocoagulation in the treatment of diabetic disc neovascularization. Part 2. Effect on colour vision. *Transactions of the Ophthalmological Society of the United Kingdom*, **101,** 93–99

Blach, R. K. and Hamilton, A. M. (1978) The technique and indications for photocoagulation in diabetic retinopathy. 1. Principles of photocoagulation. *International Ophthalmology*, **1,** 19–29

Bodansky, H. J., Cudworth, A. G., Whitelocke, R. A. F. and Dobree, J. H. (1982) Diabetic retinopathy and its relation to type of diabetes. Review of a retinal clinic population. *British Journal of Ophthalmology*, **66,** 496–499

British Multicentre Photocoagulation Group (1975) Photocoagulation in treatment of diabetic maculopathy. *Lancet*, **2,** 1110–1113

British Multicentre Photocoagulation Group (1979) Xenon arc photocoagulation in the treatment of diabetic maculopathy. *Transactions of the Ophthalmological Society of the United Kingdom*, **99,** 13–16

Colwell, J. A. (1966) Effect of diabetic control on retinopathy. *Diabetes*, **15,** 497–499

Cunha-Vaz, J. G., Faria de Abreu, J. R., Campos, A. J. and Figo, G. M. (1975) Early breakdown of the blood-retinal barrier in diabetes. *British Journal of Ophthalmology*, **59,** 649–656

Donovan, R. J. (1978) Prevalence of retinopathy in a diabetic clinic. *British Medical Journal*, **1,** 1441–1442

Duncan, L. J. P., Cullen, J. F., Ireland, J. T., Nolan, J., Clarke, B. F. and Oliver, M. F. (1968) A three-year trial of Atromid therapy in exudative diabetic retinopathy. *Diabetes*, **17,** 458–467

Engerman, R., Bloodworth, J. M. B. and Nelson, S. (1977) Relationship of microvascular disease in diabetes to metabolic control. *Diabetes*, **26,** 760–769

Eschwege, E., Job, D., Guyot-Argenton, C., Aubry, J. P. and Tchobroutsky, G. (1979) Delayed progression of diabetic retinopathy by divided insulin administration: a further follow-up. *Diabetologia*, **16,** 13–15

Fankhauser, F. and Lotmar, W. (1972) Optical attachment to the photocoagulator of Zeiss-Oberkochen for operation with the Goldmann Contact Lens. *Klinische Monatsblätter für Augenheilkunde*, **160,** 218–220

Hautecouverture, M., Monchi, A., Tchobroutsky, G., Assan, R., Slama, G. and Derot, M. (1973) Rétinopathie diabétique et sécrétion d'hormone de croissance – chez 39 diabétiques non-insulino-dépendants. *La Nouvelle Presse Médicale*, **2,** 1817–1822

Jarrett, R. J. and Keen, H. (1976) Hyperglycaemia in diabetes mellitus. *Lancet*, **2,** 1009–1012

Keen, H. (1972) The prevalence of blindness in diabetes. *Journal of the Royal College of Physicians of London*, **7,** 53–61

Kohner, E. M. (1978) The evolution and natural history of diabetic retinopathy. *International Ophthalmology Clinics*, **18,** 1–16

Lestradet, H., Papoz, L., Hellouin, D. E., Menibus, C. L., Levavasseur, F., Besse, J., Billaud, L., Battistelli, F., Tric, P. H. and Lestradet, F. (1981) Long-term study of mortality and vascular complications in juvenile-onset (type 1) diabetes. *Diabetes*, **30,** 175–179

Mauer, S. M., Steffes, M. W., Michael, A. F. and Brown, D. M. (1976) Study of diabetic nephropathy in animals and man. *Diabetes*, **25** (Supplement 2), 850–857

Patz, A., Schatz, H., Berkow, J. W., Gittleshon, A. M. and Ticho, U. (1973) Macular edema – an overlooked complication of diabetic retinopathy. *Transactions of the American Academy of Ophthalmology and Otolaryngology*, **77,** 34–42

Pettitt, D. J., Knowler, W. C., Lisse, J. R. and Bennett, P. H. (1980) Development of retinopathy and proteinuria in relation to plasma-glucose concentrations in Pima indians. *Lancet*, **2,** 1050–1052

Pirart, J. (1978) Diabetes mellitus and its degenerative complications: a prospective study of 4400 patients observed between 1947 and 1973. *Diabetes Care*, **1,** 168–188, 252–263

Sigelman, J. (1980) Diabetic macular edema in juvenile and adult-onset diabetes. *American Journal of Ophthalmology*, **90,** 287–296

Simonsen, S. E. (1966) Electroretinogram in diabetes. Vth Symposium of ISCERG (Ghent). In *The Clinical Value of Electroretinography*, 403–412. Basel: Karger

Spalter, H. F. (1971) Photocoagulation of circinate maculopathy in diabetic retinopathy. *American Journal of Ophthalmology*, **71,** 242–250

Steno study group (1982) Effect of 6 months of strict metabolic control on eye and kidney function in insulin-dependent diabetics with background retinopathy. *Lancet*, **1,** 121–124

Tchobroutsky, G. (1978) Relation of diabetic control to development of microvascular complications. *Diabetologia*, **15,** 143–152

Tso, M. O. M., Cunha-Vaz, J. G., Shih, C-Y. and Jones, C. W. (1980) Clinicopathological study of blood–retinal barrier in experimental diabetes mellitus. *Archives of Ophthalmology*, **98,** 2032–2040

Whitelocke, R. A. F., Kearns, M., Blach, R. K. and Hamilton, A. M. (1979) The diabetic maculopathies. *Transactions of the Ophthalmological Society of the United Kingdom*, **99,** 314–320

Yonemura, D., Aoki, T. and Tsuzuki, K. (1962) Electroretinogram in diabetic retinopathy. *Archives of Ophthalmology*, **68,** 19–24

# 4
# Disorders of the retinal pigment epithelium

Iain H. Chisholm

## INTRODUCTION

The exact role of the retinal pigment epithelium (RPE) in the range of inherited and metabolic diseases is often obscure. In many of these conditions, such as retinitis pigmentosa, the primary defect is undetermined. The clinical features are, however, well recognized and the retinal pigment epithelial changes characteristic. In a chapter such as this it would be inappropriate to describe these diseases in detail. Rather the intent is to concentrate on primary disorders of the retinal pigment epithelium such as age changes, conditions involving deposition of abnormal material, and disorders producing apparent retinal pigment epithelial inflammation.

The retinal pigment epithelium extends as a single layer of hexagonal cells from the optic nerve head to the ora serrata. Its apical surface is covered with cytoplasmic extensions, or microvilli, apposed to the outer segments of the retinal receptors. These processes are involved in engulfing and phagocytosing receptor material derived from the rods and cones. Disruption of this process plays a part in many degenerative and inherited disorders of the retinal pigment epithelium. The presence of pigment granules (melanosomes) within the pigment epithelium is though to serve as a 'sink', which absorbs surplus light and prevents its reflection back through the retinal receptors. This reduces spurious signals and improves visual acuity. Fluorescein stimulation and emission in the choroid is blocked by the melanin of the pigment epithelium. Forward diffusion of the dye is prevented by the tight endothelial junctions of the retinal pigment epithelial cells.

Lipofuscin accumulation is a frequent observation in disorders involving the retinal pigment epithelium. It may well account for the changes seen in Best's disease, Stargardt's disease or fundus flavimaculatus, as well as the ageing changes of drusen and central atrophy. This pigment is seen in many organs of the body and not least of all in the retinal pigment epithelium. It probably represents the non-degradable residue derived from the peroxidation of cell membrane fatty acids. It has been suggested that gradual accumulation of lipofuscin ultimately leads to mechanical disruption of intracellular organization, cellular dysfunction and death (Wing, Blanchard and Weiter, 1978).

## AGE-RELATED CHANGES OF THE PIGMENT EPITHELIUM

### Drusen and pigment epithelial changes

Drusen and pigment epithelial changes are clinical manifestations of ageing and have been linked with senile macular degeneration. Drusen are visible in at least 70% of the population over the age of 50 and histopathologically are probably universal after that age. Thinning of the pigment epithelium and local pigment hyperplasia also develop in time. Grindle and Marshall (1978) estimated that each pigment epithelial cell engulfs about 2500 receptor discs a day and commented that it is not surprising that age-related changes occur in the morphology of the pigment epithelial cell. High levels of lipofuscin are found in man from the fifth decade and in monkeys lipofuscin is shown to be derived from the inappropriate breakdown of phagosomes (Hogan, 1972). Alterations in Bruch's membrane occurring with age produce a barrier to the free transfer of outer segment debris across the membrane, resulting in a build-up of membranous and microdrusenoid deposits under the pigment epithelium. Loss of basal convolutions of the cells and thickening of the basement membrane has been described as 'basal laminar deposit' by Sarks (1976). Macrophage invasion of this region may then occur as well as phagocytic changes in the membrane itself. Light-induced free radical damage might also play a part in this gradual ageing process (Feeney-Burns, Berman and Rothman, 1980).

Two changes thus occur. Basement membrane thickening seen as banded, fibrous and amorphous material that accumulates on the outer surface of the pigment epithelium is the earliest evidence of disturbance. Drusen as localized collections of debris (*Figure 4.1*) that lie beneath the basement membrane of the pigment epithelium on the surface of, or within the outer collagenous layer of, Bruch's membrane, are seen later.

Sarks (1976) classified basement membrane changes according to the increasing amount of deposit seen and the development of pigment epithelial changes. As the deposit increases the pigment epithelium thins and reduction in the number of nuclei occurs. Proliferative changes then produce mounds of pigment granules. Later geographic atrophy with loss of the pigment epithelium is visible. At this stage the photoreceptors in the atrophic area show progressive degeneration so that the outer plexiform layer lies directly on the basal laminar material and at the same time the choroid becomes more atrophic. However, according to Gartner and Henkind (1981) the loss of nuclei in the outer nuclear layer appears to be a primary event and not necessarily correlated with changes in the retinal pigment epithelium.

As the basement membrane changes advance fibrovascular invasion from the choroid may occur. Drusen vary from small, discrete mounds of less than 50 μ to larger accumulations with diameters of several hundred μ. Their edges may be sharply or ill-defined. Some are flat whereas others displace the pigment epithelium, giving the appearance of a shallow detachment. In colour they range from white to a creamy-orange, depending on their lipofuscin content and the amount of overlying pigment. Whilst drusen are usually seen in the posterior pole they may occur in the mid-periphery and equatorial regions. When the overlying retinal pigment epithelium is thinned rather than depigment the lesions are readily

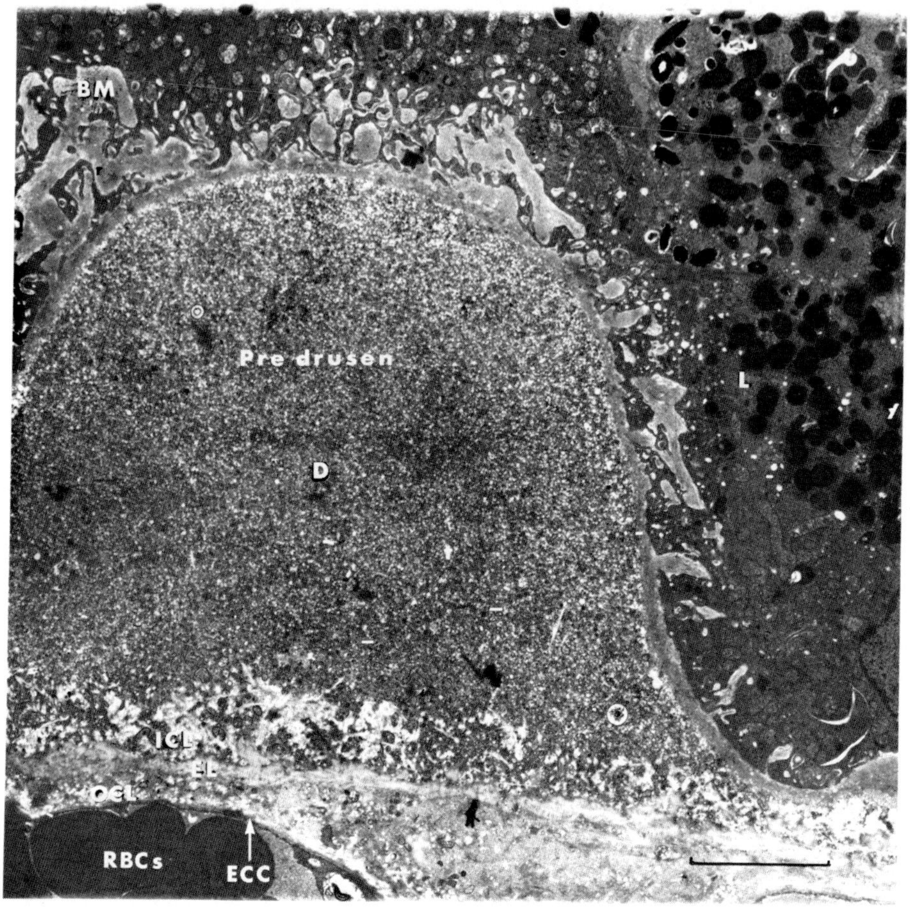


*Figure 4.1* Basement membrane thickening (basal laminar deposit) (BM) and drusen deposit (D) under the pigment epithelium of a 65-year-old subject. Lipofucsin granules (L) are seen in the outer part of the cell and the inner collagenous layer of Bruch's membrane under the drusen (ICL). The elastic layer (EL) and the outer collagenous layer (OCL) are also shown. ECC = Endothelium of choriocapillaris; RBCs = red blood cells; Bar marker = 2μ (*photograph courtesy of J. Marshall*)

recognized by retro-illumination. In each patient drusen appear to be symmetrically distributed in the two eyes (Young, personal communication). Sarks broadly groups drusen according to their apparent consistency. The hard, and often small, deposits have the staining properties of hyalinized Bruch's membrane. The softer, and usually larger, drusen are finely or coarsely granular, and on electron microscopy contain amorphous material, vesicles and other membranous debris (Sarks, 1980).

The majority of drusen are seen in patients over the age of 50. With time they appear to increase in number and become more widespread. As the retina and the pigment retinal epithelium atrophy the drusen often disappear. They also disappear when the overlying retina becomes detached. Seen early in life they are held to be a manifestation of a dominantly inherited disorder. The presence of drusen nasal to the disc and electrophysiological changes have been suggested as a method of distinguishing between the senile and inherited forms of this disorder. Gass (1973) however feels that no such differentiation can be made.

Drusen, in themselves, produce few symptoms although large mound like drusen with retinal pigment epithelial disturbance at the fovea may produce a drop in visual acuity and distortion of the Amsler grid pattern. This situation is more akin to a pigment epithelium detachment and the clinical course is one of slowly progressive visual difficulty.

The association of drusen and pigment epithelial changes with neovascularization is still not established. Gregor, Bird and Chisholm (1977) showed that small discrete drusen were less likely to be associated with neovascularization than larger indistinct lesions. Drusen themselves do not, however, seem to produce neovascularization. In a study of senile changes in Caucasian and black populations Gregor and Joffe (1978) showed an approximately equal prevalence of drusen, but a much higher incidence of disciform degeneration in the Caucasian population. This supports the suggestion that other factors are involved in neovascularization. Sarks associates neovascularization with the clinical appearance of softening and smudging of the drusen. She fails, however, to conclude whether this, the basement membrane thickening or the attendant pigment epithelial changes are the basic cause. However, the combination of these changes, together with the presence of macrophages, seems to indicate an increased risk of disciform degeneration (Sarks *et al.*, 1980). Fluorescein angiography helps to define the extent of drusen and pigment epithelial changes. Drusen usually become hyperfluorescent early and remain so due to the accumulation of dye in the substance of the drusen even after background fluorescence has faded. When the pigment epithelium is thinned, but not depigment, angiography may reveal the presence of clinically undetected drusen, particularly in the young patient with the inherited form of the disorder. Drusen that appear to accumulate dye and become less well defined as the angiogram progresses should be watched in case they are harbouring a neovascular complex. It has been shown that neovascular complexes are most likely to be treatable, on angiographic criteria, when symptoms are of less than 2 weeks' duration and visual acuity is still better than 6/12 (Grey, Bird and Chisholm, 1979). It is, therefore, the development of new symptoms, or the onset of increasing distortion, that should provoke review and angiography. When one eye has a neovascular disciform lesion there is a 12% per year, or approximately 50% 5-year risk, of the second eye following the same course, but in the absence of symptoms it is unlikely that laser photocoagulation will be indicated (Grey, Bird and Chisholm, 1979). Many eyes with drusen do not develop neovascular disciform lesions and for these the relatively benign nature of the disorder should be remembered.

## Geographic atrophy

With the passage of time drusen may give rise to atrophy of the neuroretina and retinal pigment epithelium. The development of small areas of geographic atrophy is certainly a common event and these may coalesce to form larger patches with loss of visual acuity if the fovea is involved. Gass followed 17 patients with bilateral drusen for 5 years and showed fading and disappearance of the drusen in five and geographic atrophy in five. Gass (1973) and Willerson and Aaberg (1978) reported the development of atrophy of the pigment epithelium and choriocapillaris 7 years after they had recorded heavy concentrations of drusen in the same area. In contrast, dominantly inherited central areolar choroidal sclerosis develops earlier in life and is not associated with drusen (Sorsby and Crick, 1953). All cases of central areolar choroidal sclerosis examined by Blair (1975) were bilateral, whereas only six out of 11 with geographic atrophy were bilateral at the time of their last examination.

Sarks associates the atrophy of the pigment epithelium with the basement membrane changes. The collapse of a pigment epithelial detachment might account for the sharply demarcated margins seen in some cases. Ischaemic changes in the choroid might account for the atrophy but would be less likely to produce a sharply demarcated margin. It would seem likely that several factors play a part in the clinical picture of dry macular degeneration with or without serous retinal detachment and pigment epithelial separation.

Areas of pigment epithelial loss are lighter in colour than the normal fundus and have a punched-out margin. The underlying choriocapillaris is seen and, in the later stages, large choroidal vessels are prominent.

Diffuse and geographic atrophy of the posterior pole with associated pigment clumping and drusen are common findings in the elderly. Many patients with slowly developing, dry macular degeneration accept that ageing involves failure of central vision and consequently do not consult an ophthalmologist. No specific treatment has been shown to be of value but magnification with high reading additions, simple magnifiers or more sophisticated aids may help these patients. The effect of increased illumination as an adjunct to low vision aids should not be overlooked.

## Pigment epithelial detachment

The normally tight adhesion between Bruch's membrane and the retinal pigment epithelium is maintained by the collagen fibres of the inner collagenous layer of Bruch's membrane. A disturbance of this relationship allows spontaneous separation of the two layers. The accumulation of drusen and basal laminar material may account for this disturbance, producing a serous separation of the pigment epithelium (Gass, 1967; Hogan, Alvarado and Weddell, 1971). It is unlikely that shallow retinal pigment epithelial detachments would be recognizable clinically and indeed may settle spontaneously. Higher elevations, however, produce the clinical picture of a pigment epithelial detachment. Some remain unaltered for long periods, a few flatten spontaneously, whilst others develop choroidal neovascularization through Bruch's membrane into the previously avascular detachment.

A dome-shaped elevation of the pigment epithelium, occurring in the elderly, in the presence of drusen and diffuse Bruch's membrane changes, represents the avascular form of senile macular degeneration. Gass (1967) describes this as part of the evolution of the neovascular disease, and in a small series Teeters and Bird

(1973) associated this change with a 67% risk of developing neovascularization within 19 months. In a number of eyes, however, geographic atrophy appears to follow without evidence of neovascularization (Blair, 1975; Braunstein and Gass, 1979). Two studies have shown that under the age of 56 the majority of patients retained good vision and do not develop neovascularization (Lewis, 1978; Meredith, Braley and Aaberg, 1979). This complication is seen in older patients and those with detachments larger than one disc diameter. Hoskin, Bird and Sehmi (1981) have described a further change involving the retraction of the pigment epithelium exposing bare Bruch's membrane. On fluorescein angiography this may mimic a neovascular lesion and may account for the high reported incidence of this complication. Such tearing of the retinal pigment epithelium appears to occur when it detaches without its basement membrane. It is seen earlier in patients treated with argon laser photocoagulation than in the natural history of pigment epithelial detachments (Moorfields Macular Study Group, 1982). Whilst neovascularization and pigment epithelial detachments are both seen in the elderly they may not, as was first suggested, always be directly related. There is thus a spectrum of disease with varied outcomes depending on factors such as the nature of the detachment, the age of the patient, and the presence of other changes at the level of Bruch's membrane.

The incidence of pigment epithelial detachments is much lower than that of neovascular disciform lesions. In a retrospective survey of 2000 consecutive, non-diabetic, angiograms carried out at Moorfields, 445 neovascular lesions were identified, of which 90 were considered treatable on angiographic criteria. In contrast, there were only 63 pigment epithelial detachments (Grey, Bird and Chisholm, 1979). Neovascular disciform lesions are more likely to present clinically than serous detachments of the pigment epithelium as the latter may produce relatively little visual disturbance. This fact may well indicate a higher prevalence of pigment epithelial detachments.

The dome-shaped elevation of the detachment produces an acquired hypermetropia with a disparity between the subjective and objective refraction of the eye. Blurring of the vision, distortion and micropsia are often presenting symptoms, although these are relatively mild and vision may remain good for long periods. Haemorrhage in the region of a detachment indicates the presence of neovascularization and is associated with further visual loss.

Although most recognized pigment epithelial detachments occur at the posterior pole they may also occur in the retinal periphery. Gass (1977) attributes this to the richness of the posterior pole vasculature and the greater resultant haemodynamic stress in that region. The stimulus for detachment remains unknown but presumably relates to the unique anatomical and functional characteristics of the region. Whilst the pigment epithelium remains healthy the sensory retina is applied to the surface of the detachment. Degeneration of the pigment epithelium, however, allows fluid to escape under the sensory retina and once this occurs subretinal fluid spreads more widely and diffusely.

Retinal pigment epithelial attachments vary in size, sometimes being several disc diameters across. They often have a slightly reniform configuration and are commonly unilateral. When bilateral they often have a similar appearance in each eye. The subpigment epithelial fluid may be clear or turbid and slightly yellow. The pigment epithelium itself can be seen to be spread over the surface of those with clear fluid but detail is lost when the fluid is turbid or long standing. Around the rim of clear detachments a curvilinear deposit can often be seen. This represents pigment epithelial debris deposited within the recess of the limits of the detachment. Pigment clumping and stellate figures are seen over the surface of some long standing detachments. Drusen and pigmentary disturbance usually accompany a detachment of the retinal pigment epithelium and are sometimes seen deep to the detachment, either on its back surface or at the level of Bruch's membrane. With the development of retinal and pigment epithelial degeneration, however, they usually become absorbed. Hruby or contact lens examination will show the extent of the detachment and surrounding changes. Subretinal fluid is more difficult to define as its limits merge into the flat surrounding retina, but subretinal blood has a dark, almost 'melanotic' appearance. A dark fluid level seen inferiorly within a detachment or the presence of blood or exudates around a detachment are signs of neovascularization.

The edge of a detachment may retract exposing the underlying Bruch's membrane. This event may occur rapidly and on close examination the rolled edge of the torn pigment epithelium can sometimes be seen. This event is more likely to occur when the detached pigment epithelium does not have drusen and debris on its deep surface (Hoskin, Bird and Sehmi, 1981). This led to the conclusion that the presence of basement membrane and the attached debris supports the pigment epithelium whereas its absence predisposes to sudden tearing.

Fluorescein remains strictly within the detached pigment epithelium unless there is a breakdown of the barrier, when there is a gradual spread into the space under the neurosensory retina. Not all detachments have the same characteristics on fluorescein angiography. Many fill early and evenly with dye continuing to fluoresce after the background fluorescence has faded (*Figure 4.2*). Others appear to fill evenly but more slowly, suggesting a slower rate of diffusion into the subpigment epithelial space. Masking of fluorescence within a detachment or an inferior fluid level may indicate the presence of blood. A spot that becomes brighter than the detachment itself and leaks as the angiogram progresses is suggestive of neovascularization (*Figure 4.3*). Pigment hyperplasia on the surface of a detachment indicates chronicity and will mask fluorescence. Although drusen often disappear from under a detachment some may remain on its back surface or attached to Bruch's membrane. The latter drusen may mask dye early in the study but fluoresce as they too accumulate dye. Detachments with basement membrane debris and drusen attached to their back surface fluoresce irregularly whilst in the absence of such debris this feature is absent. It is a combination of these two appearances in one detachment that seems to be associated with tearing of the pigment epithelium (*Figure 4.4*). Assessment of the level of fluorescein and other changes requires good stereoangiography and comparison with colour photographs.

Smaller detachments appear similar to multiple drusen. Some of these drusen may appear to be larger and have the angiographic characteristics of a detachment. Drusen themselves may be considered to be small focal detachments of the pigment epithelium so that their relationship to the larger lesion is close. Furthermore, both entities are at times associated with the development of neovascularization and both are flattened by photocoagulation.

Photocoagulation of disciform lesions was first reported in 1968 when the xenon arc was used (Watzke and Sneider, 1968). Later pulsed ruby laser burns were applied, and subsequently argon laser photocoagulation became the mainstay of treatment (Bird 1974; L'Esperance, 1971; Zweng, Little and Peabody, 1968).

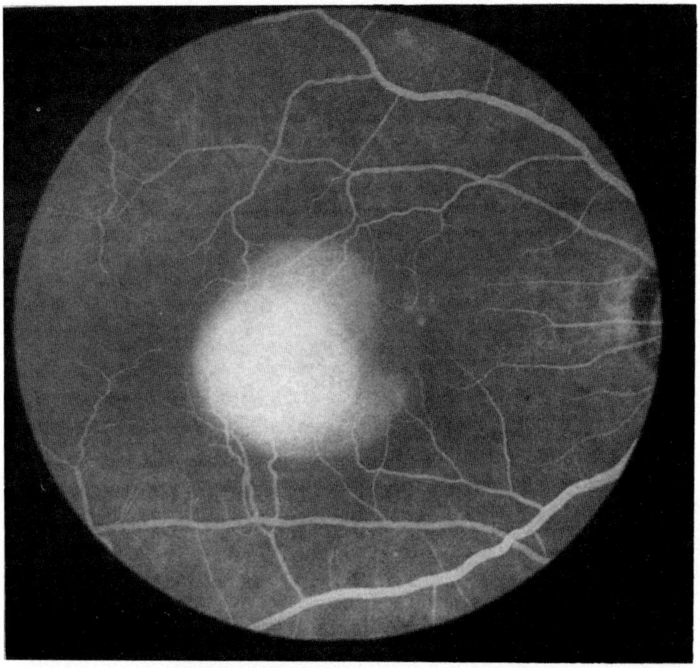

*Figure 4.2* The later phase of a fluorescein angiogram of an evenly filling pigment epithelial detachment. There is no masking within the detachment or evidence of local hyperfluorescence

Horseshoe applications around the temporal aspect of the pigment epithelial detachment were used at first and more recently a grid pattern of burns over the surface has been employed. Bird (1974) reported good results with 47 out of 53 detachments flattening after treatment and remaining so without loss of acuity during the follow-up period. This was, however, a pilot study and a prospective controlled trial (Moorfields Macular Study Group, 1982) has recently shown that treatment is not beneficial in terms of visual acuity up to 18 months after treatment. In this study the detachments were flattened in 13 out of 21 eyes. The pigment epithelium remained detached in two, a vascular disciform lesion developed in four and two developed a tear of the pigment epithelium. In contrast, the detachment persisted in 12 out of 24 untreated patients and in three flattened spontaneously. Six developed a disciform neovascular lesion, and three a tear of the pigment epithelium. This latter event occurred much earlier in treated than in untreated

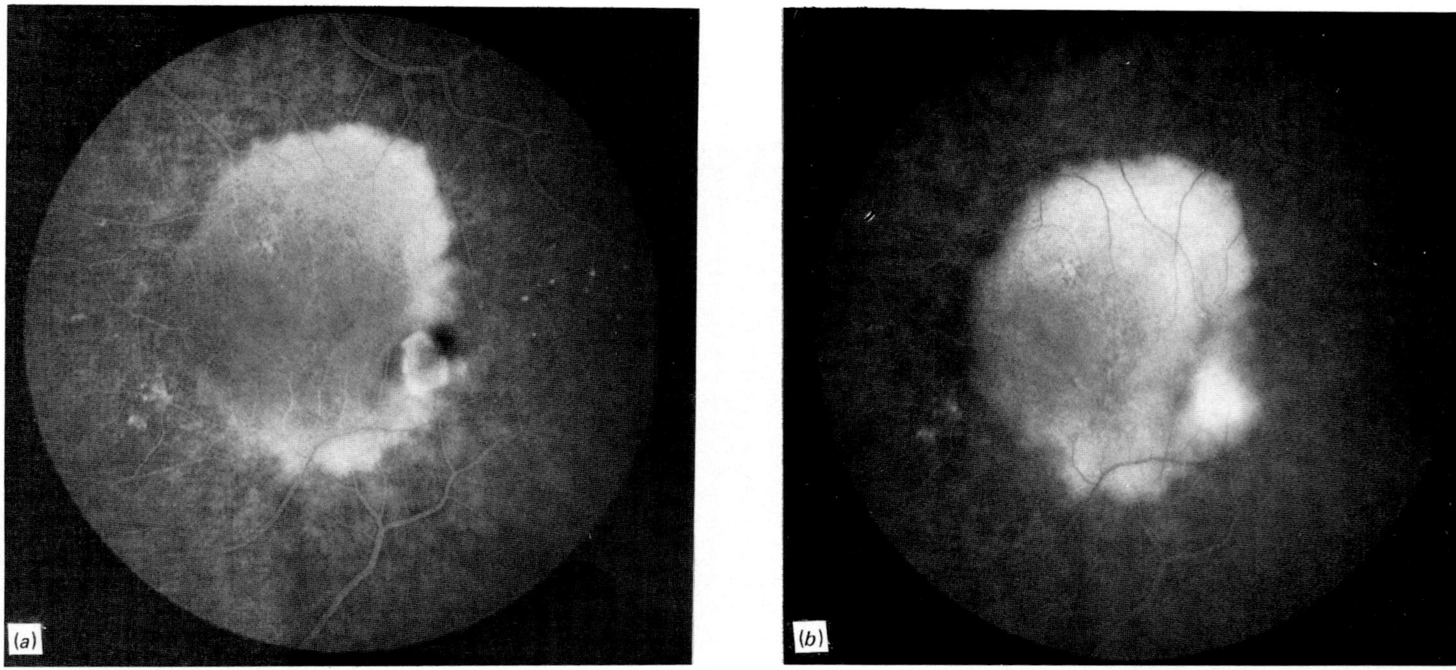

*Figure 4.3 (a) and (b)* Fluorescein angiogram of a pigment epithelial detactment showing a hyperfluorescent and a leaking spot developing as the angiogram progresses. There is also central masking and slow filling.

eyes. There was an early and sustained drop in visual acuity in treated eyes that was not seen in the untreated. Although there was a gradual drop in acuity in untreated cases it did not approach the level seen in those treated, and up to 18 months after entry there was no evidence that a crossover might occur. It was also felt that tightening of the entry criteria would not have altered the outcome of the study. No difference in the prognosis in the older and younger group of patients was found. This may, however, reflect the fact that relatively few of the patients were under

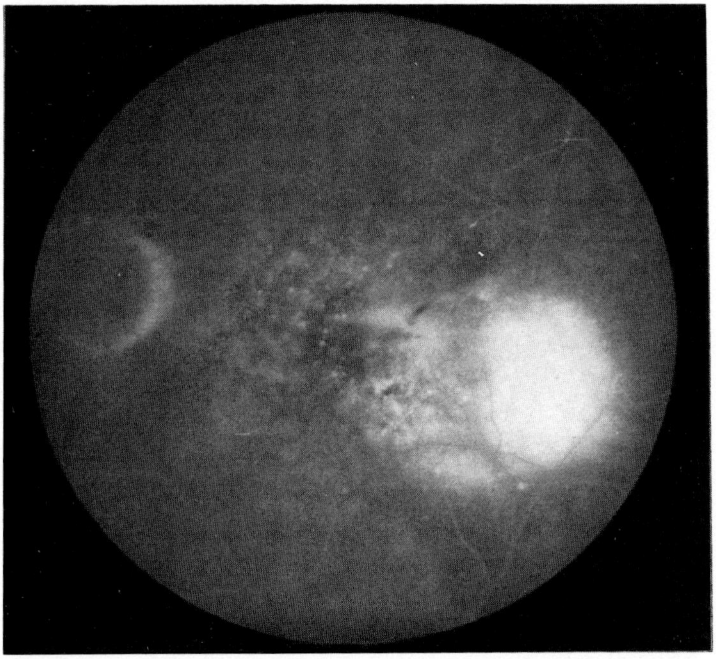

*Figure 4.4* The late phase of a fluorescein angiogram of a pigment epithelial detachment showing debris on the back surface of the detachment which fluoresces irregularly and a more even fluorescence temporally. The combination of these changes is often associated with tearing of the pigment epithelium

the age of 55 when the prognosis is thought to be better. In a number of patients there was early loss of vision even though the detachment was flattened. In these patients atrophy seemed to involve the fovea and it had to be assumed that energy had been absorbed more widely than the area of treatment. Luteal pigment absorption might have accounted for this finding. Alternatively, there might have been an inability to disperse the photic energy due to material within the detachment, or the relative remoteness of the underlying choroid to act as a heat exchanger (Parver, Auker and Carpenter, 1981).

In the natural history studies it would seem that the development of a neovascular complex poses a greater threat to vision than detachment of the pigment epithelium. Whilst photocoagulation of a new vessel complex might be considered to prevent involvement of fixation the angiographic picture is often confusing and adequate treatment extremely difficult. Modification to the treatment, either in respect of the areas treated or in the wavelength or form of energy used, might produce different results. Based on the observed good natural history in younger patients, who behave more like those with central serous retinopathy, and the observation that treatment appears to produce early visual loss, it would seem that, at present, a conservative approach to management is appropriate in pigment epithelial detachments.

## DYSTROPHIC DISORDERS OF THE RETINAL PIGMENT EPITHELIUM

A number of disorders are characterized by the deposition of material at the level of or within the pigment epithelium. The material concerned in each of these disorders is presumably different as is the morphology, inheritance and natural history of the various diseases, but a common factor may well be the disordered metabolism of lipopigment and its clearance from the sensory retina and pigment epithelium.

### Fundus flavimaculatus or Stargardt's disease

Hadden and Gass (1976) showed that this is one disease differing only in its mode of presentation. The disease is recessively inherited with approximately equal sex distribution. Its onset is thought to be in the first or second decade but visual difficulty may not become apparent until later, and in about 20% is delayed into the fourth or fifth decade (Noble and Carr, 1979). In none of Hadden and Gass' series did the vision drop below finger counting and most had better than 3/60 acuity. Normal peripheral fields and night vision are retained and only when very advanced is there much colour vision or electrophysiological loss.

Two clinical pictures are seen and these tend to combine to produce the final picture of the advanced disease: peripheral flecks and central atrophy. Peripheral flecks are seen around the macula and are prominent and yellowish in colour. Progressively the area of involvement becomes larger, affecting the more peripheral and central regions. The flecks are irregular in shape and may have a fish tail (pisciform) appearance. On fluorescein angiography, unlike drusen, they mask the background fluorescence. There is also a generalized darkening of the background (Bonnin, Passot and Triolaire, 1976) (*Figure 4.5*). With advancing disease, spots which probably represent the site of previous flecks transmit dye through the now thinned and atrophic pigment epithelium. Central atrophy of the macula, in contrast to the flecks, often has a 'beaten metal' appearance and glistens on direct illumination. There is associated pigment hypoplasia so that angiography shows a central transmission defect not unlike that seen in bull's eye maculopathy. At the onset of the disorder the peripheral flecks may predominate, or the central pigmentary disturbance and atrophy may be the dominant features. In either situation there is progression resulting in peripheral flecks with central disturbance or central atrophy with peripheral flecks.

Post-mortem findings from a 24-year-old patient with well-documented central and peripheral changes showed progressive enlargement and heterogenicity of the pigment epithelial cells from the equator posteriorly (Eagle *et al.*, 1980). Enlarged and hypomelanotic cells aggregated more posteriorly and were packed with PAS-positive material which had the properties of an abnormal form of lipofuscin. This would suggest an association with abnormal lipofuscin metabolism. The presence of lipofuscin, which will absorb the blue excitatory light, would account for the dark choroid seen on fluorescein angiograms in this condition. Fish *et al.* (1981) examined 91 patients with a variety of inherited macular dystrophies; 37 of these had dark choroids on angiography of whom 34 (92%) had flecks. The three patients without flecks had a bull's-eye pattern of pigment epithelial disease. Other conditions such as Best's disease, central areolar choroidal sclerosis, and chloroquine toxicity did not show the same change.

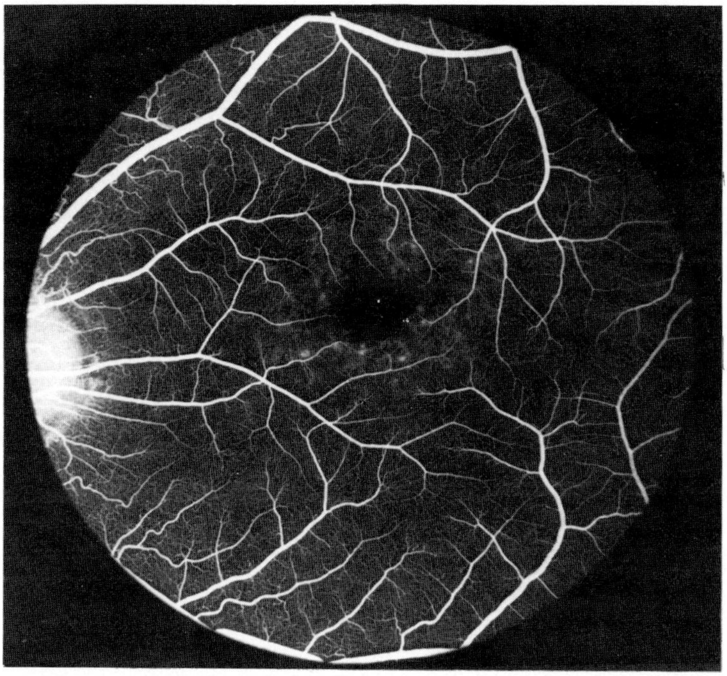

*Figure 4.5* Stargardt's disease or fundus flavimaculatus. Fluorescein angiogram showing a few hyperfluorescent spots but a generally dark background to the early stages of the study

## Pattern pigment epithelial dystrophy

Stargardt's disease is not the only condition to produce flecked retinal changes. Familial dystrophies which are dominantly or recessively inherited produce a variety of appearances. A pattern dystrophy of the retinal pigment epithelium has been reported in one family in four different forms (De Jong and Dellman, 1982). From this paper it would seem that the entities of fundus pulverulentus, horseshoe, butterfly, and reticular dystrophy are probably different manifestations of a similar disorder producing yellowish deposits at the level of the pigment epithelium. These deposits block the background fluorescence. The authors conclude that a single description as a 'pattern pigment epithelial dystrophy' would be more appropriate for these conditions.

## Best's disease

Although the clinical changes seen in Best's vitelliform macular dystrophy are usually at the posterior pole the disorder is more widespread as is shown by the marked reduction of the electro-oculogram (EOG) and the widespread retinal pigment epithelial changes seen histopathologically. The early lesion appears within the first few years of life but has been reported as late as the fifth decade or as early as the first week. It consists of a quarter to three-quarters disc diameter yellowish-orange deposit at the fovea which seems to consist of material produced in the pigment epithelium which coalesces to form an intracellular cyst. The cystoid lesion may develop a fluid level and later it may rupture, releasing yellowish material throughout the macula. This event may be followed by atrophy and hyperplasia of the pigment epithelium. Haemorrhage and neovascularization, if they occur, cause a fall of visual acuity. Multiple lesions are also seen in some patients but the majority are solitary, although bilateral. In the early stages the description of 'sunny side up egg' is sometimes used in contrast to the 'scrambled egg' stage seen later. Best's disease is dominantly inherited and is characterized by a grossly reduced EOG light rise which is not seen in other pigment epithelial disorders. Abnormal lipofuscin appears to be the material deposited (Weingeist, Kobrin and Watzke, 1982). Masking of the background fluorescence again seems to be a feature of the early angiogram. The cystoid space fills late and remains fluorescent after background fluorescence has faded. The development of neovascularization or haemorrhage produces further alteration to the angiographic picture.

## Foveomacular dystrophy

Gass (1974) described a series of elderly patients with foveomacular lesions. The lesions are usually symmetrically bilateral and are not normally associated with symptoms beyond those of mild metamorphopsia. Good vision is retained until late in life. The changes consist of a third disc diameter slightly raised, yellowish, round or oval patch with a central pigment spot. Haemorrhages and neovascularization do not appear to be associated features. Histopathologically there is thinning of the pigment epithelium which is degenerated and separated from the underlying Bruch's membrane by eosinophilic material. Angiography shows a hyperfluorescent ring surrounding the central masking. Whilst superficially it may represent a smaller version of Best's vitelliform dystrophy it is not accompanied by the later changes of that condition nor the reduced electro-oculogram. Whether the yellowish material represents lipofuscin or not is not established but the picture appears to represent a benign form of ageing at the posterior pole.

### Bull's eye maculopathy

A further change at the level of the pigment epithelium which is characteristic but which is produced by a variety of conditions is the bull's-eye appearance. A dark central area at the foveola is surrounded by a ring of apparent atrophy, around which is often a more pigment zone. Weise and Yannuzzi (1974) described a series of patients with this appearance, none of whom had taken chloroquine. Cone dystrophies, central serous retinopathy (choroidopathy), macular degeneration and Stargardt's disease have all been associated with this change. The history of chloroquine or hydroxychloroquine ingestion will point to a toxic basis in some patients whilst the history of day blindness, colour vision loss, and poor visual acuity will suggest a cone dystrophy in others. Cone dystrophies are usually sporadic although autosomal dominant and others forms also occur. In the early stages visual acuity may be preserved but the history and the presence of a perifoveal annular scotoma and the bull's eye macula should suggest the diagnosis (Grey, Blach and Barnard, 1977).

The fluorescein angiogram shows an annular transmission defect corresponding to the area of atrophy with central masking. Around this further masking occurs and in the periphery there may be a mottling of the fluorescein pattern. This indicates the more widespread nature of the disorder. As with other disorders of the pigment epithelium, the clinical changes indicate the area of maximal involvement. More widespread abnormalities will be seen on full histopathological and biochemical assessment.

## PLACOID AND GEOGRAPHIC (SERPIGINOUS) CHOROIDOPATHY

Gass (1968) first described acute posterior multifocal placoid pigment epitheliopathy (APMPPE, placoid). It typically affects young adults who present with a rapid onset of bilateral visual symptoms, sometimes following a mild systemic upset. On examination multiple, non-elevated, whitish-grey lesions are seen at the level of the pigment epithelium. These acute lesions mask the initial stages of the fluorescein angiogram but later they stain and remain hyperfluorescent after the background fluorescence has faded. If the fovea is involved there is loss of visual acuity but the prognosis for recovery otherwise is good. The individual lesions fade over the ensuing weeks and the pigment epithelium shows focal hyperplasia and atrophy.

Some cases of placoid show a temporal separation between the onset in the two eyes but recurrence does not usually occur. Others have been reported to be associated with bilateral serous detachments of the retina, raising the possibility of underlying choroidal ischaemia (Bird and Hamilton, 1972). Young, Bird and Sehmi (1980) reviewed 16 patients with acute pigment epithelial lesions, all of whom showed delayed choroidal filling. Three clinical pictures were seen. One had the appearance of placoid and it was postulated that each swollen patch represented a single non-perfused choroidal lobule. In the second, a more confluent plaque of infarction, possibly representing the occlusion of a specific submacular vessel, was noted (*Figure 4.6*). In the third group there was serous retinal detachment in the area of involvement. In contrast to the first group, the third resolved without pigmentary disturbance. Young suggested that this occurrence was due to ischaemic dysfunction rather than frank infarction of the pigment epithelium. The later pigmentary changes in placoid thus could be explained if choroidal infarction, for whatever reason, were the underlying cause.

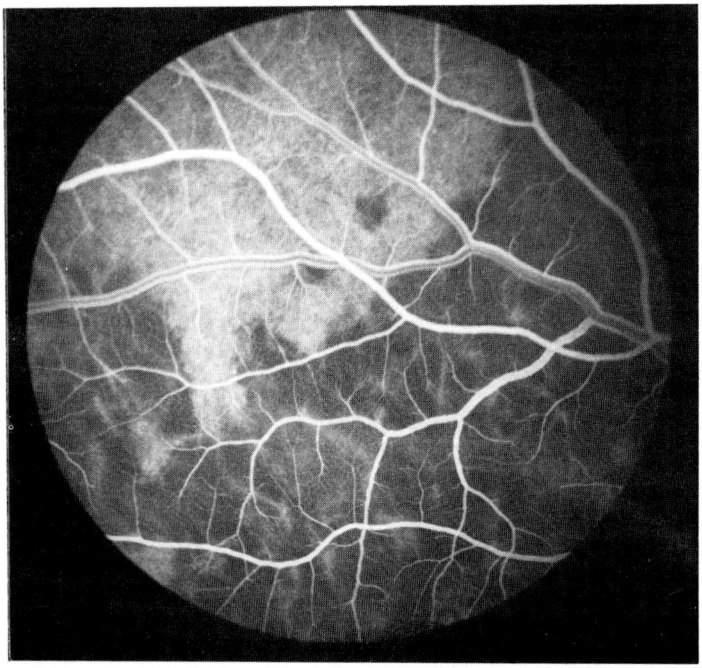

*Figure 4.6* Fluorescein angiogram of a patient with placoid showing the early venous phase. Large choroidal vessels are seen in the lower part where the choriocapillaris is non-perfused in contrast to the more normally perfused upper portion which also contains some areas of non-perfusion

Placoid affects patients in their 20s and 30s whereas geographic choroidopathy is usually a disease of the over-30s (Gass, 1977). Unlike placoid, recurrence is the rule, and bilaterality occurs but at different times. The fovea often becomes involved with consequent visual loss. Like placoid, each lesion appears to be at the level of the pigment epithelium and has a whitish-grey appearance. Subsequent acute lesions are seen in an eye with evidence of previous disturbance. Each new lesion, as in placoid, masks the early stages of the fluorescein angiogram and stains late, whereas the older lesions fluoresce early and remain so with scleral uptake of the dye. It was initially felt that the two entities were separate, but recurrence of placoid is reported and the final picture in both diseases can be similar, leading to widespread atrophy and pigment clumping. Subretinal and disc neovascularization has also been reported in a few cases (Laatikainen and Erkkila, 1982). As with placoid no definite basis has been shown for this disorder and choroidal ischaemia cannot be ruled out.

No specific treatment is effective for either placoid or geographic choroidopathy. The fact that serous detachment seen in placoid recovers spontaneously differentiates it from Harada's disease which is associated with systemic signs in addition to widespread pigment epithelial disturbance, fluorescein leakage, and retinal detachment. In this latter condition there is often rapid and complete resolution with the use of systemic cortiscosteroids.

## CONCLUSIONS

Disordered metabolism accounts for most of the clinical diseases of the retinal pigment epithelium. For some, this is the effect of ageing, whereas for others the disorder is presenile or genetically determined. In the majority of degenerative disorders, lipofuscin metabolism seems to be implicated. This also applies to the inherited dystrophies. Other disorders of the retinal pigment epithelium seem rather to be secondary manifestations of changes in adjacent structures. The interrelationship of the retinal pigment epithelium with the sensory retina and the underlying choroid must, however, be an important factor in all of these diseases.

## Acknowledgements

I should like to thank Mrs K. Church for typing the manuscript and Mr K. Sehmi for his assistance with the photographs.

## References

Bird, A. C. and Hamilton, A. M. (1972) Placoid pigment epitheliopathy presenting with bilateral serous retinal detachment. *British Journal of Ophthalmology*, **56,** 881

Bird, A. C. (1974) Treatment of senile macular degeneration by photocoagulation. *British Journal of Ophthalmology*, **58,** 367

Blair, C. J. (1975) Geographic atrophy of the retinal pigment epithelium. *Archives of Ophthalmology*, **90,** 25

Bonnin, P., Passot M. and Triolaire Cotten M Th. (1976) Le signe du silence choröidien dans les dégénérescences tapéto-rétiennes postérieures. *International Symposium on Fluorescein Angiography Documenta Ophthalmologica*, edited by De Laey, Volume **9,** pp. 461–463 *Proceedings Series*.

Braunstein, R. A. and Gass, J. D. M. (1979) Serous detachments of the retinal pigment epithelium in patients with senile macular disease. *American Journal of Ophthalmology*, **88,** 643

De Jong, P. T. V. M. and Dellman, J. W. (1982) Pigment epithelial pattern dystrophy: four different manifestations in a family. *Archives of Ophthalmology*, **100,** 1416

Eagle, R. C. Jnr., Lucier, A. C., Bernadino, V. B. and Yanoff, M. (1980) Retinal pigment epithelial abnormalities in fundus flavimaculatus: a light and electron microscopic study. *American Journal of Ophthalmology*, **87,** 1189

Feeney-Burns, L., Berman, E. R. and Rothman, H. M. . (1980) Lipofuscin of human retinal pigment epithelium. *American Journal of Ophthalmology*, **90,** 783

Fish, G., Grey, R., Sehmi, K. S. and Bird, A. C. (1981) The dark choroid in posterior retinal dystrophies. *British Journal of Ophthalmology*, **65,** 359

Gartner, S. and Henkind P. (1981) Ageing and degeneration of the human macula. 1. Outer nuclear layer and photoreceptors. *British Journal of Ophthalmology*, **65,** 23

Gass, J. D. M. (1967) Pathogenesis of disciform detachment of the neuroepithelium. 1. General concepts and classification. *American Journal of Ophthalmology*, **64,** 573

Gass, J. D. M. (1968) Acute posterior multifocal placoid pigment epitheliopathy. *Archives of Ophthalmology*, **80,** 177

Gass, J. D. M. (1973) Drusen and disciform macular detachment and degeneration. *Archives of Ophthalmology*, **62,** 547

Gass, J. D. M. (1974) A clinico-pathologic study of a peculiar foveomacular dystrophy. *Transactions of the American Ophthalmological Society*, **72,** 139

Gass, J. D. M. (1977) *Stereoscopic Atlas of Macular Diseases: Diagnosis and Treatment*, 19. St Louis: C. V. Mosby Co.

Gregor, Z., Bird, A. C. and Chisholm, I. H. (1977) Senile disciform macular degeneration in the second eye. *British Journal of Ophthalmology*, **61,** 141

Gregor, Z. and Joffe, L. (1978) Senile macular changes in the black African. *British Journal of Ophthalmology*, **62,** 547

Grey, R. H. B., Blach, R. K. and Barnard, W. M. (1977) Bull's eye maculopathy with early cone degeneration. *British Journal of Ophthalmology*, **61,** 702

Grey, R. H. B., Bird, A. C. and Chisholm, I. H. (1979) Senile disciform macular degeneration: features indicating suitability for photocoagulation. *British Journal of Ophthalmology*, **63,** 85

Grindle, C. F. J. and Marshall, J. (1978) Ageing changes in Bruch's membrane and their functional implications. *Transactions of the Ophthalmological Society of the United Kingdom*, **98,** 172

Hadden, O. B. and Gass, J. D. M. (1976) Stargardt's disease and fundus flavimaculatus. *American Journal of Ophthalmology*, **82,** 527

Hogan, M. J., Alvarado, J. and Weddell, J. E. (1971) *Histology of the Human Eye: An Atlas and Textbook*, 344. Philadelphia: Saunders

Hogan, M. J. (1972) Role of the retinal pigment epithelium in macular disease. *Transactions of the American Academy of Ophthalmology and Otolaryngology*, **76,** 64

Hoskin, A., Bird, A. C. and Sehmi, K. (1981) Tears of detached retinal pigment epithelium. *British Journal of Ophthalmology*, **65,** 417

Laatikainen, L. and Erkkila, H. (1982) Subretinal and disc neovascularization in serpiginous choroiditis. *British Journal of Ophthalmology*, **66,** 326

L'Esperance, F. A. (1971) Argon and ruby laser photocoagulation on disciform macular diseases. *Transactions of the American Academy of Ophthalmology and Otolaryngology*, **72,** 377

Lewis, M. L. (1978) Idiopathic serous detachment of the retinal pigment epithelium. *Archives of Ophthalmology*, **96,** 620

Meredith, T. A., Braley, R. E. and Aaberg, T. M. (1979) Natural history of serous detachments of the retinal pigment epithelium. *American Journal of Ophthalmology*, **88,** 643

Moorfields Macular Study Group (1982) Retinal pigment epithelial detachments in the elderly: a controlled trial of argon laser photocoagulation. *British Journal of Ophthalmology*, **66,** 1

Noble, K. G. and Carr, R. E. (1979) Stargardt's disease and fundus flavimaculatus. *Archives of Ophthalmology*, **97,** 1281

Parver, L. M., Auker, C. and Carpenter, D. O. (1981) Scleral surface temperature as a measure of reflexive increase in choroidal blood flow in response to light. *Association for Research in Vision and Ophthalmology Meeting*

Sarks, F. H. (1976) Ageing and degeneration in the macular region: a clinico-pathological study. *British Journal of Ophthalmology*, **60,** 324

Sarks, S. H. (1980) Drusen and their relationship to senile macular degeneration. *Australian Journal of Ophthalmology*, **8,** 117

Sarks, S. H., Van Driel, D., Maxwell, L. and Killingsworth, M. (1980) Softening of drusen and subretinal neovascularisation. *Transactions of the Ophthalmological Society of the United Kingdom*, **100,** 414

Sorsby, A. and Crick, R. P. (1953) Central areolar choroidal sclerosis. *British Journal of Ophthalmology*, **37,** 129

Teeters, V. W. and Bird, A. C. (1973) The development of neovascularization of senile disciform degeneration. *American Journal of Ophthalmology*, **76,** 1

Watzke, R. A. and Sneider, W. B. (1968) Light coagulation for haemorrhagic disciform degeneration in the macula. *Translations of the American Academy of Ophthalmology and Otolaryngology*, **72,** 389

Weingeist, T. A., Kobrin, J. L. and Watzke, R. C. (1982) Histopathology of Best's macular dystrophy. *Archives of Ophthalmology*, **100,** 1108

Weise, E. W. and Yannuzzi, L. A. (1974) Ring maculopathies mimicking choroquine retinopathy. *American Journal of Ophthalmology*, **78,** 204

Willerson, D. and Aaberg, T. M. (1978) Senile macular degeneration and geographic atrophy of the retinal pigment epithelium. *British Journal of Ophthalmology*, **62,** 551

Wing, G. L., Blanchard, G. C. and Weiter, J. J. (1978) The topography and age relationship of lipofuscin concentration in the retinal pigment epithelium. *Investigative Ophthalmology and Visual Science*, **17,** 601

Young, N. J. A., Bird, A. C. and Sehmi, K. (1980) Pigment epithelial diseases with abnormal choroidal perfusion. *American Journal of Ophthalmology*, **90,** 607

Zweng, H. C., Little, H. L. and Peabody, R. R. (1968) Laser photocoagulation of macular lesions. *Transactions of the American Academy of Ophthalmology and Otolaryngology*, **72,** 377

# 5
# Evaluation and treatment of subretinal neovascular membranes

Peter H. Morse and Janet V. Burch

## ETIOLOGY

A subretinal neovascular membrane is a tissue response to injury or disease. Subretinal neovascular membranes have been observed idiopathically in both young and old patients. They have also been associated with many conditions (*Table 5.1*)

Table 5.1 Diseases associated with subretinal neovascular membranes

| | |
|---|---|
| Presumed ocular histoplasmosis syndrome | |
| Severe myopia | |
| Healed disseminated chorioretinitis | |
| Toxoplasmosis | |
| Toxocariasis | |
| Sarcoidosis | |
| Drusen of the optic nerve head | Henkind (1978) |
| Hereditary drusen of Bruch's membrane | Cleasby (1976) |
| Angioid streaks | Cantrill and Burgess (1980) |
| Pseudotumor cerebri | Sheffer *et al.* (1980) |
| Choroidal folds | Troost, Sufit and Grand (1979) |
| Best's vitelliruptive macular dystrophy | Jamison (1978) |
| Fundus flavimaculatus | Morse *et al.* (1981) |
| Rubella retinopathy | Friberg and Grove (1980) |
| Choroidal nevi | Miller, Bresnick and Chandra (1976) |
| Choroidal melanoma | Deutman and Grizzard (1978) |
| Choroidal hemangioma | Frank and Purnell (1978) |
| Harmatoma of the retinal pigmented | Waltman *et al.* (1978) |
| epithelium | Michelson, Michelson and Chisari (1980) |
| Metastatic tumor | Jampol *et al.* (1979) |
| Coccidioidomycosis | Smith, Kelley and Harbin (1974) |
| Harada's disease | Hilton (1975) |
| Acute multifocal posterior placoid pigment epitheliopathy | |
| Behçet's disease | |
| Geographic (helicoid, serpiginous) choroiditis | |
| Choroidal rupture | |
| Excessive photocoagulation | |

Subretinal neovascular membranes may be single or multiple and be particularly likely to occur as a secondary complication of idiopathic diseases of the retinal pigmented epithelium and Bruch's membrane, or as a sequela of a disseminated chorioretinitis which has damaged Bruch's membrane and the retinal pigmented epithelium (RPE). Predisposing factors are a dehiscence in Bruch's membrane, physical deformation of anatomical boundaries and, conceivably, focal ischemia (Goldberg, 1976). Subretinal neovascular membrane formation may be further enhanced by the phagocytosis or enzymatic lysis of tissues by macrophages or lymphocytes.

## CLINICAL FEATURES

Unless a subretinal neovascular membrane compromises central vision or the visual field, the patient will be asymptomatic. However, the majority of patients seen by the ophthalmologist complain of diminished or blurred central vision, a positive or relative central or paracentral scotoma, metamorphopsia or a diminished appreciation of colors. There may be periods of exacerbation and remission of the patient's symptoms. A disease process with a natural history such as that of a subretinal neovascular membrane may cause a diminution of visual acuity as a result of transient serous or hemorrhagic separation of the foveola. After resorption of the fluid, the visual acuity may be restored to its previous level.

The location of a subretinal neovascular membrane is of critical importance, not only with respect to the symptoms experienced by the patient but also with respect to the potential for treatment. The commonest locations for symptomatic lesions are paramacular, macular, foveolar, or juxtapapillary.

The clinical appearance of subretinal neovascular membranes is widely variable, often depending upon the manifestations of the underlying disease. For example, a very small subretinal neovascular membrane may appear as a minute serous elevation of the retinal pigmented epithelium, resembling a druse and undergo its natural history with the deposition of a small amount of hard yellow exudate and ultimately cholesterol crystals after resorption of the fluid. So-called drusen may predispose to or signify diseases of the retinal pigmented epithelium, and it must be remembered that all yellow-colored lesions at the level of the retinal pigmented epithelium are not drusen. Such yellow deposits often represent a diseased or malfunctioning retinal pigmented epithelium. Such deposits or an alteration in the metabolism of the retinal pigmented epithelium may cause a secondary compromise of adjacent tissues, such as the photoreceptors, Bruch's membrane or the choriocapillaris since these tissues are anatomically, physiologically and functionally interrelated and interdependent. Any patient over 45 years of age with the symptoms and signs of a disease resembling central serous choroidopathy should arouse suspicion as showing manifestations of the very earliest subretinal neovascular membrane. A macular or juxtapapillary serous or hemorrhagic elevation of the retinal pigmented epithelium or sensory retina may be an early manifestation of a subretinal neovascular membrane before it has enlarged to a sufficient size to be discernible by either ophthalmoscopy or fluorescein angiography. Patients demonstrating these findings, especially those with diseases known to be associated with subretinal neovascular membrane, should be examined every 1–3 months. Clinically, subretinal neovascular membranes initially appear as serous or hemorrhagic elevations of the retinal pigmented epithelium or sensory retina. Frequently there is a marginal subsensory retinal hemorrhage, which, after it breaks through the retinal pigmented epithelium, is red in color. Almost invariably the subretinal neovascular membrane is located beneath these grey–green or yellow–pink colored lesions. Depending upon the location, duration and secondary manifestations of the disease, it may temporarily or permanently alter the function of the involved tissues.

The ophthalmoscopic appearances of the growth and natural history of a subretinal neovascular membrane are quite distinct. Once it becomes manifest, the greatest unknown is its potential for enlargement, the rapidity of its growth and the stimuli for such growth. Some subretinal neovascular membranes may remain stationary for years and then suddenly enlarge (*Figures 5.1 and 5.2*). The presence of a subretinal neovascular membrane located beneath the foveola, even without serous transudation or hemorrhage, may compromise the metabolism and function of the photoreceptors and retinal pigmented epithelium, which are essential for central vision. If the integrity of the retinal pigmented epithelium is disturbed one may see a mottling of hypopigmentation and hyperpigmentation or areas that are relatively depigmented with clumping of the melanin granules as a result of the physical disruption of the retinal pigmented epithelial cells. The melanin granules, which have previously been more or less evenly dispersed within the cells, are cast out and clump together once the cell is anatomically destroyed.

Diseases which are associated with subretinal neovascular membranes may also have manifestations of alterations in the retinal pigmented epithelium such as mottled hypopigmentation and hyperpigmentation indistinguishable from secondary changes in the retinal pigmented epithelium. The buds of capillaries initiating subretinal neovascular membrane growth usually originate from the choriocapillaris but occasionally originate from larger choroidal vessels and are accompanied by mesenchymal fibrous tissue. In the initial phases the vascular component is predominant and transudes plasma or hemorrhages.

The early stage is superseded by the intermediate or chronic phase in which the vascular tissue involutes and the fibrous component opacifies and becomes more visible. During the stages of transudation and hemorrhage, the retinal pigmented epithelium and sensory retina may be elevated to a variable extent, either by plasma or hemorrhage. Intermediate-to-chronic manifestations may be represented by subretinal hemorrhage, resorbing subretinal hemorrhage, which is yellow in color, hard yellow exudates in the retina, cholesterol crystals, subretinal fibrosis, chorioretinal atrophy, clumping of melanin granules, areas of hypopigmentation and hyperpigmentation, chronic serous separation of the central retina and overlying cystoid macular edema. Hemorrhage from subretinal neovascular membranes may break through into the vitreous, obscuring fundus details. In the chronic stages one observes subretinal fibrosis, which is largely the residual mesenchymal tissue àcompanying the growth of the subretinal neovascular mem-

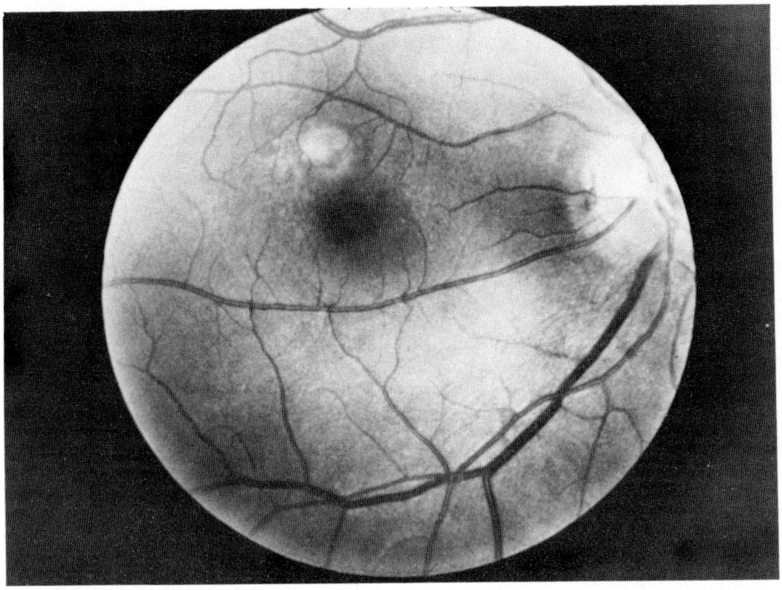

*Figure 5.1* Right fundus of a patient with a small subretinal neovascular membrane above the foveola seen in December 1976

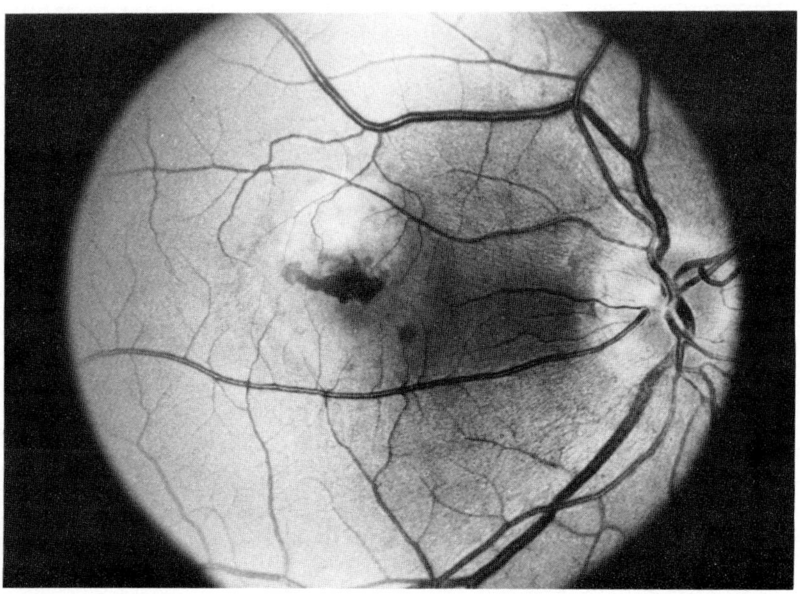

*Figure 5.2* Right fundus of the same patient as in *Figure 5.1* as he appeared at the end of March 1981 showing a rapid enlargement of the subretinal neovascular membrane which had remained quiet for over 4 years

brane. Some subretinal fibrosis may be the result of metaplasia of the retinal pigmented epithelium. The smaller retinal vessels in the fibrous tissue transude serous fluid which may lead to a chronic separation of the central retina. This chronic serous or sometimes recurrent hemorrhagic separation of the sensory retina predisposes to continuous atrophy of the photoreceptors and a deleterious effect on the retinal pigmented epithelium. The degeneration and atrophy is a consequence of the altered anatomical, physiological, and metabolic function of the retinal pigmented epithelium and contiguous tissues. As a consequence of chronic serous separation of the retina there may also be dilatation and tortuosity of the overlying retinal vessels (Gass, 1967a, 1967b, 1967c, 1967d; Chandra *et al.*, 1974; Patz, Fine and Orth, 1976; Small *et al.*, 1976; and Teeters and Bird, 1973)

## FLUORESCEIN ANGIOGRAPHY

One of the indications for retinal fluorescein angiography is to delineate the extent of a subretinal neovascular membrane. Fluorescein angiography is not a diagnostic modality, but rather a useful therapeutic guideline. Photographs should be sharply focused and be taken in all phases of dye transit.

The earliest manifestations of a subretinal neovascular membrane, because of its small size, may not be clearly definable, but only appear as a small enlarging hyperfluorescent dot. Hemorrhage or turbid subretinal fluid may also obscure the presence or extent of a subretinal neovascular membrane. A small one creating a serous separation of the retinal pigmented epithelium may be hidden by the turbidity of the subretinal fluid. Once a subretinal neovascular membrane has attained sufficient size to be defined by fluorescein angiography in the early stage of development when the vascular component is predominant, a characteristic lacy pattern appears in the early phases of fluorescein angiography (*Figures 5.3, 5.4, 5.5 and 5.6*).In the later stages the details of the vascular patterns are obscured by extravasation of the dye. In the late stages of the natural history of subretinal neovascular membranes when the fibrous tissue predominates, fluorescein angiography reveals a staining or low-grade leaking from the minute, ophthalmoscopically invisible blood vessels within the fibrous tissue. Fluorescein angiography is of no value in an eye in which the subretinal neovascular membrane appears in its end-stage involuted subretinal fibrous condition with marked disruption of the retinal pigmented epithelium. Fluorescein angiography should be done on the eye with better vision or more acute manifestations of a subretinal neovascular membrane in the hope of being able to apply treatment at a more propitious time. Once photocoagulation has been applied, a fluorescein angiogram immediately following treatment is of little value because the hyperfluorescence and staining is intensified, often blurring fine detail and obviating clear interpretation. Fluorescein angiograms to determine the obliteration of the subretinal neovascular membrane if they are necessary should be obtained 7–14 days following photocoagulation when healing has begun. The rapidity of the healing may depend upon the intensity of the photocoagulation (Fine, 1977; Schatz, 1977).

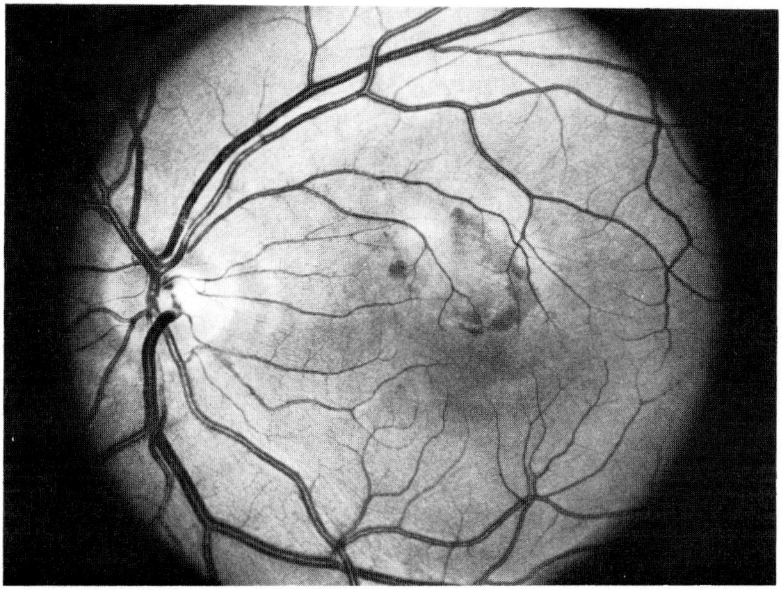

*Figure 5.3* Left fundus of a patient whose subretinal neovascular membrane underwent a sudden enlargement threatening his central vision. The darker surrounding area is caused by subretinal hemorrhage

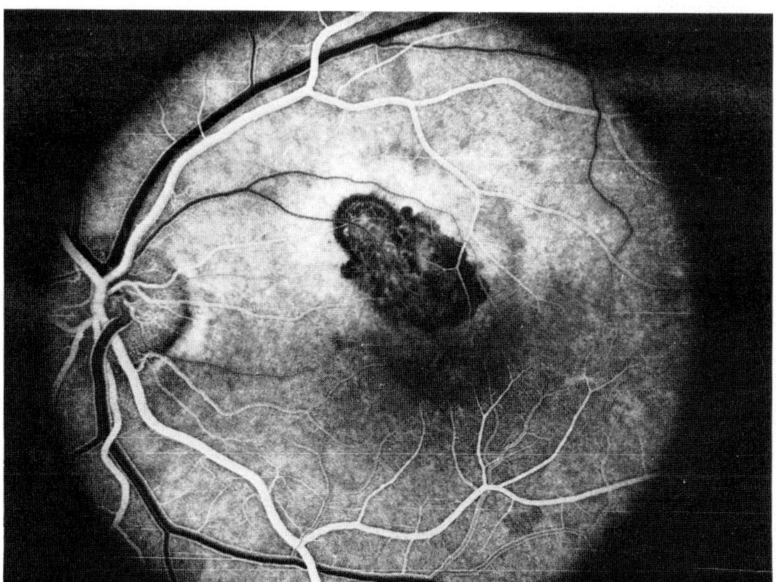

*Figure 5.4* Early-stage fluorescein angiogram of the same patient as in *Figure 5.3* showing the characteristic lacy configuration of the early vascular stage of the subretinal neovascular membrane

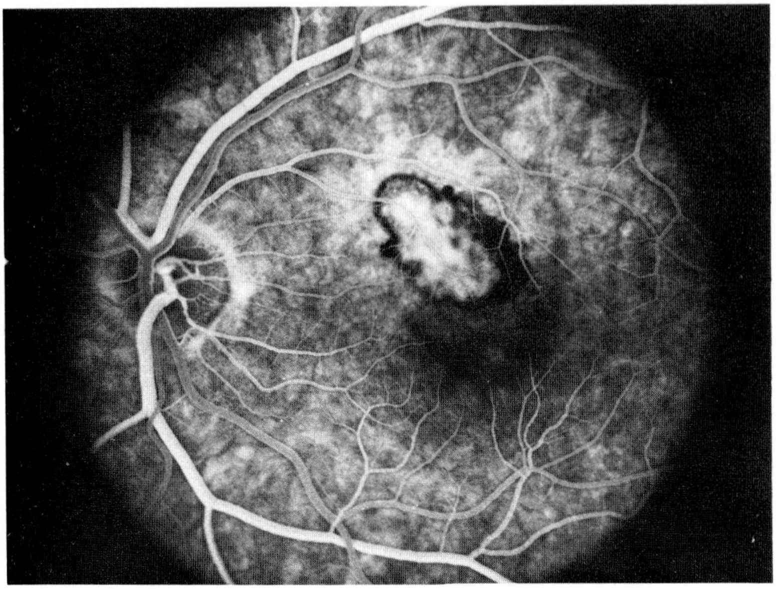

*Figure 5.5* Later stage fluorescein angiogram of the same patient as in *Figures 5.3* and *5.4* showing a diffuse leaking of the dye. Note that the surrounding hemorrhage which outlines the lesion remains dark in color

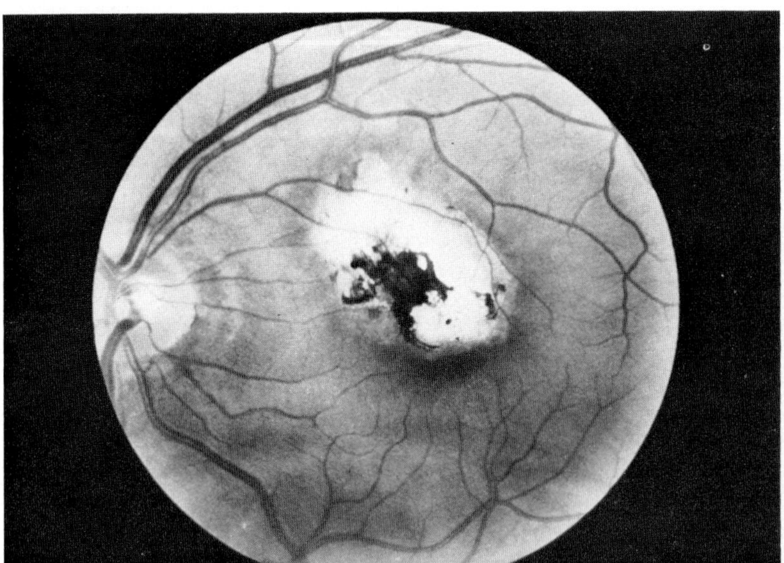

*Figure 5.6* Left fundus of the same patient as in *Figures 5.3, 5.4* and *5.5* showing the chorioretinal atrophy with hypopigmentation and hyperpigmentation 2 years following laser treatment. The chorioretinal atrophic area is larger than the acute laser lesion and the patient retained 6/6 and 4 point central vision

## TREATMENT TECHNIQUE

Photocoagulation is currently the most effective therapeutic modality to obliterate subretinal neovascular membranes. The success of the therapy and the visual outcome will depend upon the location, size, and amount of secondary damage such as disruption of the integrity of the retinal pigmented epithelium or the presence of chronic serous separation of the macula created by the subretinal neovascular membrane. Predisposing degenerative diseases may have caused irreparable damage to the patient's central vision prior to the complications imposed by the subretinal neovascular membrane.

A good quality fluorescein angiogram may be used as a guide during photocoagulation. Frequently the outlines of lesions are not seen with good definition ophthalmoscopically or using the slit-lamp and contact lens. In such cases the retinal vascular pattern on the fluorescein angiogram may be used to delineate the extent of the subretinal neovascular membrane when the eye is photocoagulated. If photocoagulation is done with a contact lens and a slit-lamp delivery system, a topical anesthetic only is used. On occasion, because of pain experienced by the patient, anxiety, or the desire for akinesia because of treatment near the foveola, a retrobulbar anesthetic may be necessary.

Any modality of photocoagulation may be used in treatment, including the xenon arc, argon, or krypton lasers. However, in lesions close to the foveola, the choice of wavelength is important. The blue wavelengths of the argon laser are deleterious as they are intensely absorbed by xanthophyll. The green wavelengths of the argon laser and the red wavelengths of the krypton laser are the most useful and effective. The red wavelengths of the krypton laser penetrate to the deeper layers from whence subretinal neovascular membranes originate and they also are not absorbed by blood. Greater absorption of certain wavelengths by blood may lead to a conduction of the thermal effect of the photocoagulation which will create more damage to adjacent tissues. Commonly, following treatment, the size of the resultant spot of chorioretinal atrophy enlarges. This may be disastrous if the pigmented epithelium beneath the foveola is damaged. The intensity of the photocoagulation must be adjusted, using three variables – spot size, duration of exposure, and power to ensure adequate but not excessive treatment. It has been found that heavy or intense treatment originally advocated for the treatment of subretinal neovascular membranes is frequently unnecessary. Often two to three treatments of a lesser intensity will be better than one heavy treatment.

In general, one tries to avoid treatment closer than 125 μ to the circle of terminal retinal capillaries which surround the capillary-free zone, or within the papillomacular bundle. Laser burns spread to a greater extent if there is an increase in the power or duration of the treatment time. If the duration of the treatment time is shortened to less than 0.01 sec the greater impact may create a rupture of retinal or choroidal vessels. To estimate the distance for safe treatment, in order to avoid the capillary-free zone, one takes one half of the diameter of the capillary-free, zone which is 500 μ, and adds to it 125 μ, which is the diameter of a retinal vein on the disc. This gives a figure of 375 μ from the umbo, leaving a margin of 125 μ from the capillaries forming the capillary-free zone. One may also estimate sizes by sharply focusing the attenuated laser beam on the retina and observing the size of the spot. In an attempt to locate the point of the patient's fixation one may ask him or her to look at the blue dot. However, patients with markedly reduced central visual acuity may be unable to visualize the spot.

The objective is to treat a subretinal neovascular membrane in its entirety, and sometimes it is not possible to avoid treatment within the papillomacular bundle or in an area 375 μ or more from the umbo. On occasion, one may treat only a portion of the membrane. Rapid photographs of the earliest phases of fluorescein dye transit during the angiogram may identify feeder vessels to which the more intense photocoagulation should be directed.

Using a 50–100 μ spot size, one outlines the extent and location of the subretinal neovascular membrane. An area of uninvolved tissue surrounding the outlined membrane should also be lightly treated. Once the membrane has been demarcated the spot size may be enlarged to 200 or 500 μ and the central portion of the membrane photocoagulated.

The treatment spot size, which is the attenuated laser beam, should be focused at the level of the lesion being treated. This is particularly true when there is overlying subretinal fluid and the beam should be focused on the subretinal neovascular membrane underlying the secondary serous separation. When one is treating juxtapapillary membranes lying beneath the papillomacular bundle, overlying subretinal fluid is beneficial for its insulating effect. The treatment should not create a white reaction in the retina within the papillomacular bundle (*Figures 5.7, 5.8, 5.9, 5.10, 5.11 and 5.12*).

The reaction to the laser should be grey to grey–white in color. If a krypton laser is used an adequate lesion is obtained with a less visible reaction.

As the acute laser burn heals it is replaced by a variable amount of chorioretinal atrophy with hypopigmentation and hyperpigmentation. The appearance of a grey–green or yellow–pink-colored elevation at the margin of the chorioretinal atrophy signifies a recurrence of the subretinal neovascular membrane and is an indication for immediate retreatment.

Patients should be examined weekly for 1 month following photocoagulation. Thereafter they should be seen every 3–6 months or annually depending upon whether or not they have a predisposition to further subretinal neovascular membrane growth.

Adequate and successful treatment with photocoagulation limits the size of a subretinal neovascular membrane and aborts its growth potential. The natural history of the process is accelerated by photocoagulation by obliterating the vascular component and leaving the residual fibrosis. If photocoagulation is used on smaller membranes in the earlier stages the resultant scotoma will be smaller and the amount of subretinal fibrosis, which increases in size as the membrane grows, will be minimal. With satisfactory obliteration of neovascularization the risk of hemorrhage and chronic serous fluid transudation is also eliminated (Fine *et al.* 1976, 1977: Leveille, Morse and Burch, 1981; Schatz and Patz, 1973a, 1973b; Schlaegel, 1977).

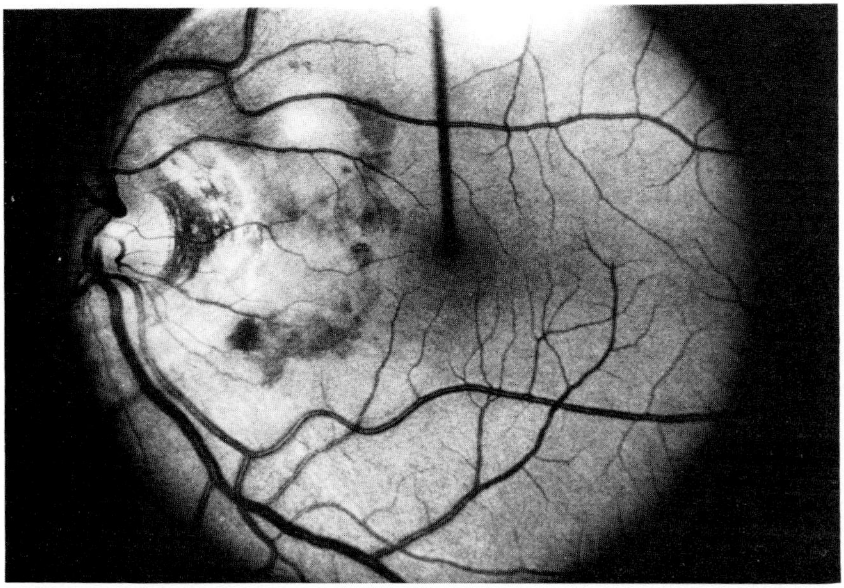

*Figure 5.7* Left fundus of the patient with peripapillary chorioretinal atrophy as a result of healed chorioretinitis. There is a large subretinal neovascular membrane with a margin of subretinal hemorrhage spreading toward the foveola (see fixation marker)

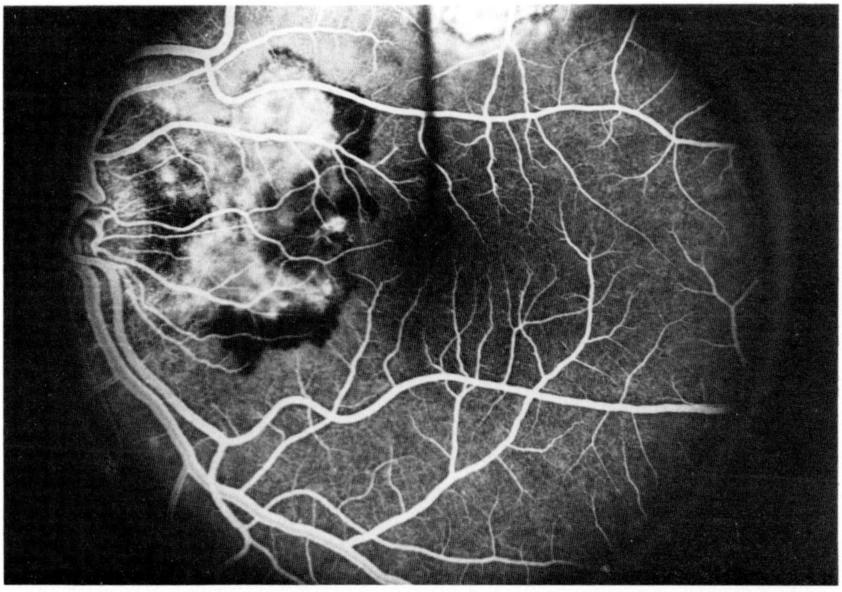

*Figure 5.8* Fluorescein angiogram of the patient illustrated in *Figure 5.2* showing the hyperfluorescence of the subretinal neovascular membrane and the darker margin of the hemorrhage

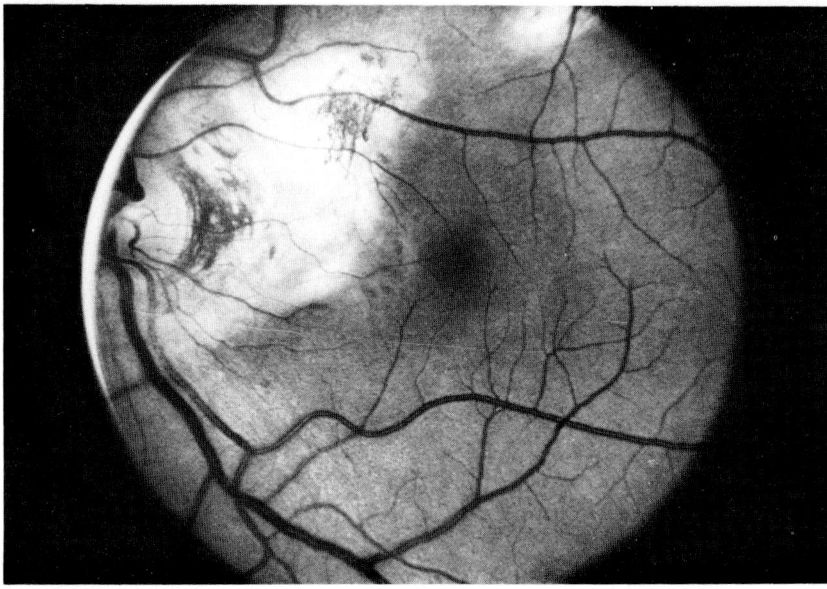

*Figure 5.9* Fundus of the same patient as in *Figures 5.7* and *5.8*, 7 months following obliteration of the original subretinal neovascular membrane with the argon laser. At the inferior margin of the chorioretinal atrophy there was a grey–green-colored elevation indicative of a subretinal neovascular membrane recrudescence approaching the foveola

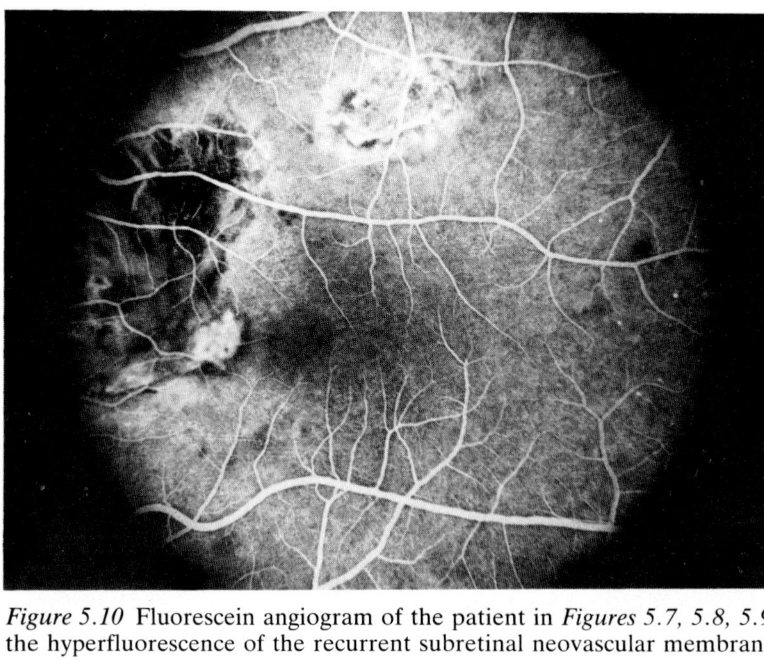

*Figure 5.10* Fluorescein angiogram of the patient in *Figures 5.7, 5.8, 5.9* and *5.10* showing the hyperfluorescence of the recurrent subretinal neovascular membrane

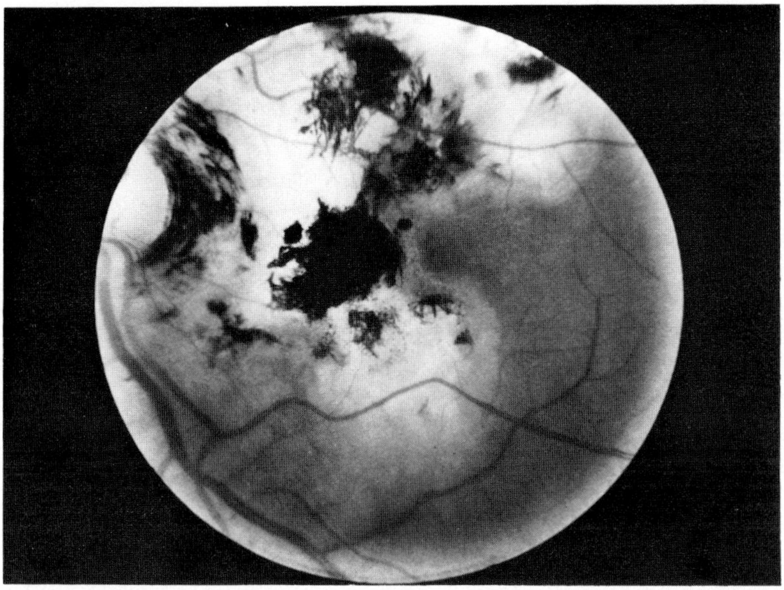

*Figure 5.11* Fundus photograph of the patient in *Figures 5.7, 5.8, 5.9* and *5.10* showing successful obliteration of the subretinal neovascular membrane after further argon laser treatment. The patient retained 6/12 and 6 point visual acuity

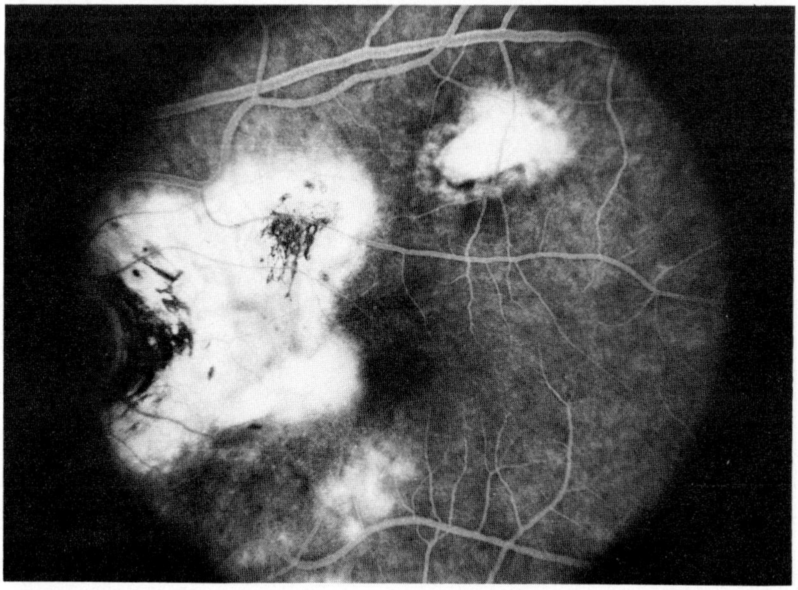

*Figure 5.12* Fluorescein angiogram of the patient illustrated in *Figures 5.7, 5.8, 5.9, 5.10* and *5.11* confirming the obliteration of the subretinal neovascular membrane and the intactness of the retinal pigmented epithelium underlying the foveola. The hyperfluorescence is from residual fibrosis and the exposed sclera

## Complications

Inadequate, incomplete or excessive treatment may each cause failure. There may be a regrowth of the subretinal neovascular membrane from within the photocoagulated area at its margin and elsewhere, particularly in a patient with a predisposing disease, such as senile macular degeneration or the presumed ocular histoplasmosis syndrome. Excessive photocoagulation may create chorioretinal atrophy and dehiscences in Bruch's membrane which may lead to the appearance of another subretinal neovascular membrane. Excessive impact of the laser beam, especially when using shorter duration of exposure and higher power, may cause a rupture of retinal or choroidal vessels. Prior to the healing of the lesion created by the laser, there is often a greater amount of transudate or edema which may temporarily decrease visual acuity. If the amount of fibrous tissue in the membrane is large, its contraction during the healing process may create retinal folds or striae. If these folds or striae affect the foveola, there may be a decrease in central visual acuity or the patient may experience metamorphopsia. Photocoagulation may also create scotoma or sectoral visual field defects, depending upon the location and intensity of its application. Other complications of photocoagulation include damage to the cornea, lens, and iris. These are quite rare and may be avoided by care during the treatment. Combined or choroidal separation is sometimes seen as a complication of extensive photocoagulation, and preretinal or vitreoretinal membranes have also been noted, usually after heavy photocoagulation.

## PROGNOSIS AND COMMENT

The natural history of subretinal neovascular membranes is unpredictable with respect to their appearance, rapidity of growth, and ultimate size. The symptoms may not occur in a patient until the membrane has extended beneath the foveola, making effective treatment difficult if not impossible. Subretinal neovascular membranes occurring in areas that are safe for treatment may undergo spontaneous involution without therapy. However, it is impossible to predict at this time which patients will have this favorable outcome and which will lose central vision by the enlargement of these membranes. Even in patients who are well informed, intelligent, and aware of their condition, a rapid enlargement of a subretinal neovascular membrane may threaten or destroy central vision. The ultimate prognosis depends upon the location of the lesion, the efficacy of the treatment, and the secondary changes caused by the complication of subretinal neovascular membrane growth or the underlying diseases which predispose to such neovascularization.

## Acknowledgement

This work was supported in part by an unrestricted grant from Research to Prevent Blindness, New York.

## References

Cantrill, H. L. and Burgess, D. (1980) Peripapillary neovascular membranes in presumed ocular histoplasmosis. *American Journal of Ophthalmology*, **89,** 192

Chandra, S. R., Gragoudas, E. S., Friedman, E., van Buskirk, E. M. and Klein, M. L. (1974) Natural history of disciform degeneration of the macula. *American Journal of Ophthalmology*, **78,** 579

Cleasby, G. W. (1976) Idiopathic focal subretinal neovascularization. *American Journal of Ophthalmology*, **81,** 590

Deutman, A. F. and Grizzard, W. S. (1978) Rubella retinopathy and subretinal neovascularization. *American Journal of Ophthalmology*, **85,** 82

Fine, S. L., Patz, A., Orth, D. H., Klein, M. L., Finkelstein, D. and Yassur, Y. (1976) Subretinal neovascularization developing after prophylactic argon laser photocoagulation of atrophic macular scars. *American Journal of Ophthalmology*, **82,** 352

Fine, S. L. (1977) Fluorescein angiography in ocular histoplasmosis with an introduction on principles of angiographic interpretation. *Perspectives in Ophthalmology*, **1,** 111

Fine, S. L., Klein, M. L., Patz, A. and Finkelstein, D. (1977) Criteria for photocoagulation of neovascular membranes in ocular histoplasmosis. *Perspectives in Ophthalmology*, **1,** 125

Frank, K. E. and Purnell, E. W. (1978) Subretinal neovascularization following rubella retinopathy. *American Journal of Ophthalmology*, **86,** 462

Friberg, T. R. and Grove, A. S. Jr. (1980) Subretinal neovascularization and choroidal folds. *Annals of Ophthalmology*, **12,** 245

Gass, J. D. M. (1967a) Pathogenesis of disciform detachment of the neural epithelium. I. General concepts and classification. *American Journal of Ophthalmology*, **63,** 573

Gass, J. D. M. (1967b) Pathogenesis of disciform detachment of the neural epithelium. III. Senile disciform macular degeneration. *American Journal of Ophthalmology*, **63,** 617

Gass, J. D. M. (1967c) Pathogenesis of disciform detachment of the neural epithelium. IV. Fluorescein angiographic study of senile disciform macular degeneration. *American Journal of Ophthalmology*, **63,** 645

Gass, J. D. M. (1967d) Pathogenesis of disciform detachment of the neuroepithelium. V. Disciform macular degeneration secondary to focal choroiditis. *American Journal of Ophthalmology*, **63,** 661

Goldberg, M. F. (1976) Bruch's membrane and vascular growth. *Investigative Ophthalmology*, **15,** 443

Henkind, P. (1978) Ocular neovascularization. The Krill Memorial Lecture. *American Journal of Ophthalmology*, **85,** 287

Hilton, G. F. (1975) Late serosanguineous detachment of the macula after traumatic choroidal ruptures. *American Journal of Ophthalmology*, **79,** 997

Jamison, R. R. (1978) Subretinal neovascularizaton and papilledema associated with pseudotumor cerebri. *American Journal of Ophthalmology*, **85,** 78

Jampol, L. M., Orth, D., Daily, M. J. and Rabb, M. F. (1979) Subretinal neovascularization with geographic (serpiginous) chroiditis. *American Journal of Ophthalmology*, **88,** 683

Leveille, A. S., Morse, P. H. and Burch, J. V. (1981) Subretinal neovascular membranes. *Perspectives in Ophthalmology*, **4,** 313

Michelson, J. B., Michelson, P. E. and Chisari, F. V. (1980) Subretinal neovascular membrane and disciform scar in Behçet's disease. *American Journal of Ophthalmology*, **90,** 182

Miller, S. A., Bresnick, G. H. and Chandra, S. R. (1976) Choroidal neovascular membrane in Best's vitelliform macular dystrophy. *American Journal of Ophthalmology*, **82,** 252

Morse, P. H., Leveille, A. S., Antel, J. P. and Burch, J. V. (1981) Bilateral juxtapapillary subretinal neovascularization associated with pseudotumor cerebri. *American Journal of Ophthalmology*, **91,** 312

Patz, A., Fine, S. L. and Orth, D. H. (1976) *Diseases of the Macula*, 12–22. St Louis; C. V. Mosby Co.

Schatz, H. and Patz, A. (1973a) Exudative senile maculopathy. I. Results of argon laser treatment. *Archives of Ophthalmology*, **90,** 183

Schatz, H. and Patz, A. (1973b) Exudative senile maculopathy. II. Complications of argon laser treatment. *Archives of Ophthalmology*, **90,** 197

Schatz, H. (1977) Subretinal neovascularization: clinical findings and fluorescein angiographic characteristics. *Perspectives in Ophthalmology*, **1,** 59

Sheffer, A., Green, W. R., Fine, S. L. and Kincaid, M. (1980) Presumed ocular histoplasmosis syndrome. A clinicopathologic correlation of a treated case. *Archives of Opthalmology*, **98,** 335

Schlaegel, T. F. (1977) The principles of partial photocoagulation of the presumed ocular histoplasmosis syndrome. *Perspectives in Ophthalmology*, **1,** 119

Small, M. L., Green, W. R., Alpar, J. J. and Drewry, R. E. (1976) Senile macular degeneration. *Archives of Ophthalmology*, **94,** 601

Smith, R. E., Kelley, J. S. and Harbin, T. S. (1974) Late macular complications of choroidal ruptures. *American Journal of Ophthalmology*, **77,** 650

Teeters, V. W. and Bird, A. C. (1973) The development of neovascularization of senile disciform macular degeneration. *American Journal of Ophthalmology*, **76,** 1

Troost, B. T., Sufit, R. L. and Grand, M. G. (1979) Sudden monocular visual loss in pseudotumor cerebri. *Archives of Neurology*, **36,** 440

Waltman, D. D., Gitter, K. A., Yannuzzi, L. and Schatz, H. (1978) Choroidal neovascularization associated with choroidal nevi. *American Journal of Opthalmology*, **85,** 704

# 6
# The retina in metabolic diseases in childhood

Alistair Fielder and David Taylor

## INTRODUCTION

Although rare, the disorders described in this chapter are of more than purely academic interest as they can masquerade as more common conditions without the same systemic impact or genetic implications. The correct diagnosis is not only relevant from the genetic point of view as in certain cases treatment is now available.

## JUVENILE BATTEN'S DISEASE (NEURONAL CEROID LIPOFUSCINOSIS)

Batten's disease is the commonest neurodegenerative disorder seen at the Hospital for Sick Children in London (Spalton, Taylor and Sanders, 1980). It can be divided into infantile, late infantile, and juvenile types on clinical, electrophysiological, and ultrastructural grounds.

The infantile and late infantile types usually develop visual problems in the course of the disease, but it is the juvenile variant which is of greatest importance to the ophthalmologist as it may present with visual failure early in its clinical course.

### Retinopathy

In juvenile Batten's disease visual failure begins between the ages of 4 and 8 years (most commonly in the 6th and 7th year). The typical ophthalmoscopical picture is that of a bull's eye maculopathy (*Figure 6.1*). Later, a more widespread pigmentary disturbance develops with thinning of the arterioles and atrophy of the retinal nerve fibre layer (*Figure 6.2*). Occasionally a peripheral 'bone corpuscle' type of pigmentation is seen. Leakage of fluorescein from the retinal circulation may occur in actively degenerating retina (Spalton, Taylor and Sanders, 1980).

The electroretinogram is absent from an early stage. At the time of presentation, visual impairment is usually profound and the apparently rapid deterioration that

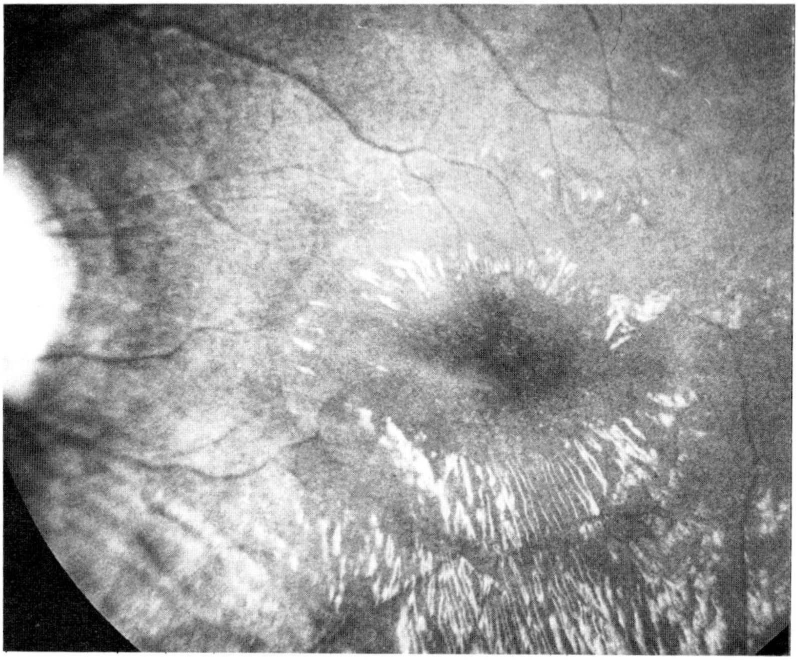

*Figure 6.1* Bull's-eye maculopathy in juvenile Batten's disease

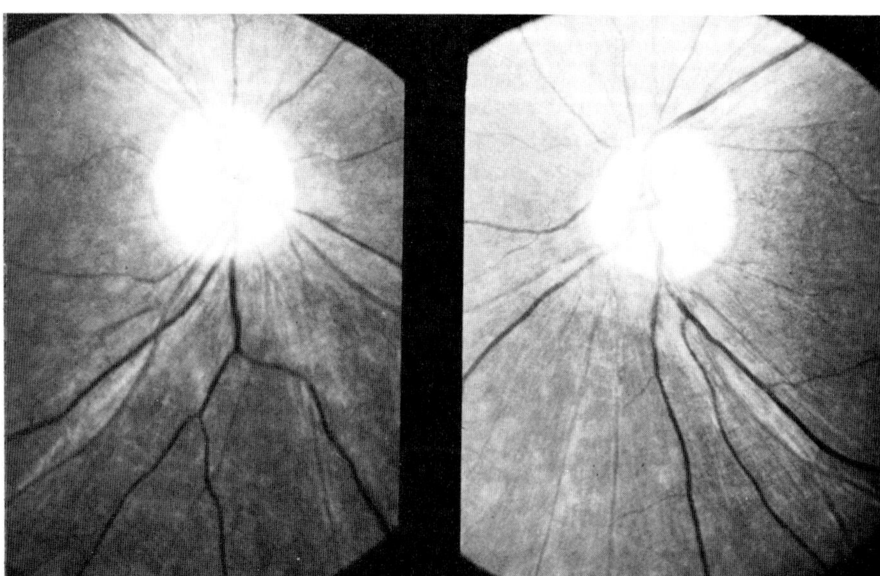

*Figure 6.2* Juvenile Batten's disease – late stage showing vascular attenuation and retinal nerve fibre atrophy

has been recorded in some cases may well be due to its late discovery, since young children tend to compensate well for a visual handicap until it becomes incapacitating.

Some children with central scotomas tend to look above a fixation target (Spalton, Taylor and Sanders, 1980). This is due to the fact that the inferior field of vision is preserved, perhaps because photoxicity affects the inferior retina more severely than the superior retina. It has been suggested that visual deterioration might be delayed by the wearing of dark glasses or by occluding an eye.

## Systemic features

Abnormal behavioural changes are common at the time of presentation, and not infrequently the child has been rather slower than his peers at school. However, obvious mental deterioration is usually delayed until after the onset of visual symptoms, and occurs between the 6th and 12th year, but occasionally earlier or later.

Seizures tend to develop 2 and 4 years after the onset of visual problems; they are usually of the grand mal type but are easily controlled and infrequent. The disease follows a prolonged course with gradual intellectual deterioration with death occurring many years after the onset of visual failure.

## Special investigations

Electroencephalography may provide good evidence of underlying cerebral dysfunction. The characteristic EEG abnormalities described by Pampiglione and Harden (1977) should lead the clinician to search for vacuolated lymphocytes (*Figure 6.3*) and subsequently 'fingerprint body' neuronal inclusions (*Figure 6.4*) which are the hallmark of this disease.

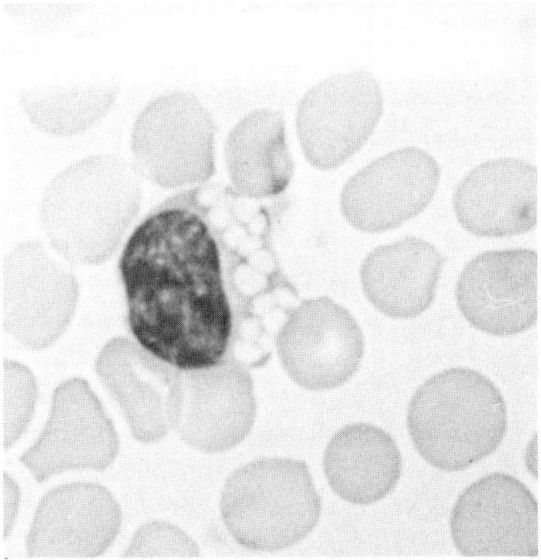

*Figure 6.3* Juvenile Batten's disease. Vacuoles are found in the cytoplasm of lymphocytes at the edges of peripheral blood smears

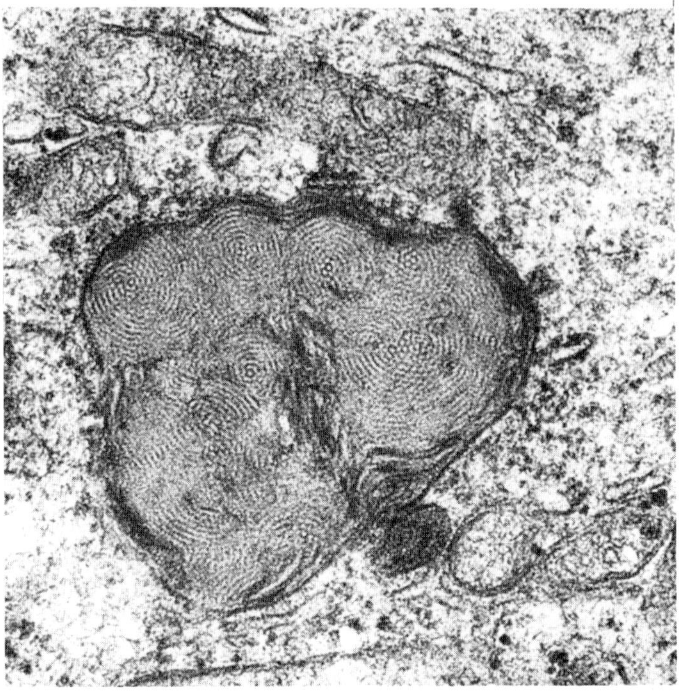

*Figure 6.4* Juvenile Batten's disease. A fingerprint body intraneuronal inclusion

The diagnosis of juvenile Batten's disease is frequently delayed for several years since the most common initial diagnosis is that of a purely retinal disorder and the systemic nature of the disorder is overlooked until the patient develops fits.

## THE CHERRY-RED SPOT

The presence of a cherry-red spot at the macula indicates storage of a variety of abnormal substances in the retinal ganglion cells. Since the ganglion cells are absent from the fovea and multilayered at the macula, the normal central red spot contrasts with the abnormal white surrounding tissue.

This appearance is seen at some stage in virtually every patient with Tay–Sachs' disease ($GM_2$ $type_1$ and $GM_1$ $type_1$) as well as the Sandhoff variant ($GM_2$ $type_2$), and sometimes in older onset types of $GM_2$ gangliosidosis. It also occurs in some patients with the commonest form of Niemann–Pick disease – the acute neuronopathic type A. Cherry-red spots have also been described in patients with metachromatic leucodystrophy (Cogan, Kuwabara and Moser, 1970; Libert *et al.*, 1979), in Farber's disease, and in one patient with ophthalmoplegic lipidosis (Taylor *et al.*, 1981). In metachromatic leucodystrophy and ophthalmoplegic lipidosis the appearance of the spot is usually less pronounced and has been described as a macular greying.

## Sialidosis (the cherry-red spot myoclonus syndrome)

This is one of the few cherry-red spot syndromes that may present to the ophthalmologist. Bilateral cherry-red spots may be found on routine examination (*Figure 6.5*). However, visual difficulties soon supervene and may become severe as the ganglion cells die and the cherry spot fades, so that ultimately the fundus shows only atrophy of the optic nerve and retinal nerve fibre layer.

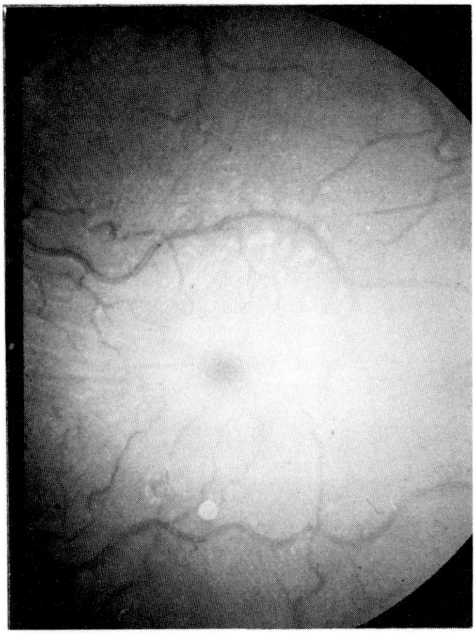

*Figure 6.5* Cherry-red spot in the cherry-red spot myoclonus syndrome (sialidosis)

The disease is inherited in an autosomal recessive manner. The diagnosis is made by finding low levels of sialidase in cultured fibroblasts. O'Brien and Warner (1980) have identified two subgroups of this disorder, both having bilateral cherry-red spots and sialidase deficiency.

### Type 1

Type 1 patients present from about 8 years of age. They have normal intellect and facies, and a normal β-galactosidase activity (Lowden and O'Brien, 1979; Rapin, Katzman and Engel, 1975; Thomas *et al.*, 1979). The myoclonus is progressive and ultimately disabling.

### Type 2

Type 2 patients tend to present earlier with intellectual deterioration. They have coarse facies, short stature, bony abnormalities suggestive of a mucopolysaccharidosis (*Figure 6.6*) (Goldberg *et al.*, 1971) and low levels of β-galactosidase. Some also have a faint clouding of the cornea.

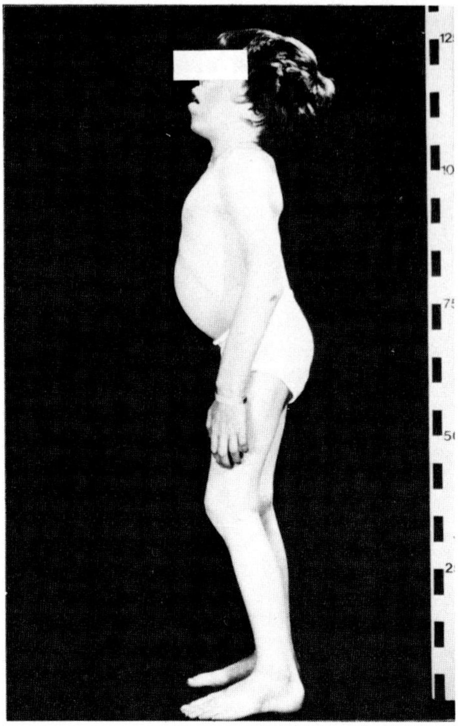

*Figure 6.6* Sialidosis type 2. The patients are intellectually retarded, have coarse features, kyphoscoliosis and other skeletal abnormalities, as well as mild corneal clouding

## LEBER'S AMAUROSIS

This condition was first described by Leber in 1869. Inheritance is autosomal recessive. The disease exhibits considerable clinical variation, probably partly because it embraces more than one disorder. The following criteria must be fulfilled for the diagnosis to be established: blindness or severe visual impairment from birth, an absent or markedly reduced electroretinogram (ERG) in the presence of normal or nearly normal fundus.

### Retinopathy

Classically Leber's amaurosis presents with severely reduced vision or nystagmus during the first few months of life. Occasionally the mother (particularly if there has been a previously affected child) may be aware of unusual behavioural reactions to activities such as being carried down stairs or being bathed within the first few weeks of life. Although most patients have very poor vision, a relatively mild form of the disease has been described (Stanley, MacDonald and Flynn, 1977; Vaizey *et al.*, 1977). However, even in mild cases the electroretinogram is absent or severely diminished.

Alstrom and Olson (1957) observed that over the years gradual deterioration of any remaining vision occurs, although whether this is inevitable is still unknown. This functional deterioration is reflected in the changing fundal appearance, and recognition of this progression is obviously important to the ophthalmologist who may see a patient for the first time in adult life for genetic counselling.

The essentially normal fundus in a blind infant may be responsible for the frequency and great variety of incorrect diagnoses. The diverse retinal appearance seen in Leber's amaurosis has been reviewed recently (Stanley, MacDonald and Flynn, 1977; Keast-Butler, 1982), although initially often normal, slow evolution to a typical retinitis pigmentosa picture can often occur. Other changes include peripheral or central granularity 'salt and pepper' pigmentation, vascular attenuation, peripheral white spots, and optic atrophy. Stanley, MacDonald and Flynn (1977) reported two cases with bull's eye macular changes.

Since Schappert-Kimmijser, Henkes and van den Bosch (1959) reported pseudopapillitis, swollen discs showing late staining on fluorescein angiography have been seen in a number of cases. These changes are probably due to stasis oedema as there is no evidence of capillary dilatation (Flynn and Cullen, 1975). Rarely macular 'colobomas' are seen in Leber's amaurosis (Leighton and Harris, 1973).

## Other ocular features

Nystagmus is usually but not invariably present. Strabismus and photophobia may also occur, and the oculodigital sign, or eye poking, is characteristic but not pathognomonic of this condition. Constant eye poking in these infants may lead to atrophy of orbital fat and enophthalmos.

Keratoconus occurs more frequently than in the normal population (Alstrom and Olson, 1957; Karel, 1968; Schappert-Kimmijser, Henkes and van den Bosch, 1959; Waardenburg, 1957). Acute changes appear to be more common than in isolated keratoconus. Cataract and keratoglobus similarly have an increased incidence.

## Systemic associations

The frequent occurrence of systemic abnormalities in association with Leber's amaurosis has only recently been acknowledged. As these children often present initially to the ophthalmologist it is important to be aware of the existence of these abnormalities.

Neurodevelopmental disorders include a variable subnormality, epilepsy, EEG abnormalities, disequilibrium and occasionally deafness (Dekaban, 1969; Vaizey *et al.*, 1977). The clinician involved in assessing the retarded infant should be aware of this association, as all too often visual impairment is incorrectly labelled as 'cortical blindness'.

A variety of skeletal abnormalities have been described and a Leber's-like picture may be seen in Jeune's syndrome (Bard *et al.*, 1978). The association with renal abnormalities is now well known, particularly in the triad of juvenile nephronophthisis, congenital hepatic fibrosis and Leber's amaurosis (Keast-Butler, 1982). Occasionally the renal lesions may dominate the clinical picture (Delaney, Mullaney and Bourke, 1978).

The pathophysiology of Leber's amaurosis is unknown, but it has been postulated that there is a developmental failure affecting the neurosensory retina that later shows secondary degenerative changes (Mizuno *et al.*, 1977). Should this dysgenetic disturbance affect both renal and retinal tissues simultaneously, the concurrence of ocular and renal defects could then be explained (Dekaban, 1969).

## BASSEN–KORNZWEIG SYNDROME (ABETALIPOPROTEINAEMIA)

Abetalipoproteinaemia is inherited as an autosomal recessive trait; approximately a quarter of affected individuals are Ashkenazi Jews. Obligate heterozygotes cannot be identified. Although the exact metabolic defect is unknown, lipoprotein synthesis and thus transport of dietary fat from the intestine to the tissues of the body is defective. Plasma lipids are less than 50% of the normal level; triglycerides, phospholipids, and particularly cholesterol are all reduced. Jejunal biopsy is pathognomonic.

### Retinopathy

A pigmentary retinopathy develops towards the end of the first decade of life (Carr, 1976; Herbert, Gotto and Fredrickson, 1978). However, the pigment clumping is often larger than in classical retinitis pigmentosa, and is not confined to the equatorial regions. Peripheral white dots representing retinal pigment epithelial atrophy, macular pigmentary changes, vascular attenuation, and optic atrophy may also occur. The visual fields are constricted and the electro-oculogram, electroretrogram and dark adaptation are all abnormal.

### Other ocular features

Disturbances of ocular motility and ptosis are common. Yee, Cogan and Zee (1976) have studied three patients in whom they observed a characteristic pattern of progressive paresis of the medial rectus muscles, acquired exotropia, and dissociated nystagmus on lateral gaze. Electronystagmography revealed slow saccades. These abnormalities are almost certainly central in origin and quite unlike those encountered in chronic progressive external ophthalmoplegia.

### Systemic features

Fat malabsorption is present from birth. This improves with time but during the first decade a devastating neuropathy becomes evident. It is characterized by loss of deep tendon reflexes as well as loss of both position and vibration sense. Cerebellar signs result from spinal and brain stem involvement rather than from primary cerebellar disease.

Acanthocytes constitute between 50 and 70% of the peripheral blood film, and anaemia is common in children. Death usually occurs before middle age.

## Treatment

Due to the malabsorption of fat, there is a deficiency of fat soluble vitamins. Treatment with vitamin A was at first encouraging (Carr, 1976), but a patient developed pigmentary retinopathy despite normal vitamin A levels (Wolff, Lloyd and Tonks, 1964). Vitamin E is an antioxidant which helps to maintain membrane stability and is profoundly deficient in abetalipoproteinaemia. If vitamin E is given during the first year of life it has been found to delay the development of neurological and retinal lesions. Treatment started later in life arrests the progression and also leads to some improvement of retinal function (Muller, Lloyd and Bird, 1977; Muller and Lloyd, 1982).

# REFSUM'S SYNDROME

In 1946 Refsum reported a new syndrome characterized by retinitis pigmentosa, peripheral neuropathy, cerebellar ataxia and a high CSF protein in the absence of pleocytosis. Originally the condition was called heredopathia atactica polyneuritiformis, but with the discovery that phytanic acid accumulates in tissues it has become known as phytanic acid storage disease or simply Refsum's syndrome. The disease is inherited as an autosomal recessive trait and is not confined to any particular ethnic group, although most patients are said to have Scandinavian ancestry.

Many tissues of the body, including the eye (Cummings, 1971; Toussaint and Danis, 1971) become infiltrated by phytanic acid. This substance is found only in trace amounts in the plasma of normal individuals, but in patients with Refsum's syndrome it may constitute between 5% and 30% of the total plasma fatty acids.

## Retinopathy

Although Refsum's syndrome is rare, the ophthalmologist should be aware of its existence as the first symptom is night blindness. Furthermore, as treatment is now available, a precise diagnosis is not simply academic.

Night blindness commences early in childhood and is present in all affected individuals. The retinopathy is progressive and is characterized by a generalized 'salt and pepper' appearance (*Figure 6.7*) rather than the bone corpuscular changes of classical retinitis pigmentosa (Hansen, Bachen and Flage, 1979; Spaeth, 1971). Macular involvement is common and retinal vascular attenuation and optic atrophy may occur.

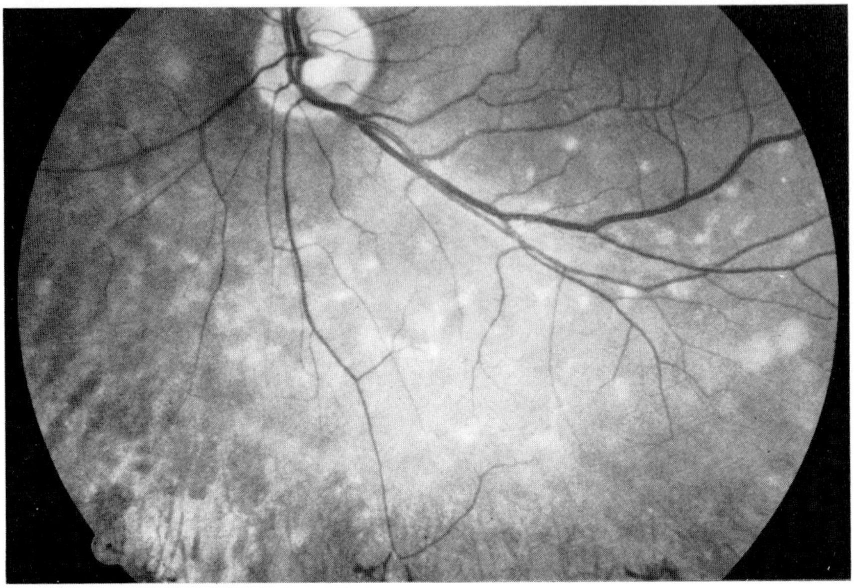

*Figure 6.7* Refsum's syndrome. White dots around main vascular arcade and mid-peripheral bone-corpuscular pigmentation. Note good calibre of retinal arterioles despite the presence of tubular visual fields

## Other ocular features

Miosis with poor pupillary dilatation is frequent and it may influence dark-adaptometry (Hansen, Bachen and Flage, 1979); so that despite the presence of a pigmentary retinopathy dark-adaptation may be normal. Lens opacities are common and cataract surgery may be necessary.

## Systemic features

Systemic features seen in phytanic acid storage disease include: symmetrical motor and sensory peripheral neuropathy, cerebellar ataxia, raised CSF proteins without pleocytosis, nerve deafness, anosmia, ichthyosis, epiphyseal dysplasia, and ECG changes. Untreated, the clinical course is one of slow progression with the patient becoming increasingly sensorially isolated. Remissions, sometimes long-lasting, with almost complete alleviation of symptoms are characteristic, as are exacerbations typically associated with pregnancy, surgery, or a febrile illness. Sudden death may occur at any stage of the disease but is rare in childhood.

## Treatment

The mechanism by which the clinical manifestations of Refsum's syndrome develop is unknown (Steinberg, 1978). The aim of treatment is to eliminate the stored phytanic acid and, as this is exogenously derived, a phytanic-free, high-calorie diet has been useful (Refsum, 1981). Plasma exchange is a useful adjunct (Gibberd *et al.*, 1979). Although improvement of visual function is not expected, treatment with follow-up of many years has been shown to prevent further ocular and systemic progression.

## GYRATE ATROPHY

Gyrate atrophy of the choroid and retina with hyperornithinaemia was first described in 1973. Since that time various studies have demonstrated low values of the enzyme ornithine ketoacid aminotransferase in lymphocytes, fibroblasts and liver (Kaiser-Kupfer, Valle and Valle, 1978; Sipila, Simell and O'Donnell, 1981). Ornithine plasma levels are increased by 10 to 20 times. Aqueous and CSF levels are also increased (Takki and Simell, 1976). Other plasma amino acid levels are also altered, albeit to a lesser extent. The disease is inherited as an autosomal recessive trait. Heterozygotes may be detected by using an oral ornithine loading test. Antenatal diagnosis is now possible.

### Retinopathy

Impairment of night vision commences in early childhood and progresses to blindness by the fifth decade. The first ophthalmoscopic changes occur in the mid-periphery with the appearance of round areas of chorioretinal atrophy and obliteration of the choriocapillaris (*Figure 6.8*). Initially discrete, they later coalesce and extend towards the posterior pole. Pigment dispersion around these patches is observed and peripapillary atrophy may also occur. The fine 'velvety' pigmentation at the macula, obscuring the underlying choroidal vessels, is seen particularly well on fluorescein angiography and helps to differentiate gyrate atrophy from choroideraemia. Colour vision is unaltered, but concentric peripheral field constriction is always present. Dark adaptation is normal but the EEG is either subnormal or extinguished, the scotopic response being affected first. The electro-oculogram is flat. Recently a milder variant of gyrate atrophy has been identified with a later onset and slower progression (Kaiser-Kupfer, Valle and Bron, 1980).

### Other ocular features

High myopia, cataract, and vitreous degeneration are seen in all patients.

### Systemic features

It is surprising that hyperornithaemia does not produce more systemic disturbances than the clinically insignificant but consistently observed atrophy of type 2 skeletal muscle fibres (McCulloch and Marliss, 1975), and EEG changes.

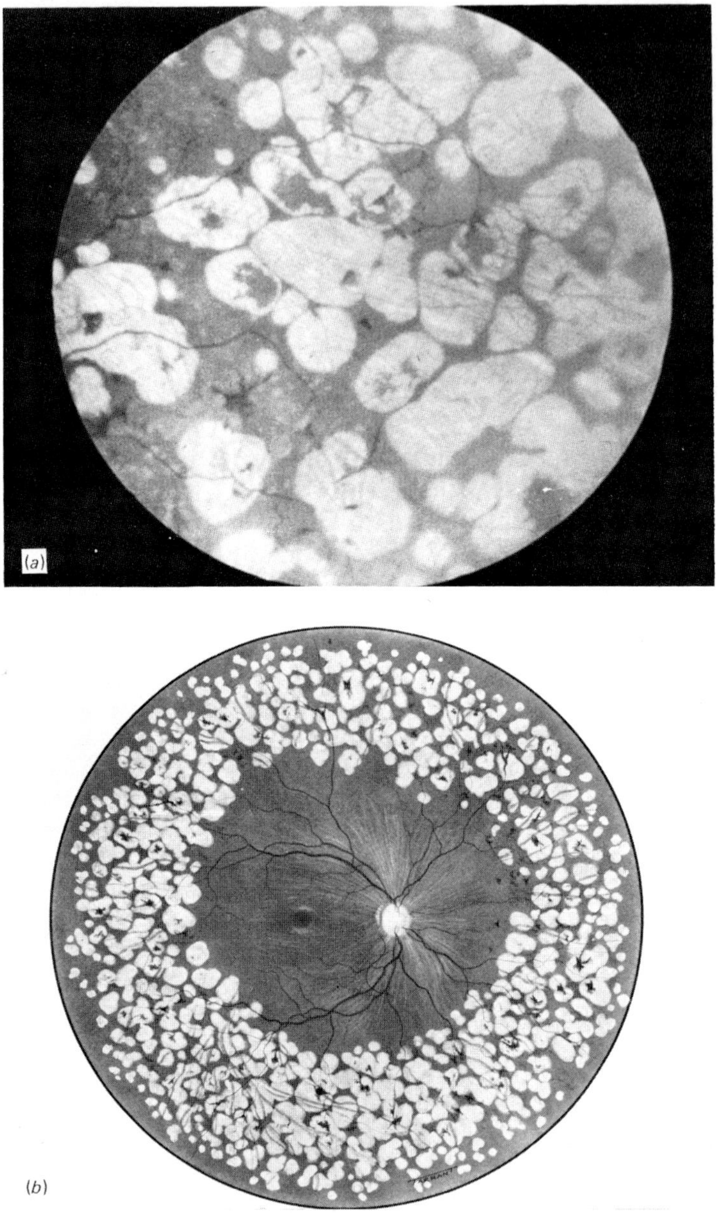

*Figure 6.8 (a) and (b)* Typical appearance in gyrate atrophy of choroid and retina

## Treatment

Treatment aimed at correcting the hyperornithaemia is difficult. A low arginine diet, lysine hydrochloride, supplemental creatinine and pyridoxine (vitamin $B_6$) have all been tried. The variable response to vitamin $B_6$ therapy has been attributed to genetic heterogeneity (Kaiser-Kupfer, Valle and Bron, 1980). Further consideration of therapeutic possibilities is not appropriate at this relatively early stage of our knowledge of this condition.

## CYSTINOSIS

Cystinosis is an autosomal recessively inherited condition characterized by widespread tissue crystal deposition. Three clinical types are recognized:

(1) Nephropathic cystinosis is the most severe form. It presents in the first few months of life, the clinical picture being dominated by diminished renal function with death occurring usually before the second decade.
(2) Benign cystinosis is asymptomatic and is usually detected on routine ocular examination.
(3) The intermediate form has variable features; the onset is later (18 months to 17 years) and renal function is not as severely compromised as in the nephropathic form (Schneider, Schulman and Seegmiller, 1978).

### Retinopathy

The retinopathy is characterized by patchy peripheral depigmentation, particularly involving the temporal retina and occasionally extending posteriorly to involve the macula (Wong, 1976). It is found in all patients with nephropathic cystinosis, sometimes in the intermediate form but never in the benign. The retinal changes can precede involvement of the cornea. Until recently it was thought that retinal function was unaffected in eyes with retinopathy, but with extensive involvement electroretinogram abnormalities and visual field constriction may occur (Yamamoto *et al.*, 1979).

### Other ocular features

Crystal deposition may occur in the conjunctiva and cornea as well as the retina, and the ophthalmologist has an important diagnostic role. The beautiful corneal appearance is due to homogeneous crystal deposition (*Figure 6.9*). Peripherally they involve the entire stromal thickness whilst centrally only the anterior two-thirds are affected. Crystals deposited in the bulbar and forniceal conjunctiva give rise to a ground glass appearance. Conjunctival biopsy is a simple and accurate diagnostic test. Severe photophobia is a frequent feature which is probably due to corneal light scatter.

### Treatment

Specific treatment using dimercaprol (BAL), DL penicillamine, diet and ascorbic acid has been ineffective (Schneider, Schulman and Seegmiller, 1978; Segal, 1979).

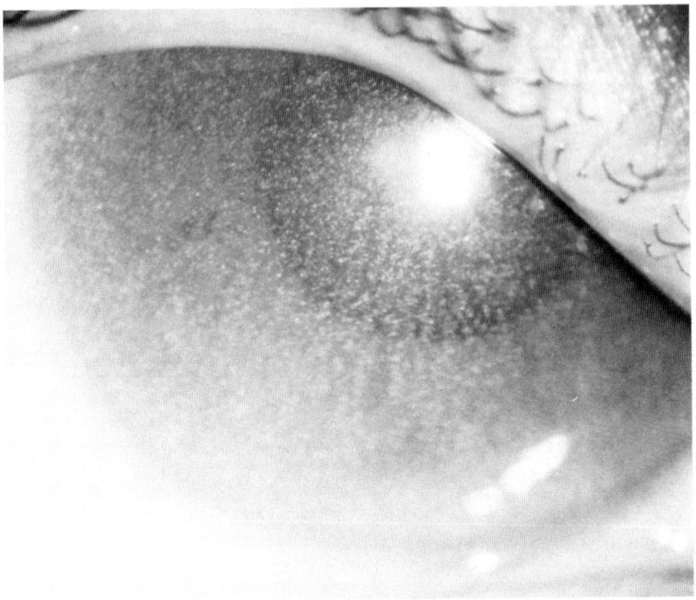

*Figure 6.9* Cystinosis – corneal crystalline deposits

Renal transplantation is now being used but although the transplanted kidneys do not develop cystinotic changes, in other body tissues cystine accumulation continues unabated. Clinically this means that ocular involvement may be more extensive than previously seen in untreated patients. Thus maculopathy and generalized full-thickness corneal deposition may be observed more frequently in the future.

## OXALOSIS

Tissue deposition of oxalate crystals in the eye occurs under two conditions. The first is in degenerate tissue such as the lens in phacolytic glaucoma and Morgagnian cataract, or in long-standing retinal detachments; the second is in primary or secondary hyperoxaluria. Secondary oxaluria results from ingestion of oxalic acid or its precursor, hyperabsorption, sarcoidosis and renal failure. Primary hyperoxaluria is a rare autosomal recessive inherited condition which can be of two types. Type 1 is due to a deficiency of the cytoplasmic enzyme α-ketoglutarate: glyoxylate carboligase. Onset is usually in childhood with renal involvement dominating the clinical picture. Type 2 is extremely rare, more benign, and without ocular manifestations.

### Retinopathy

Clinical ocular involvement in primary Type 1 oxaluria is confined to the retina. Initially small white flecks are noted at the posterior pole (*Figure 6.10*). Later they

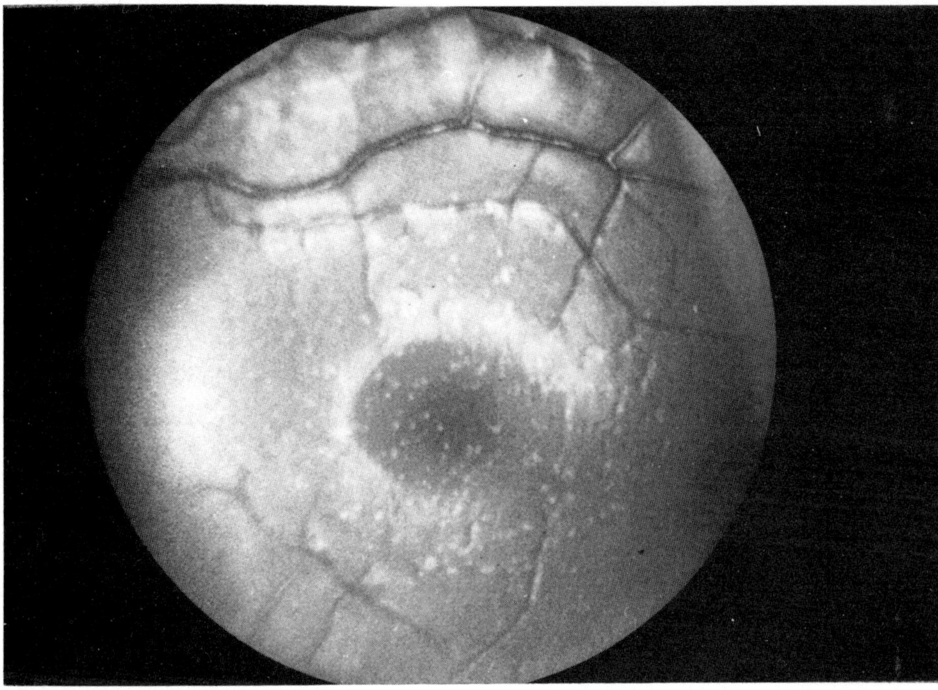

*Figure 6.10* Oxalosis – flecked retina

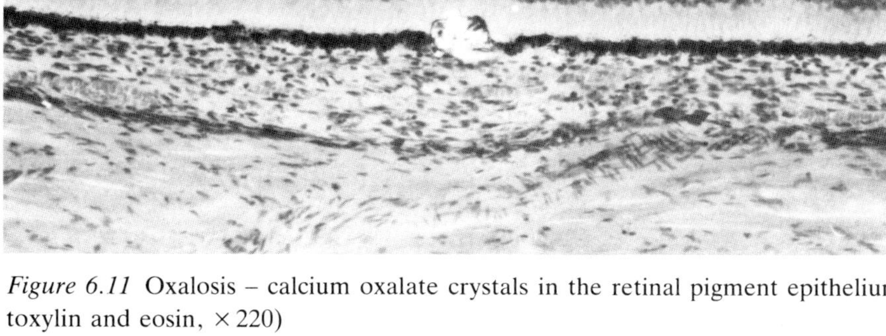

*Figure 6.11* Oxalosis – calcium oxalate crystals in the retinal pigment epithelium (haematoxylin and eosin, ×220)

spread peripherally (Bullock and Albert, 1975; Fielder, Garner and Chambers, 1980). Only one case has been reported with visual impairment due to macular involvement (Gottlieb and Ritter, 1977). Retinopathy is a manifestation of advanced oxalosis paralleling crystal deposition in other tissues. Histopathologically, calcium oxalate crystals are observed in the retinal pigmented epithelium (*Figure 6.11*). They probably originate intracellularly, but later grow and disrupt the cell.

## Treatment

Pyridoxine (vitamin $B_6$), is the only effective treatment for this condition.

## Acknowledgements

The authors would like to thank Dr R. G. Godwin-Austen for allowing Mr Fielder to study his patients with Refsum's syndrome, and the departments of Medical Illustrations at the Hospital for Sick Children, Great Ormond Street and the Derbyshire Royal Infirmary. Mr Alan Mushin supplied *Figures 6.8a* and *b*. Miss Josephine Lace and Mrs Anna Taylor prepared the manuscript.

## References

Alstrom, C. H. and Olson, O. (1957) Heredo-retinopathia congenitalis monohybrida recessiva autosomalis. *Hereditas*, **43,** 1–177

Bard, L. A., Bard, P. A., Owens, G. W. and Hall, B. D. (1978) Retinal involvement in thoracic-pelvic-phalangeal dystrophy. *Archives of Ophthalmology*, **96,** 278–281

Bullock, J. D. and Albert, D. M. (1975) Flecked retina. *Archives of Ophthalmology*, **93,** 26–31

Carr, R. E. (1976) Abetalipoproteinaemia and the eye. In *The Eye and Inborn Errors of Metabolism, Birth Defects XXII, No 3*, edited by D. Bergsma, A. J. Bron and E. Cotlier. New York: Alan R. Liss

Cogan, D. G., Kuwabara, T. and Moser, H. (1970) Metachromatic leucodystrophy. *Ophthalmologica*, **166,** 2–17

Cummings, J. N. (1971) Inborn errors of metabolism in neurology (Wilson's disease, Refsum's disease and lipidoses). *Proceedings of the Royal Society of Medicine*, **64,** 313–322

Dekaban, A. S. (1969) Hereditary syndrome of congenital retinal blindness (Leber), polycystic kidneys and maldevelopment of the brain. *American Journal of Ophthalmology*, **68,** 1029–1037

Delaney, V., Mullaney, V. and Burke, E. (1978) Juvenile nephronophthisis, congenital hepatic fibrosis and retinal hypoplasia in twins. *Quarterly Journal of Medicine*, **186,** 281–290

Fielder, A. R., Garner, A. and Chambers, T. L. (1980) Ophthalmic manifestations of primary oxalosis. *British Journal of Ophthalmology*, **64,** 782–788

Flynn, J. T. and Cullen, R. F. (1975) Disc oedema in congenital amaurosis of Leber. *British Journal of Ophthalmology*, **59,** 497–502

Gibberd, F. B., Billimoria, J. D., Page, N. G. R. and Retsas, S. (1979) Heredopathia atactica polyneuritiformis (Refsum's Disease) treated by diet and plasma-exchange. *Lancet*, **1,** 575–578

Goldberg, M. F., Cotlier, E., Fichenscher, L. G., Kenyon, K., Enat, R. and Borowsky, S. A. (1971) Macular cherry-red spot, corneal clouding and β-galactosidase deficiency; clinical, biochemical, and electronmicroscopic study of a new autosomal recessive storage disease. *Archives of Internal Medicine*, **128,** 387–398

Gottlieb, R. P. and Ritter, J. A. (1977) Flecked retina – an association with primary hyperoxaluria. *Journal of Pediatrics*, **90,** 939–942

Hansen, E., Bachen, N. I. and Flage, T. (1979) Refsum's disease. *Acta Ophthalmologica (Kbh.)*, **57,** 899–913

Herbert, P. N., Gotto, A. M. and Fredrickson, D. S. (1978) Familial lipoprotein deficiency. In *The Metabolic Basis of Inherited Disease*, edited by J. B. Stanbury, J. B. Wyngaarden and D. S. Fredrickson, 544–588. New York: McGraw Hill

Kaiser-Kupfer, M. I., Valle, D. and Valle, L. A. (1978) A specific enzyme defect in gyrate atrophy. *American Journal of Ophthalmology*, **85,** 200–204

Kaiser-Kupfer, M. I., Valle, D. and Bron, A. J. (1980) Clinical and biochemical heterogeneity in gyrate atrophy. *American Journal of Ophthalmology*, **89,** 219–222

Karel, I. (1968) Keratoconus in congenital diffuse tapetoretinal degeneration. *Ophthalmologica*, **155,** 8–15

Keast-Butler, J. (1983) Congenital retinal blindness. In *Current Aspects of Paediatric Ophthalmology*, edited by K. C. Wybar and D. S. I. Taylor. New York: Marcel Dekker Inc. (in press)

Leighton, D. A. and Harris, R. (1973) Retinal aplasia in association with macular coloboma, keratoconus and cataract. *Clinical Genetics*, **4,** 270–274

Libert, J., Van Hoof, F., Toussaint, D., Roozitalab, H., Kenyon, K. and Green, R. (1979) Ocular findings in metachromatic leucodystrophy. *Archives of Ophthalmology*, **97,** 1495–1504

Lowden, J. A. and O'Brien, J. S. (1979) Sialidosis; a review of human neuraminidase deficiency. *American Journal of Human Genetics*, **31,** 1–18

McCulloch, C. and Marliss, E. B. (1975) Gyrate atrophy of the choroid and retina with hyperornithaemia. *American Journal of Ophthalmology*, **80,** 1047–1057

Mizuno, K., Takei, Y., Sears, M. L., Peterson, W. S., Carr, R. E. and Jampol, L. M. (197) Leber's congenital amaurosis. *American Journal of Ophthalmology*, **83,** 32–42

Muller, D.P. R., Lloyd, J. K., and Bird, A. C. (1977) Long-term management of abetalipoproteinaemia. *Archives of Disease in Childhood*, **52,** 209–214

Muller, D. P. R. and Lloyd, J. K. (1982) Effect of large oral doses of vitamin E on the neurological sequelae of patients with abetalipoproteinaemia. *Annals of the New York Academy of Science* (in press)

O'Brien, J. S. and Warner, T. G. (1980) Sialidosis; delineation of subtypes by neuraminidase assay. *Clinical Genetics*, **17,** 35–38

Pampiglione, G. and Harden, A. (1977) So-called neuronal ceroid lipofuscinosis; neurophysiological studies in 60 children. *Journal of Neurology, Neurosurgery and Psychiatry*, **40,** 232–330

Rapin, I., Katzman, R. and Engel, J. Jr. (1975) Cherry red spots and progressive myoclonus without dementia: a distinct syndrome with neuronal storage. *Archives of Neurology (Chicago)*, **32,** 349

Refsum, S. (1981) Heredopathia atactica polyneuritiformis. *Archives of Neurology*, **38,** 605–606

Schappert-Kimmijser, J., Henkes, H. E. and van den Bosch, J. (1959) Amaurosis congenita (Leber). *Archives of Ophthalmology*, **61,** 221–218

Schneider, J. A., Schulman, J. D. and Seegmiller, J. E. (1978) Cystinosis and the Fanconi syndrome. In *The Metabolic Basis of Inherited Disease*, edited by J. B. Stanbury, J. B. Wyngaarden and D. S. Fredrickson, 1660–1682. New York: McGraw Hill

Segal, S. (1979) Editorial: Cystinosis and its therapy. *New England Journal of Medicine*, **300,** 789–790

Sipila, I., Simell, O. and O'Donnell, J. J. (1981) Gyrate atrophy of the choroid and retina with hyperornithemia. *Journal of Clinical Investigation*, **67,** 1805–1807

Spaeth, G. L. (1971) Ocular manifestations of the lipidoses. In *Retinal Diseases in Children*, edited by W.Tasman, 127–206. New York: Harper and Row

Spalton, D. J., Taylor, D. S. I. and Sanders, M. D. (1980) Juvenile Batten's disease: an ophthalmological assessment of 26 patients. *British Journal of Ophthalmology*, **64,** 726–732

Stanley, J. H., MacDonald, J. and Flynn, J. T. (1977) Leber's congenital amaurosis: a clinical study. In *Neuro-ophthalmology Update*, edited by J. L. Smith, 91–97. New York: Masson Publ. USA Inc.

Steinberg, D. (1978) Phytanic acid storage disease: Refsum's syndrome. In *The Metabolic Basis of Inherited Disease*, edited by J. B. Stanbury, J. B. Wyngaarden and D. S. Fredrickson, 688–706. New York: McGraw-Hill

Takki, K. and Simell, O. (1976) Gyrate atrophy of the choroid and retina with hyperornithemia (HOGA). In *The Eye and Inborn Errors of Metabolism, Birth Defects 12, no. 3*, edited by D. Bergsma, A. J. Bron and E. Cotlier, 373–384. New York: Alan R. Liss

Taylor, D., Lake, B. D., Marshall, J. and Garner, A. (1981 Retinal abnormalities in ophthalmoplegic lipidosis. *British Journal of Ophthalmology*, **65,** 484–488

Thomas, P. K., Abrams, J. D., Swallow, D., and Stewart, G. (1979) Sialidosis type I. Cherry-red spot myoclonus syndrome with sialidase deficiency and altered electrophoretic mobilities of some enzymes known to be glycoproteins. *Journal of Neurology, Neurosurgery and Psychiatry*, **42,** 873–880

Toussaint, D. and Danis, P. (1971) An ocular pathologic study of Refsum's syndrome. *American Journal of Ophthalmology*, **72,** 342–347

Vaizey, M. J., Sanders, M. D., Wybar, K. C. and Wilson, J. (1977) Neurological abnormalities in congenital amaurosis of Leber. *Archives of Disease in Childhood*, **52,** 399–402

Waardenburg, P. J. (1957) Does agenesis or dysgenesis neuroepithelial retinae, whether or not related to keratoglobus, exist? *Ophthalmologica*, **133,** 454–461

Wolff, O. H., Lloyd, J. K. and Tonks, E. L. (1964) Abetalipoproteinaemia with special reference to the visual defect. *Experimental Eye Research*, **3,** 439–442

Wong, V. G. (1976) Ocular manifestations in cystinosis. In *The Eye and Inborn Errors of Metabolism, Birth Defects 12, no. 3*, edited by D. Bergsma, A. J. Bron and E. Cotlier, 181–186. New York: Alan R. Liss

Yamamoto, G. K., Schulman, J. D., Schneider, J. A. and Wong, V. G. (1979) Long-term ocular changes in cystinosis: observations in renal transplant recipients. *Journal of Pediatric Ophthalmology and Strabismus*, **16,** 21–25

Yee, R. D., Cogan, D. G. and Zee, D. S. (1976) Ophthalmoplegia and associated nystagmus in abetalipoproteinemia. *Archives of Ophthalmology*, **94,** 571–575

# 7
# Human chorioretinal biopsy

David Taylor

## INTRODUCTION

As we approach an era where many previously blinding retinal diseases may be treatable and even curable, the need for a safe technique of chorioretinal biopsy increases.

Diseases such as herpes simplex or cytomegalovirus retinitis as well as a larger group of other viral, fungal and bacterial infections and leukaemic infiltrations are becoming increasingly within therapeutic range. In addition to this, with the greater knowledge of the underlying metabolic abnormalities in some of the inherited retinal dystrophies we may soon need to have a method for histopathological diagnosis.

At present the indications are difficult to define but it is certainly indicated in a blind eye when a definitive diagnosis would lead to treatment which would either prevent blindness in the fellow eye or arrest a life threatening systemic process (Taylor *et al.*, 1981). With increasing evidence of a low incidence of complications it is now reasonable to operate on eyes with residual vision. Peyman, Juarez and Raichand (1981) who had a low incidence of complications, considered that a reasonable indication is 6/60 acuity or less in patients with substantial retinal disease.

Peyman's technique, based on methods of removing choroidal melanomas, involves supporting the eye in a special wire basket, trephining a disc of sclera, cauterizing the choroid and then removing a trephined area of choroid and retina with corneoscleral scissors. He performed a vitrectomy after the sclera was closed in order to prevent the formation of a scaffold for tissue ingrowth and subsequent vitreous traction. The only one of nine patients who did not have a vitrectomy developed a traction detachment but in Peyman's series there were no other serious complications.

Constable *et al.* (1980), in work on human eyes about to be enucleated or blind and being operated on for glaucoma, used transient systemic arterial hypotension to prevent choroidal bleeding, but this may not be necessary and must increase the risk of the biopsy. In dogs, Constable, Slater and Horne (1980) prevented vitreous loss by the use of mannitol and controlled hyperventilation together with transient systemic hypotension. Cryotherapy may be used around the site of biopsy but this is probably not necessary especially if there is already substantial chorioretinitis (Taylor *et al.*, 1981).

## A TECHNIQUE FOR CHORIORETINAL BIOPSY

Preoperatively the patient can be assured that the procedure is no more painful than a squint operation. However, the risks and possible benefits should be fully detailed. Since in most cases the biopsy specimen will be divided, the appropriate laboratories must be forewarned, and glutaraldehyde fixative and appropriate culture plates must be sent to the operating room before the operation is started.

An hour before the operation, a weight-appropriate maximal dose of mannitol is given intravenously and the pupils maximally dilated.

Conjunctiva and Tenon's capsule are turned back on a fornix-based trapezium-shaped flap and the two muscles bordering the site are transfixed with a holding suture. If the proposed biopsy site is under a muscle it is necessary to make a larger flap and temporarily remove the muscle. The site to be biopsied is largely determined by the site of the lesion. It is best to chose an active area if the disorder is patchy, and to avoid areas that may be necrotic; therefore in cases of retinitis the edge of a lesion should be biopsied. The vortex veins and long posterior ciliary arteries should be avoided where possible. At the start of the operation the site should be confirmed by indirect ophthalmoscopy and marked with a suture.

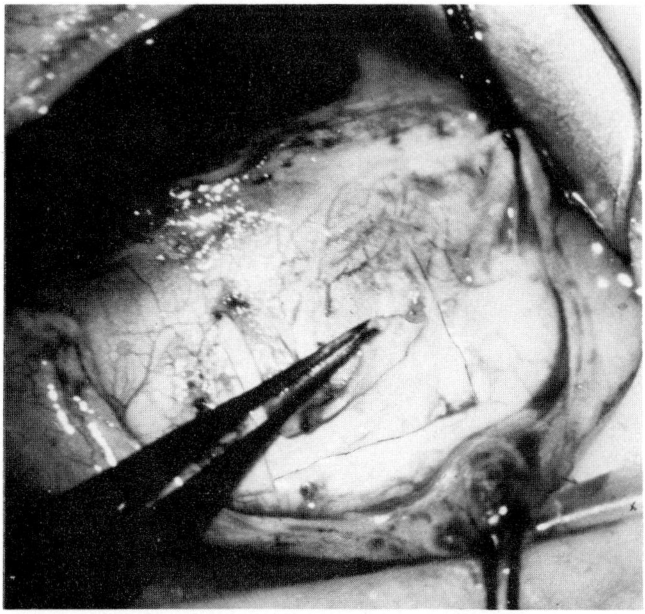

*Figure 7.1* Retinal biopsy. A 5 or 6 mm square partial thickness scleral flap is fashioned with a full-thickness central square of 2 or 3 mm

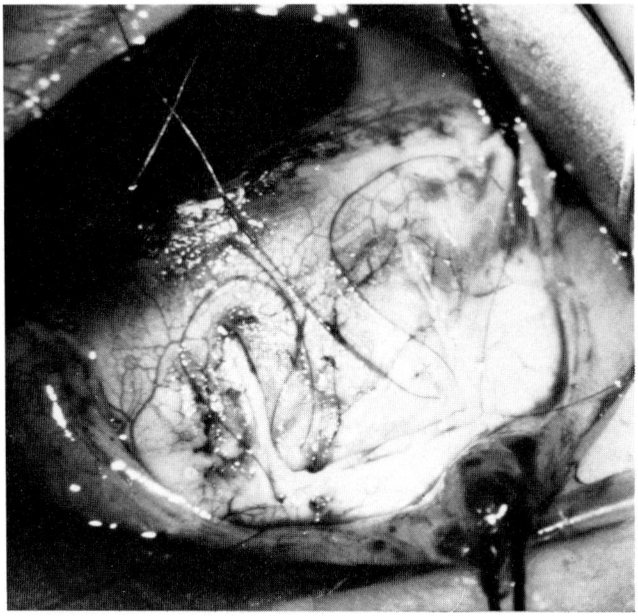

*Figure 7.2* Pre-placed sutures are inserted

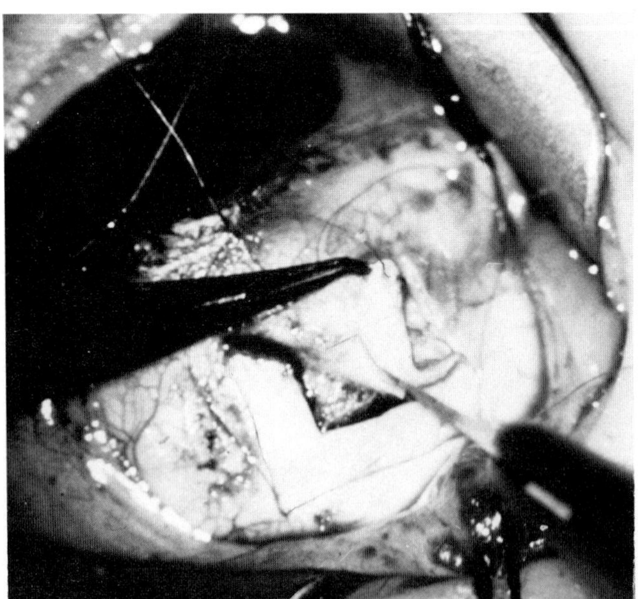

*Figure 7.3* The full-thickness central area is defined, revealing the underlying choroid

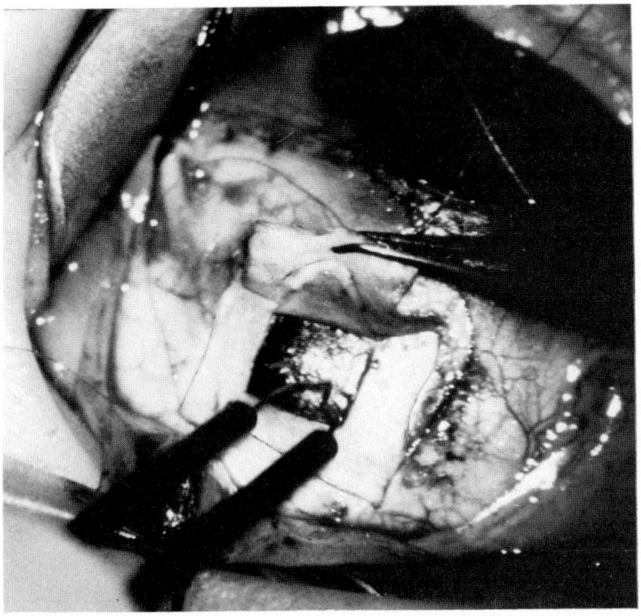

*Figure 7.4* Large vessels and the area around the biopsy may be cauterized

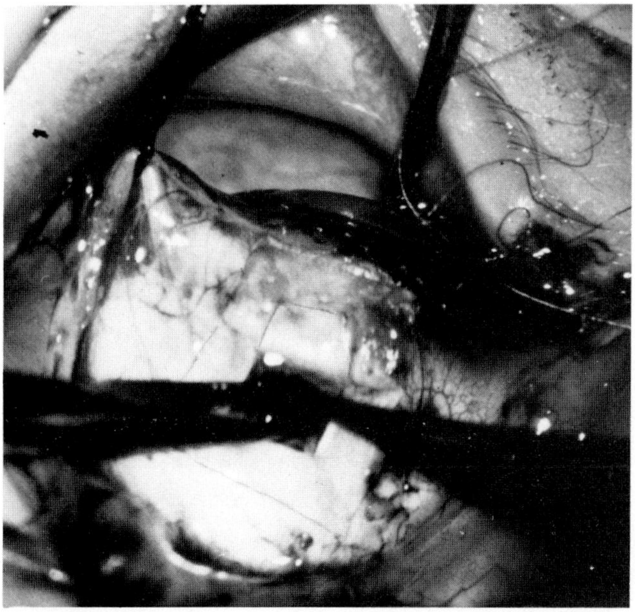

*Figure 7.5* The biopsy is taken with a diamond or steel knife and scissors; removing a triangular piece is the easiest method

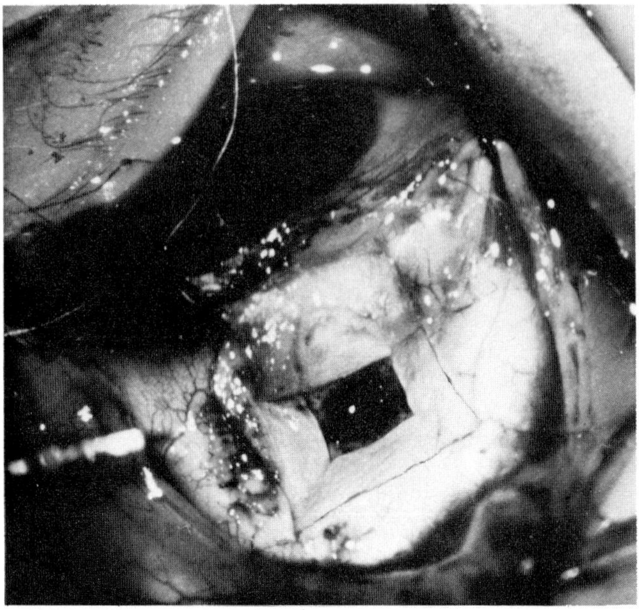

*Figure 7.6* The vitreous may be left intact, providing the preoperative preparation and the anaesthetic technique are adequate

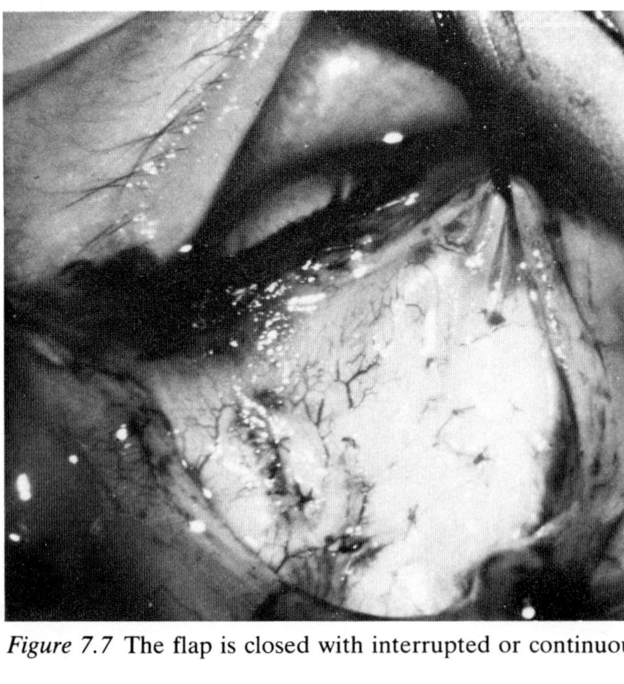

*Figure 7.7* The flap is closed with interrupted or continuous sutures

If cryotherapy is to be used, it may be applied around the site at this stage. The procedure is carried out under the operating microscope. A 5 or 6 mm half-thickness flap is turned back (*Figure 7.1*). Two pre-placed sutures are put at the two free corners (*Figure 7.2*); a 2 or 3 mm full thickness area is fashioned (*Figure 7.3*).

The sclera separates easily from the suprachoroidal space. The perimeter may be lightly cauterized (*Figure 7.4*). The choroid and retina are penetrated with a fine, sharp-pointed knife and a wide 'V' fashioned in the choroid and retina. The base of the 'V' is cut with sharp pointed scissors (*Figure 7.5*) and the biopsy removed (*Figure 7.6*). If a vitrectomy is performed it can be done at this stage or after closure. The trapdoor is then closed with interrupted sutures (*Figure 7.7*) and intraocular pressure restored with saline. The conjunctiva and Tenon's are closed and if a muscle has been removed this is replaced. Subconjunctival antibiotics and corticosteroids may be injected.

The technique described is by no means the only method and will undoubtedly become further refined. Perhaps the best techniques for the future will be in the hands of vitreoretinal surgeons who already perform fragmentary retinal biopsies with vitrectomy machines. It is easy to conceive a technique for an *ab interno* punch biopsy, but no easy feat to perform with safety at the moment . . . but in the future?

## References


Constable, I. J., Slater, D. H. and Horne, R. (1980) Chorioretinal biopsy in dogs. *Investigative Ophthalmology and Visual Science,* **19,** 603–609

Constable, I. J., Chester, G. H., Horne, R. and Harriot, J. F. (1980) Human chorioretinal biopsy under controlled systemic hypotensive anaesthesia. *British Journal of Ophthalmology,* **64,** 559–564

Peyman, G. A., Juarez, C. P. and Raichand, M. (1981) Full-thickness eye-wall biopsy: long-term results in 9 patients. *British Journal of Ophthalmology,* **65,** 723–726

Taylor, D., Day, S., Tiedemann, K., Chessels, J., Marshall, W. C. and Constable, I. J. (1981) Chorioretinal biopsy in a patient with leukaemia. *British Journal of Ophthalmology,* **65,** 489–493

# 8
# Management of proliferative diabetic retinopathy

A. M. Peter Hamilton, Rolf K. Blach and Rodger Whitelocke

## INTRODUCTION

Proliferative diabetic retinopathy may lead to blindness from vitreous haemorrhage, retinal detachment, and neovascular glaucoma. The underlying cause of proliferative diabetic retinopathy is retinal ischaemia due to capillary non-perfusion. The two most common sites of capillary closure are the peripheral retina and the area temporal to the macula.

Preretinal new vessels, also sometimes referred to as 'new vessels elsewhere' (NVE), arise from retinal veins adjacent to areas of capillary non-perfusion. Intraretinal new vessels appear as small vascular projections from retinal veins. They may ultimately grow into the non-perfused area, giving the appearance of a modified attenuated capillary bed (*Figure 8.1*). It has been estimated that if over a quarter of the retina is non-perfused the scene is set for the development of disc new vessels (NVD). The ophthalmoscopic clues suggesting the presence of retinal ischaemia are listed in *Table 8.1*. Preretinal new vessels are visible ophthalmoscopically although they are much more striking on fluorescein angiography, showing clearly in the early stages of the angiogram and later giving rise to leakage (*Figure 8.2*).

*Table 8.1* Clinical feature of capillary non-perfusion

| | |
|---|---|
| (*a*) | Intraretinal haemorrhages, either large diffuse haemorrhages or blot haemorrhages, occurring in clusters |
| (*b*) | Oedematous semi-opaque retina frequently associated with the cluster blot haemorrhages |
| (*c*) | Cottonwool spots |
| (*d*) | White sheathed arteries and veins |
| (*e*) | Venous abnormalities – beading (sausage-like veins) or looping |
| (*f*) | Neovascularization |

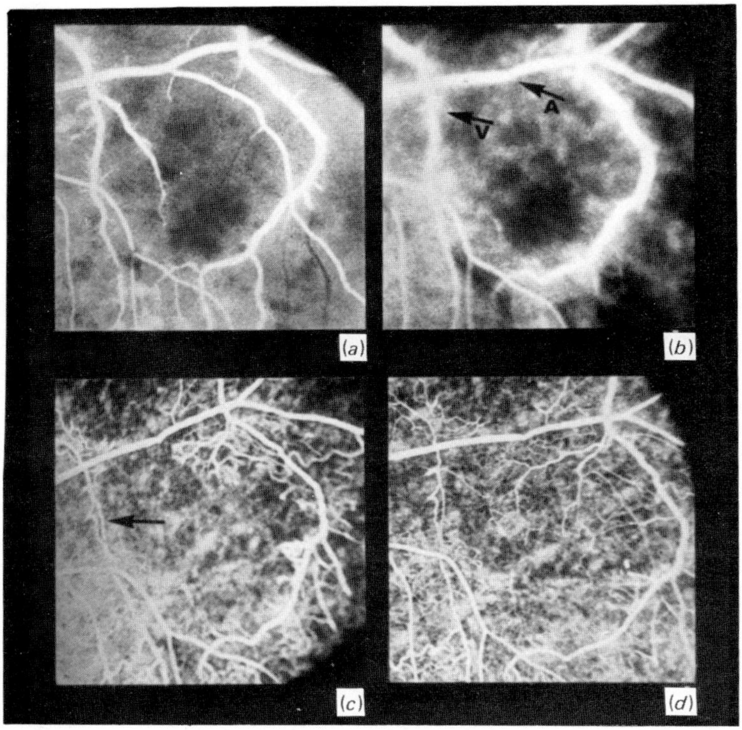


*Figure 8.1* Fluorescein angiograms taken (*a*) 6 weeks, (*b*) 3 months, (*c*) 6 months, and (*d*) 9 months after the development of an area of capillary non-perfusion showing the growth of intraretinal new vessels. V = vein; A = artery

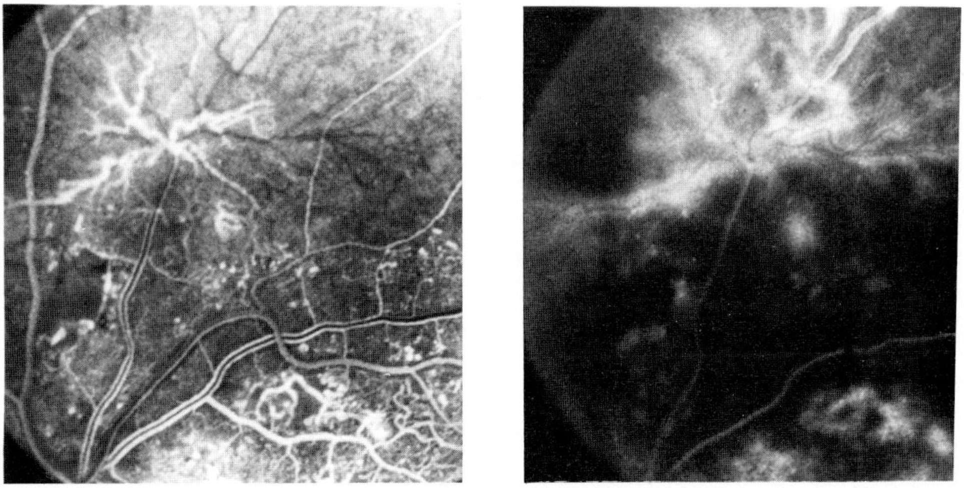

*Figure 8.2* Early (*left*) and late (*right*) phases of the angiogram showing late leakage of dye from preretinal new vessels

## PROGNOSIS

The prognosis of proliferative diabetic retinopathy depends on the severity of neovascularization and degree of fibrosis. The prognosis in early cases is uncertain, but it has been estimated that without treatment blindness occurs within 1 year in 4 per cent of cases, whereas up to 35 per cent of patients with more severe retinopathy are blind within 5 years. There is one particularly severe type of proliferative diabetic retinopathy which occurs in juvenile-onset diabetics after about 10–15 years of diabetes in which the proliferation advances at an alarming rate, resulting in blindness within 3–6 months.

The rate of progression of proliferative diabetic retinopathy is variable and a number of factors have been implicated in causing advancement (*Table 8.2*). We feel that although these factors are important a stage is reached when the retinopathy becomes self-perpetuating and correction of aggravating factors does not result in improvement.

*Table 8.2* Factors considered responsible for advancement of retinopathy

| |
|---|
| (*a*) Poor diabetic control |
| (*b*) Hypertension |
| (*c*) Uraemia |
| (*d*) Pregnancy |
| (*e*) Contraceptive pill |
| (*f*) Smoking |
| (*g*) Coagulative diseases such as leukaemia, Waldenstrom's macroglobulinaemia |

The classification and subclassification of diabetic retinopathy is shown in *Figure 8.3*.

## TREATMENT

### Objectives

Treatment of proliferative diabetic retinopathy is aimed at reversing neovascularization and preventing sight-threatening complications. Although the efficacy of photocoagulation is now established what is still unclear is the best modality and technique. The currently used techniques are outlined in this chapter. However, it is almost certain that these will improve in the future as a result of careful clinical studies.

### Instruments

Xenon arc photocoagulation was first introduced in 1959 by Professor Meyer-Schwickerath and because many of the major studies have been carried out with this instrument its efficacy is well established. Its major disadvantages are: the

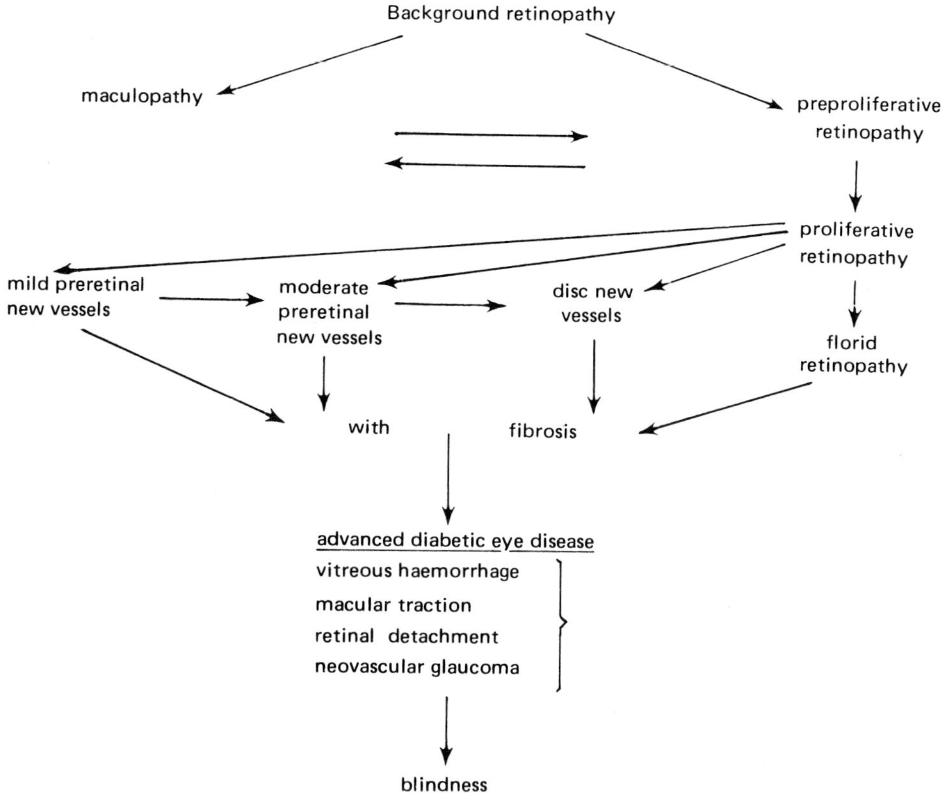


*Figure 8.3* Classification and subclassification of diabetic retinopathy

necessity to use a retrobulbar injection of anaesthetic, the limited view of the fundus, the inability to coagulate close to the macula, and the difficulty in obtaining an even burn. Its major advantages are its proven effectiveness and patient preference. The side-effects, although frequently transient, such as nyctalopia, reduced visual field and impairment of colour vision are more marked with the xenon light coagulator than with the argon laser. Finally, of some controversy is the effect of xenon burns on retinal fibrosis. It has been our feeling that xenon may induce contraction of fibrous tissue particularly if heavy burns are applied, while gentle argon burns have less of an effect.

Argon laser, on the other hand, can be applied close to the macula with relative safety; it usually needs no retrobulbar injection, there is a wide field of view, and the range of safety is considerable. The main disadvantages are lack of patient co-operation and in some cases pain, particularly following retreatment adjacent to or over previously treated areas.

More recently, krypton laser photocoagulation has been shown to produce a burn that penetrates deeper into the choroid than an argon burn. It has also been shown to be transmitted more effectively through the foveal pigment. However, neither of these advantages apply to the treatment of retinal vascular disease, and indeed in clinical practice the krypton laser was equally effective as the argon in producing resolution of disc new vessels. It has the disadvantage of causing more pain, and the safety margin of burn intensity is reduced due to the increased likelihood of choroidal haemorrhage.

In general, the argon laser has become the instrument of choice in the treatment of proliferative diabetic retinopathy. Its ease of use is particularly important when retreatment is required. Its lack of side-effects such as myopia, nyctalopia, colour defects and reduced visual field is important as many patients have minimal if any pretreatment symptoms. Its ease of application and wide margin of safety make it the most effective treatment modality.

However, xenon arc photocoagulation is still a useful method of treatment which we now confine to patients who have not responded to extensive argon photocoagulation, and in those with either poor compliance or insuperable pain with the laser.

## Technique

### Preproliferative retinopathy

The presence of capillary non-perfusion and intraretinal new vessels may lead to sight-threatening proliferative diabetic retinopathy. However, these findings do not represent any immediate threat to vision and any treatment at this stage may be a greater threat than merely regular observation. Therefore, the presence of capillary non-perfusion and intraretinal new vessels are not an indication for photocoagulation, but attention should be paid to eliminating or treating any of the aggravating factors listed in *Table 8.2*. Having said this, we would consider that if there is poor patient compliance as far as regular attendance is concerned, treatment should be seriously considered. In these cases areas of non-perfusion are identified by fluorescein angiography and photocoagulated using burns of 500 μ spot size and short duration (approximately 0.02–0.20 sec) with a power that just produces blanching of the retinal pigment epithelium. The burns should be spaced approximately ½–1 burn diameters apart. The importance of a gentle burn cannot be overstressed (*Figure 8.4*). Heavy burns will almost certainly produce full thickness damage to the retina, possible disruption of Bruch's membrane, and occasionally choroidal neovascularization.

### Proliferative retinopathy

#### PRERETINAL NEW VESSELS (NVE)

Mild new vessels, that is a few scattered areas lying flat on the internal limiting membrane, are treated by applying laser burns around and under the lesions (*Figure 8.5*). The burns should be of 200–500 μ spot size, 0.02–0.20 sec duration, confluent and of an intensity that produces minimal blanching of the retinal pigment epithelium. No attempt is made to close the new vessels but merely to treat

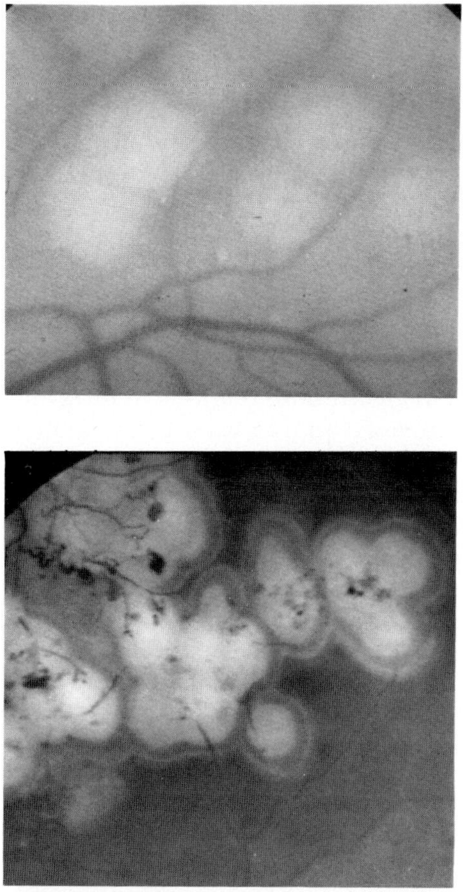

*Figure 8.4* Appearance of gentle photocoagulation burns (*above*) and heavy burns showing a halo around the burn (*below*)

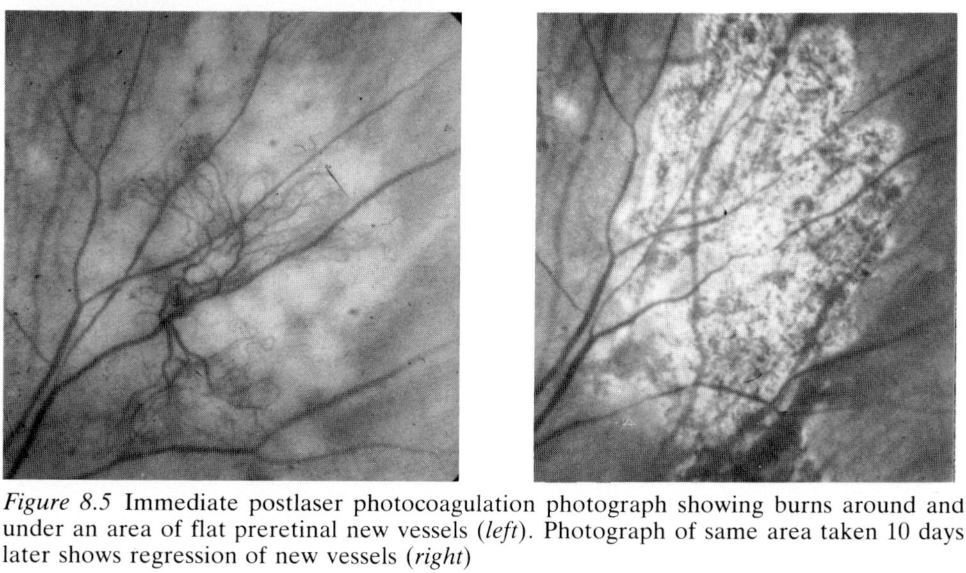

*Figure 8.5* Immediate postlaser photocoagulation photograph showing burns around and under an area of flat preretinal new vessels (*left*). Photograph of same area taken 10 days later shows regression of new vessels (*right*)

the underlying retinal pigment epithelium. The adjacent vein from which the new vessel is derived should be carefully avoided as its closure may aggravate the situation and cause bleeding. The intensity of burn required to produce this minimal or gentle reaction varies among individuals as well as in different parts of the fundus. Care should therefore be taken to adjust the intensity of the burn accordingly.

Following the initial treatment the patient should be re-examined within 4–6 weeks to evaluate the result. If regression is complete, then re-examination should be made in approximately 3–4 months. If the new vessels have only partially regressed or show no signs of regression, then further photocoagulation is carried out in exactly the same way as the initial treatment. If after a further 4–6 weeks the vessels still persist, then scatter photocoagulation is applied to the peripheral area of retina in the quadrant exhibiting capillary non-perfusion. If after 4–6 weeks the vessels still persist, then retreatment of the peripheral retina is carried out, filling in any gaps.

In some cases the new vessels will have already been pulled forward by the contracting vitreous. In these cases the initial treatment is the same as in the case of mild flat new vessels. However, not infrequently the neovascularization persists in these eyes, even after adequate treatment. If this occurs then there are two further options: (*a*) If the vessels do not directly overlie a major vein they can be closed by direct treatment; (*b*) If they directly overlie the feeding veins it will be impossible to occlude them by direct treatment. In this case photocoagulation has to be applied to the peripheral supplying veins so that they are gradually occluded down and through the new vessel complex to the next venous tributary. The spot size used is 200–500 μ with a duration of 0.20–0.50 sec with an intensity that will occlude the vein. Although this form of treatment may seem drastic it is usually extremely effective, and there is usually no additional field loss.

If the peripheral new vessels are moderate to severe and are associated with a small amount of fibrosis or even a mild tractional retinal detachment, then panretinal photocoagulation should be carried out to the entire peripheral retina. Additional burns are applied around and under any new vessels in a more confluent manner. The spot size should be approximately 500 μ and the duration 0.02 sec. Areas of tractional retinal detachment should be surrounded by several rows of gentle burns. There is no evidence that laser photocoagulation increases contraction of existing fibrous tissue and there is apparently no further contraction of fibrous tissue that has already undergone spontaneous contraction. If areas of the retina are masked by haemorrhage, visible areas are treated and then the remaining areas if and when the haemorrhage absorbs. Any additional neovascularization should be treated as outlined above in the previous section with similar intervals between examinations.

### DISC NEW VESSELS

Disc new vessels present the greatest threat to vision. Treatment is by panretinal photocoagulation (*Figure 8.6*). A 500 μ spot size is used, with a duration of 0.02–0.20 sec with an intensity that just blanches the retinal pigment epithelium.

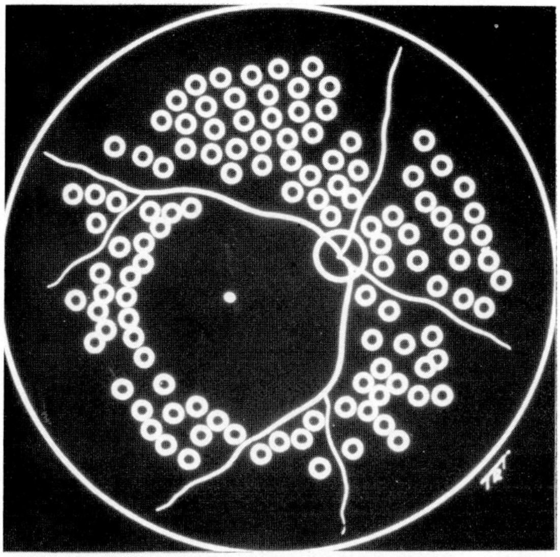

*Figure 8.6* Schematic representation of panretinal photocoagulation (PRP)

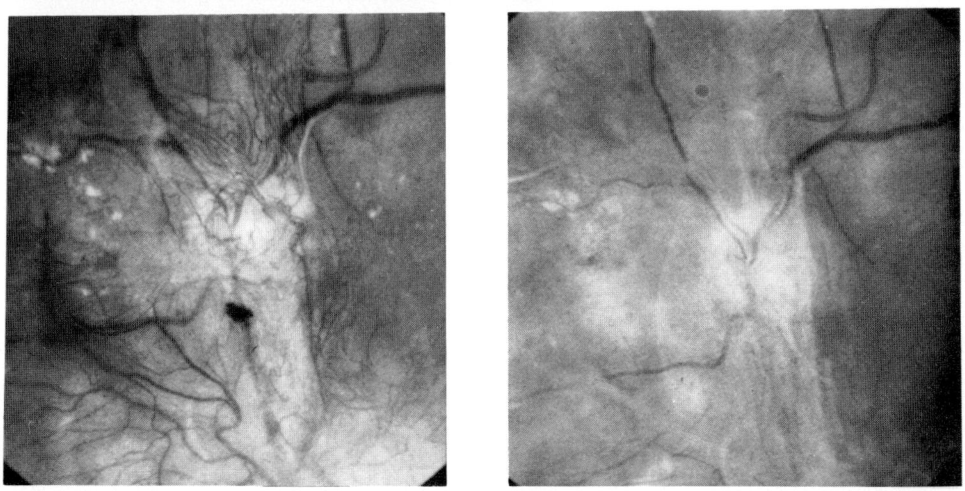

*Figure 8.7* Disc new vessels with accompanying fibrous tissue. (*Left*) pretreatment appearance, (*right*) post-treatment appearance shows regression of new vessels but no change in fibrous tissue

A total of between 2000 and 3500 burns should be applied (*Figure 8.7*). Although some have suggested that the more peripheral parts of the retina should be treated with larger burns, we have found that this causes pain, and we prefer to keep the spot size at 500 μ. It has been suggested that this amount of treatment at one sitting frequently causes macular oedema. In our experience this is extremely rare and is usually associated with heavy burns, particularly when they are applied over previously treated areas.

Any residual neovascularization should be retreated as outlined in the previous sections and the patient reviewed at 3–4 monthly intervals. If disc new vessels persist despite adequate and repeated panretinal photocoagulation, then direct treatment should be considered if they do not overlie a major artery or vein. In direct treatment a spot size (usually between 50 and 200 μ) that just straddles the thickness of the vessel is used with a duration of 0.20–0.50 sec and an intensity that produces either direct closure, blanching or darkening of the red cell column. The aim of treatment is to close off the new vessel. This may well need to be repeated and the patient must be examined at hourly intervals throughout the day. Once closure has been maintained for over an hour, reopening is unlikely to occur. In some cases direct photocoagulation will cause the entire vessel to contract, leaving only a fibrous knot (*Figures 8.8 and 8.9*). When commencing direct photocoagulation the early burns should be applied to the finest most distal vessels and then the larger or feeding vessels should be occluded. However, if new vessels overlie major vessels then repeated panretinal photocoagulation using the xenon arc should be considered over the top of the argon burns (*Figures 8.10, 8.11, 8.12 and 8.13*).

Because eyes with disc new vessels carry the worst prognosis, treatment should be considered an emergency. Photocoagulation should be started adjacent to the nasal side of the disc and then above and below the disc, just outside the superior and inferior temporal vascular arcades. Burns should then be applied temporal to the macula to areas of capillary non-perfusion. Having applied between 500 and 600 burns to the posterior pole, a three-mirror contact lens or a panfunduscopic lens is used to treat the peripheral retina just anterior to the equator. It is our experience that the younger the patient the more peripheral the treatment has to be placed.

With practice, panretinal photocoagulation can be carried out in about 30 minutes. However, with the recent modification which allows the application of burns in rapid succession, this time can be reduced by half.

In the presence of vitreous or subhyaloid haemorrhage as much treatment as possible should be applied during the first session and then at subsequent occasions the treatment completed if and when the haemorrhage absorbs. There is no evidence that haemorrhage alters the outcome of treatment, although a higher power may be necessary to produce the required burn. In the presence of lens opacities it will also be necessary to increase the power and it may also be necessary to manipulate the three-mirror lens or fundus lens to get around the opacities.

### FLORID PROLIFERATIVE DIABETIC RETINOPATHY

The course of this rare type of proliferative diabetic retinopathy has been described as rapid, bloody and blinding. Once established, the retinopathy is extremely difficult to eliminate. For this reason it is our view that photocoagulation should be carried out early. If the patient is seen with the second eye in the preproliferative stage, we perform prophylactic panretinal photocoagulation although at present we have no evidence that this has any advantages over conventional therapy.

### PROLIFERATIVE DIABETIC RETINOPATHY AND PREGNANCY

The effect of pregnancy on the course of the disease is variable. In some cases the progression of proliferation can be as rapid as in florid proliferative diabetic retinopathy and it is therefore important to follow these patients very closely. Once

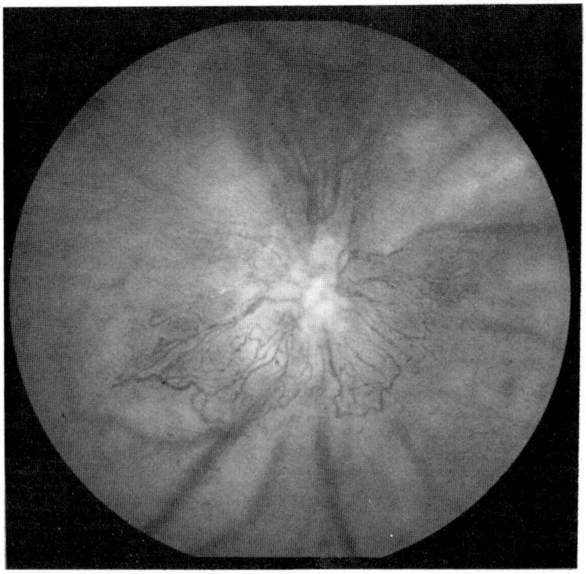

*Figure 8.8* Persistent disc new vessels after adequate panretinal photocoagulation

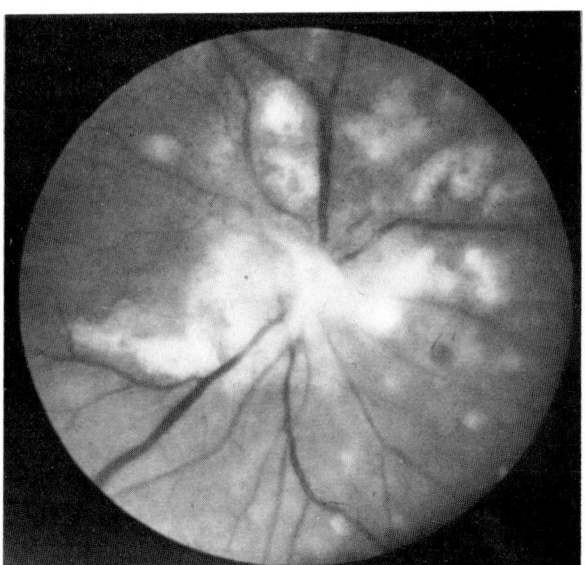

*Figure 8.9* Post-treatment appearance of *Figure 8.7*. The new vessels have been successfully occluded after multiple sessions of direct photocoagulation. Note the residual knot of fibrous tissue on the disc

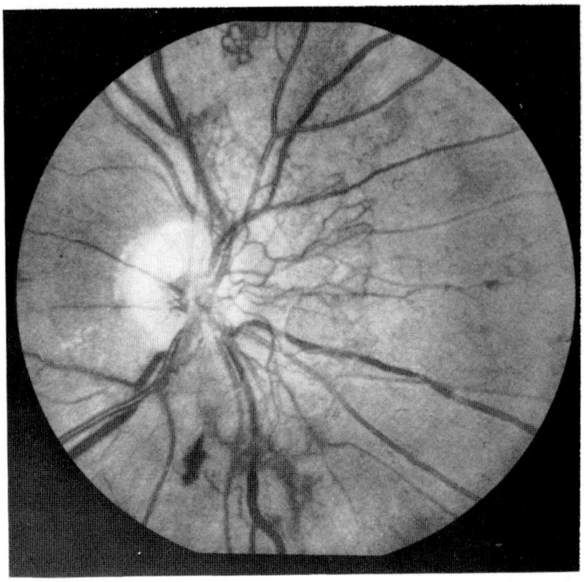

*Figure 8.10* Pretreatment appearance of new disc vessels

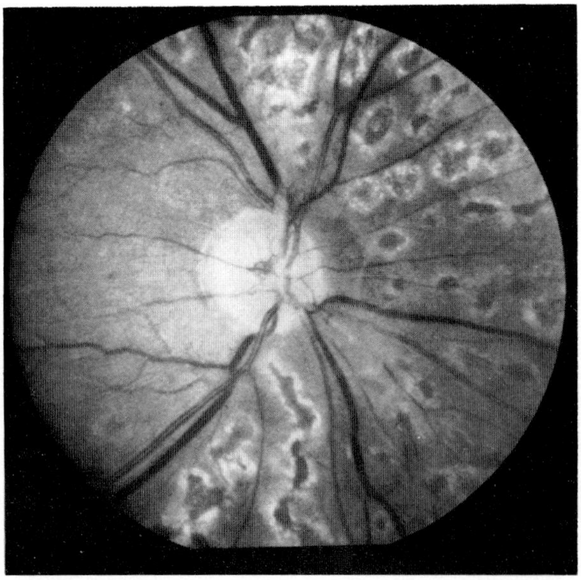

*Figure 8.11* Almost complete regression of disc vessels after 3500, 500 μ argon laser burns

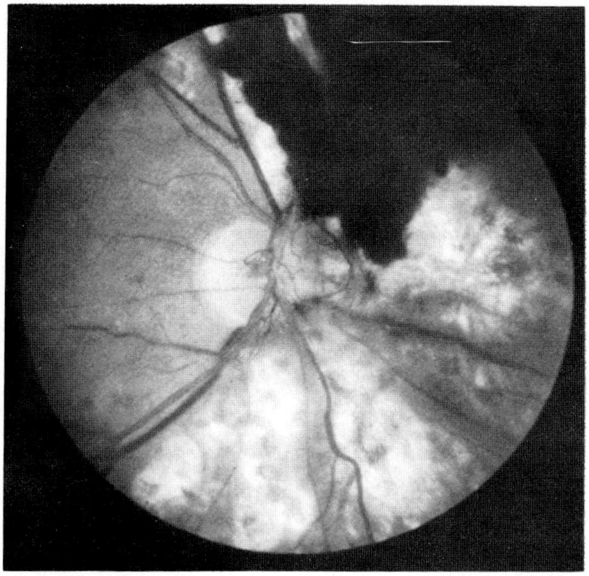

*Figure 8.12* Recurrence of new vessels with vitreous haemorrhage

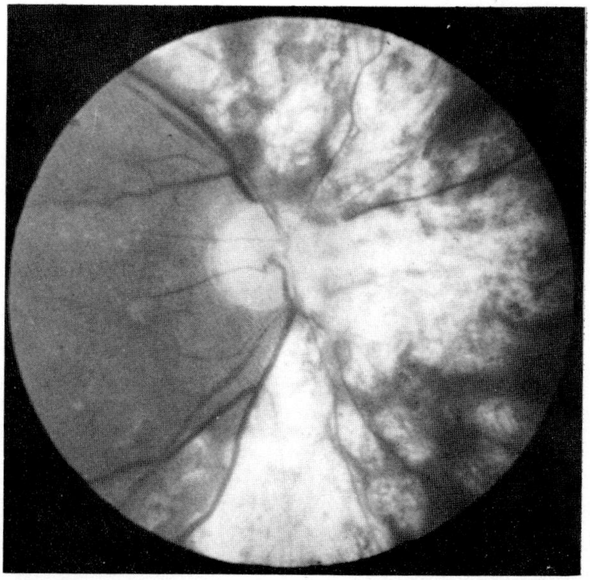

*Figure 8.13* Complete regression of new vessels after 880, 4.5 degree burns using the xenon arc photocoagulator (*Figures 8.9, 8.10, 8.11 and 8.12* are of the same eye)

neovascularization has been successfully treated there is no reason why subsequent pregnancies should be discouraged as frequently there is no further advancement of the retinopathy. Indeed, we have seen several successful pregnancies in the presence of extensive laser treatment.

## ADVERSE EFFECTS OF PHOTOCOAGULATION

### Side-effects

#### Immediate and transient

Within the first 48 hours patients may notice blurring of vision. Examination may reveal a peripheral annular choroidal detachment associated with a variable degree of myopia, shallowing of the anterior chamber with an anterior displacement of the iris–lens diaphragm. Severe shallowing may cause angle closure and elevation of intraocular pressure. Treatment of elevated intraocular pressure is with acetazolamide. Topical corticosteroids appear to be ineffective. The severity of these changes is not directly related to the amount of photocoagulation and their exact mechanism is unknown. They are fortunately transient and usually resolve after about 10 days.

#### Long lasting effects

These are more common following xenon than laser photocoagulation. The main effects include blurred vision, night blindness, altered colour perception, constricted visual fields, micropsia, and a darkening of overall vision, as though looking through a neutral density filter. These effects last for 6–18 months and in some cases visual acuity may be reduced by a line or so. Visual field changes are common following extensive photocoagulation and are at their maximum within 1 week following treatment. Thereafter they gradually improve, and by 3 months they return to normal. The effects on visual field following panretinal photocoagulation are more marked after xenon photocoagulation but minimal following laser. Indeed, following 2000 argon laser burns many patients are unaware of any field defect and may even say that their field of vision has improved. However, if burns are arranged in a confluent fashion the field defect is more obvious.

Many diabetics with extensive retinopathy exhibit colour defects even in the presence of normal visual acuity. Following photocoagulation with both xenon and argon photocoagulation the blue end of the spectrum is lost, and indeed in some patients there may be complete loss of colour vision. The degree of recovery of colour vision is variable and usually incomplete.

These symptoms tend to recover and within 6 months the majority disappear.

## Complications

As in all surgical procedures, photocoagulation is associated with major complications. Each stage of the procedure has its own group of complications and in addition there may be delayed effects due to the photocoagulation.

### Immediate complications

Complications associated with retrobulbar injections are as follows: perforation of the eyeball, retrobulbar haemorrhage, injection into the dural sheath with subsequent damage to the optic nerve, or possibly tracking of the anaesthetic into the subarachnoid space. If the contact lens is improperly applied it is possible to produce a corneal abrasion and oedema.

The most disastrous complication of light application is a foveal burn. To avoid this, careful examination of the macula and paramacular region is made prior to commencing photocoagulation, and during the course of photocoagulation constant reference to these areas is made. Photocoagulation should be started at the posterior pole with constant reference to the disc and macula and thereafter applied to the more peripheral retina.

Immediate complications are occlusion of a retinal vein or artery. Occlusion of a vein may aggravate the retinopathy. If the vein is still closed by the end of the photocoagulation session, then photocoagulation in a panretinal technique should be applied to the area of drainage of the vein peripheral to the occlusion. Closure of a retinal arteriole will result in an infarct in the distribution of that arteriole.

Applications of light may accidentally hit the iris and result in atrophy or the development of late posterior synechiae or iris haemorrhages. If there is pigment on the surface of the lens, either in the form of broken synechiae or epicapsular stars, it is possible to produce small focal burns within the anterior lens substance surrounding the areas of pigment. High energy applied to the retina with a small spot size may give rise to superficial burns in the cornea. These heal within a matter of hours.

With heavy and confluent photocoagulation scotomata and nerve bundle defects may be produced.

### Delayed effects

Inadequate photocoagulation may aggravate the retinopathy. In addition, fibrous tissue may proliferate and give rise to a preretinal traction membrane. Contraction of fibrous tissue may lead to retinal detachment or macular traction. Small high-energy burns may rupture Bruch's membrane and give rise to haemorrhage and the 'disciform' response.

## SUMMARY

Photocoagulation is an established and proven form of treatment of proliferative diabetic retinopathy. Technique and experience are important for achieving good results. It is hoped that the fundamental action of photocoagulation will soon be discovered and a rational and scientific approach to the treatment be established. For the time being we are left with a technique which has become established as a result of many trials and errors. Finally, in order to overcome the problem of retinopathy careful screening is necessary to identify those at risk.

## Further reading

Haut, J., Limon, S., Masson, M. and Perdriel, G. (1981) *Le Laser en Ophtalmologie*. Paris: Masson

Constable, I. and Lim, A. (1981) *Laser – Its Clinical Uses in Eye Diseases*. Edinburgh: Churchill Livingstone

L'Esperance, F. A. and James, W. (1981) *Diabetic Retinopathy: Clinical Evaluation and Management*. St Louis: C. V. Mosby

# 9
# Retinal vein occlusion

John S. Shilling

## ANATOMY OF VENOUS CIRCULATION

The tributaries of the central retinal vein show a fairly standard distribution from the four quadrants. The macula is drained by a number of small veins into the superior and inferior temporal veins, and smaller tributaries drain the areas of retinal periphery into the four major veins. The central retinal vein enters the optic nerve, passes through the lamina cribrosa and thence, having passed through the optic nerve sheath, drains into the orbital veins.

The retinal veins may be occluded at a number of sites and the area of retina involved is determined by the site of occlusion. Central retinal vein occlusion involves the whole retina; hemisphere vein occlusions involve either the upper or lower half of the retina; occlusion of a major temporal or nasal vein involves a quadrant of retina, and minor tributaries either involve a small area of retinal periphery or the macula. The clinical pattern and symptoms produced by retinal vein occlusion are determined by the area of retina involved and therefore by the site of occlusion. It is, however, recognized that the responses of the retina to occlusive diseases are limited and some features are common to all types of occlusion.

## AETIOLOGY OF RETINAL VEIN OCCLUSION

The aetiologies of retinal vein occlusion are multiple. Some are well understood but others are only partially so, and in others the cause remains obscure. *Systemic hypertension* is recognized as a cause of quadrantic and some peripheral occlusions in which the vein is occluded as it crosses the diseased artery in its common sheath. The arterial wall is thickened by the hypertensive disease and therefore there is a tendency to nipping of the vein and occlusion. *Inflammation of the vein wall (periphlebitis)* is unquestionably the cause of some peripheral and major venous occlusions. The role of inflammation in central vein occlusion, however, remains in doubt; although some authorities believe that this is an important cause of occlusion in young patients, and classify this disease separately as 'central retinal vasculitis'.

The role of blood constituents also remains somewhat of an enigma. It is well known that abnormalities of plasma proteins can cause venous dilatation and the clinical picture of 'slow flow' retinopathy. Overt venous occlusions are, however, rather less common than might be expected on theoretical grounds. Waldenstrom's macroglobulinaemia is the best example of this. Lipid abnormalities have been shown by some to be present in a number of patients with venous disease, but their exact role is not fully understood. Polycythaemia rubra vera, and other diseases in which the cellular constituents of the blood are increased or abnormal, have been implicated in some patients. In general, investigations of blood viscosity have been disappointing and have failed to add much to the understanding of the cause of occlusion in an individual patient.

Local ocular disease is undoubtedly important. Glaucoma is an important cause of central retinal vein occlusion, and also of hemisphere occlusion, when the upper or lower half retinal drainage is impeded at the edge of a glaucomatous cupped disc. Some believe that hemisphere occlusions represent a variant of central retinal vein occlusion. It is thought that the involvement of half the retina occurs because of a congenital variant of the retinal venous drainage, in which the drainage from the upper and lower halves of the retina remain separate within the optic nerve for a longer distance than is normal. It is doubtful whether raised intraocular pressure plays any part in quadrantic or smaller occlusions in which the block is away from the optic disc.

## EFFECTS ON THE RETINA

Various changes occur in the area of retina drained by an occluded vein, and in general differ only in the area involved. The early appearance is that of retinal haemorrhage. The blood may be located primarily in the superficial nerve fibre layer, but it may also involve deeper retinal layers in more severe cases. If the macular area is involved the haemorrhage will cover this important area. The retinal veins are dilated and may be more tortuous than normal. In central retinal vein occlusion the optic disc is hyperaemic.

Fluorescein angiography at the acute stage of the disease demonstrates leakage, but much of the detail is obscured by the blood which masks underlying choroidal fluorescence. Subsequently, the haemorrhage absorbs and more details of the retina become visible. It is then possible to define the vasculature in detail, and to follow the natural course of the vascular changes with repeated fluorescein angiography.

Changes are seen in the arteries, capillaries and veins and the appearances of each component of the vasculature may change with time.

### Arteries

Following a venous occlusive episode the arterioles may progressively narrow, and late sheathing is a common occurrence. This is thought to represent a secondary event and does not necessarily imply arterial disease as a cause of the original vascular occlusive pattern. Fluorescein may leak from arteries as they pass through areas of retinal ischaemia.

## Veins

The retinal veins may also progressively occlude or narrow and become sheathed. Veins which were initially demonstrated to be perfusing fairly normally may eventually fail to do so.

## Capillaries

Changes in the state of the capillary microvasculature in retinal vein occlusion have proved to be the most useful features in assessing the ultimate visual prognosis, and also in deciding the best approach to treatment. There are two basic responses in the capillary network.

The first response is that of hyperpermeability in which the capillaries in the affected parts of the retina are dilated and fluorescein angiography demonstrates incompetence of the vessels with leakage of dye in the late angiographic photographs. It is common for the abnormal permeability to affect the macula and the

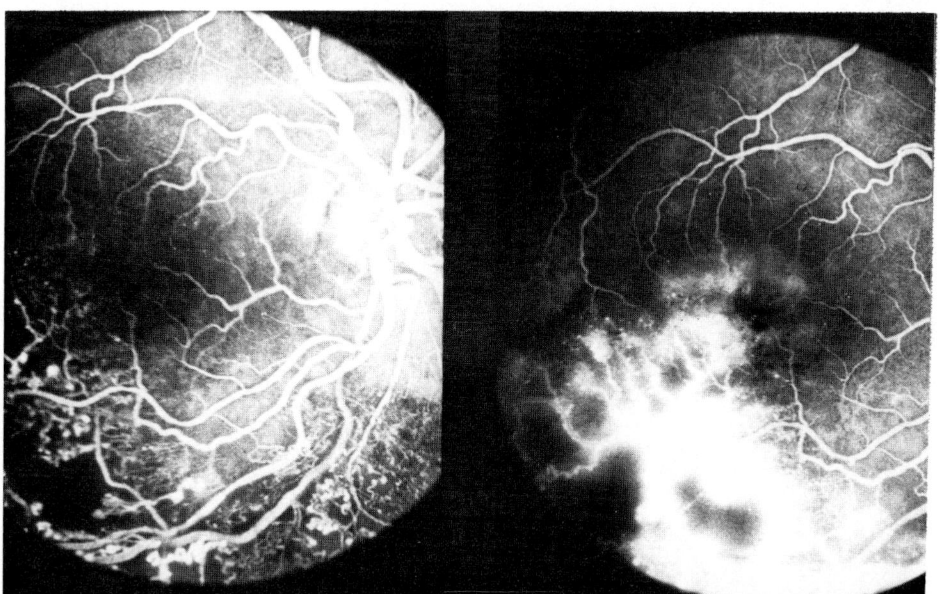

*Figure 9.1* Right eye with an inferotemporal retinal branch vein occlusion. Early (*left*) and late (*right*) phases of a fluorescein angiogram show some capillary closure, but predominantly a hyperpermeability response with macular oedema

clinical appearance of macular oedema therefore results (*Figure 9.1*). The disturbance of central vision that results from macular oedema is variable, and it is very difficult to correlate the clinical and fluorescein angiographic appearance of the macula with visual acuity in an individual.

In some cases oedema of the retina is accompanied by the formation of intraretinal hard exudate (*Figure 9.2*). This is usually in a circinate pattern in retinal disease, as opposed to the stellate pattern of exudate that occurs with optic disc oedema. Visual acuity in these patients may be permanently reduced due to macular oedema. In a few cases progressive loss of central vision occurs, and when this happens a plaque of exudate on the fovea is an important aetiology. In others, atrophy of the retinal pigment epithelium is the cause or, rarely, a new haemorrhage at the macula is responsible. A preretinal traction membrane at the macula is a further cause of macular dysfunction.

The second retinal response is the result of ischaemia leading to neovascularization of the posterior or anterior segment of the eye. The new vessel formation in the posterior segment may be followed by recurrent vitreous haemorrhage, and may also progress to fibrosis and traction retinal detachment. It has been shown clearly that large areas of capillary closure are a necessary precursor to the

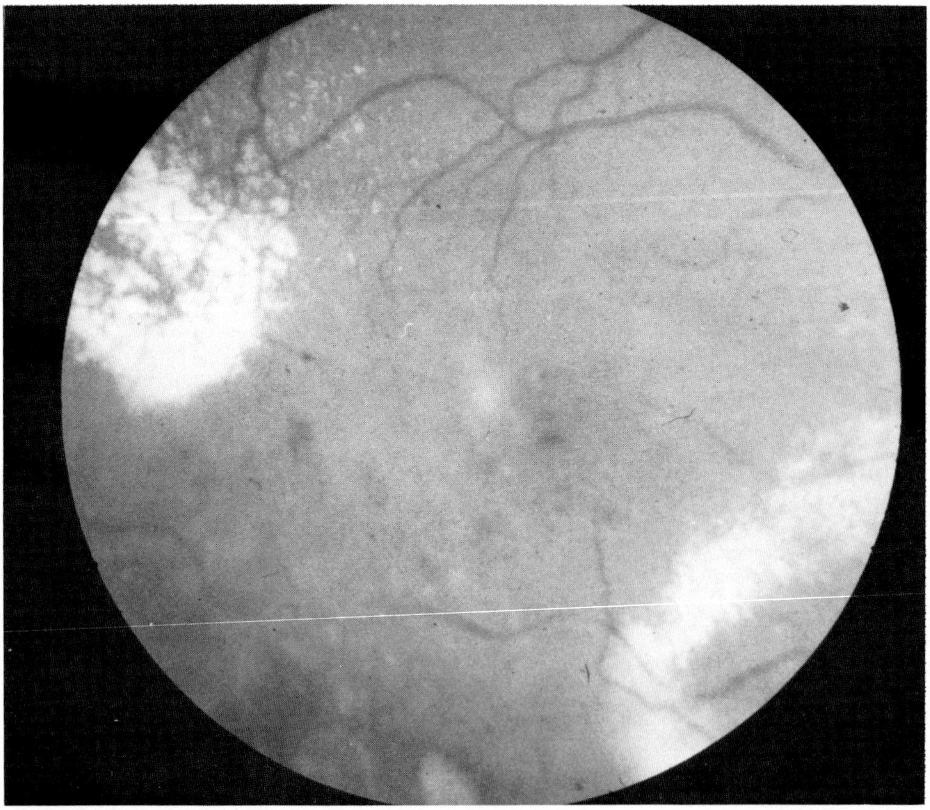

*Figure 9.2* Photograph of same patient showing haemorrhages, chronic macular oedema and intraretinal exudates

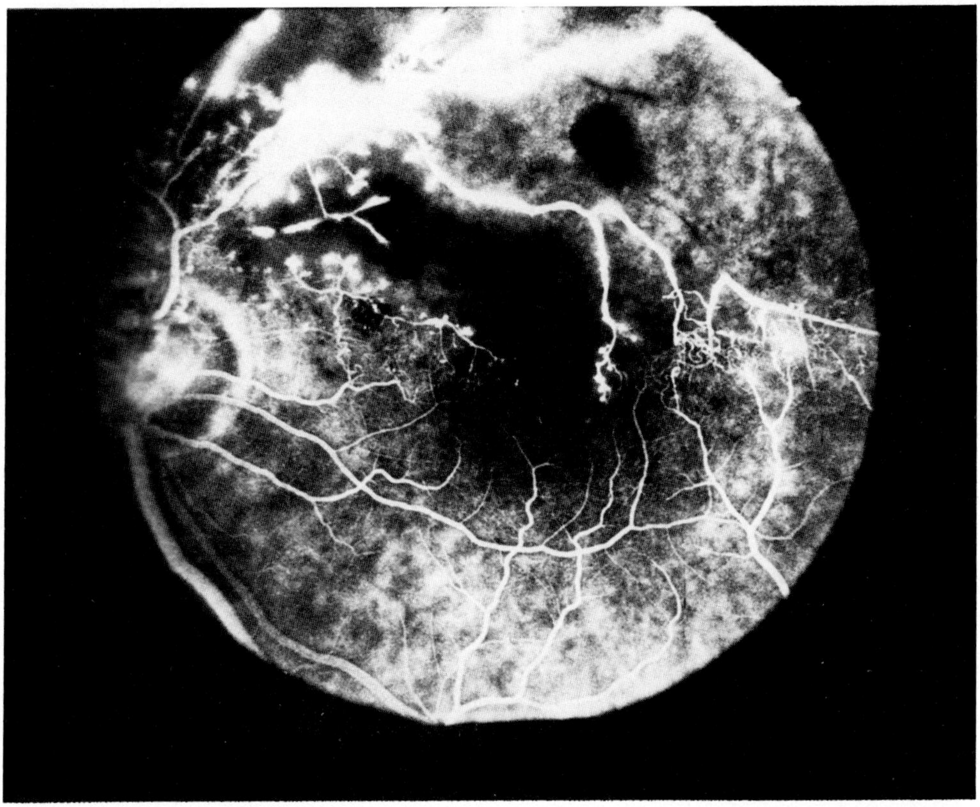

*Figure 9.3* Superotemporal retinal branch vein occlusion. Midphase fluorescein angiogram shows extensive quadrantic capillary closure, intraretinal and preretinal new vessels and early disc neovascularization

development of neovascularization (*Figure 9.3*). This finding correlates well with other neovascular retinopathies and a generalization may be made which states that whatever the underlying aetiology of retinal vascular disease, new vessels will only form when there is significant capillary closure extending to the retinal periphery. In some diseases it may be difficult to document closure satisfactorily, diabetes being one example of this. A rider should be added to the hypothesis of neovascularization of the retina. Inflammatory vascular disease may sometimes cause new vessel formation in the absence of recognizable capillary closure. These new vessels like any other may develop from the optic disc or peripheral retina, and their particular characteristic is that they may spontaneously regress with control of inflammation. It is not known why these vessels form. It may be that the capillary bed closes intermittently, or alternatively that a quite different aetiology is responsible for the promotion of new vessels in this situation.

Rubeosis iridis and subsequent neovascular glaucoma may occur following a central retinal vein occlusion. Although rubeosis may occasionally develop following a branch vein occlusion, neovascular glaucoma is rare.

## TREATMENT

### Systemic

The various drugs used in the treatment of retinal vein occlusion include anticoagulants, fibrinolysins, corticosteroids and immunosuppressives. The former two have been particularly disappointing. There are, of course, certain situations in which systemic therapy is specifically indicated for an underlying disease process such as hypertension or an inflammatory disorder. Corticosteroids may be necessary in patients with sarcoidosis and immunosuppressives in Behçet's disease.

### Photocoagulation

#### Maculopathy

Cystoid macular oedema usually responds poorly to photocoagulation and at present there is no good evidence that visual acuity can be improved by this form of treatment.

Exudative maculopathy, on the other hand, although rare, may be helped by photocoagulation, with maintenance of good visual acuity so long as treatment is applied before the fovea is involved by hard exudates. However, because the number of cases of exudative maculopathy requiring treatment is small, it has not been possible to carry out statistically meaningful controlled studies. There is, however, no doubt that patients with increasing hard exudate deposition at the posterior pole should be considered for treatment.

#### Posterior segment neovascularization

In general, photocoagulation for neovascularization is more successful than for maculopathy. Prior to treatment the area of capillary closure can be identified by fluorescein angiography and then the affected area can be ablated with accuracy. Disc new vessels usually respond well to treatment but the effect on peripheral vessels is variable. Although peripheral vessels may partially shrink, complete regression is less common.

Direct treatment to peripheral new vessels may be effective, but heavy photocoagulation is necessary to achieve this, and there is a danger of subsequent preretinal traction. It is therefore not recommended in the first place, although sometimes required as a secondary treatment if indirect photocoagulation fails.

The special indications for applying this treatment in patients with retinal branch vein occlusion differ a little from those in diabetes, because it is thought that the risk of permanent loss of vision is less. Vitreous haemorrhage tends to clear spontaneously, and progressive traction retinal detachment is not common. Photocoagulation is therefore rarely urgent. It is, however, agreed that photocoagulation treatment is indicated if disc new vessels are present and in all cases if vitreous haemorrhage has occurred.

## Anterior segment neovascularization

Photocoagulation for anterior segment neovascularization is perhaps less well established. It is, however, recognized that rubeosis of the iris may resolve following photocoagulation of ischaemic retina. *In patients with central retinal vein occlusion* studies have shown that neovascular glaucoma may be prevented by panretinal photocoagulation, and although these patients very rarely regain vision, the development of a painful and blind eye may be aborted. The timing of the treatment is arguable. Fluorescein angiography performed within 3 months of the occlusion will identify capillary closure, so long as the amount of retinal haemorrhage is not too extensive to obscure details, and in the presence of this feature the risk of glaucoma is considerable. Treatment may be applied at this stage, or alternatively, the patient may be kept under regular surveillance for early rubeosis, and treated only if new vessels start to appear. The early diagnosis of new vessels may, however, be difficult, especially with deeply pigmented irides and glaucoma may occur too quickly for satisfactory treatment. It must be stressed that it is necessary to examine these patients with regular gonioscopy because neovascularization of the angle may be the first indication of progressive disease. For these reasons it is our policy to treat the retinal capillary closure with photocoagulation at an early stage in this group of patients.

# 10
# Management of choroidal melanoma and retinoblastoma

Devron H. Char

## INTRODUCTION

Recent studies have altered some of our concepts and increased our understanding of the pathogenesis, pathophysiology and management of intraocular tumors. The emphasis of this chapter is on the clinical management of these two common primary intraocular neoplasms; the indications, contraindications, advantages and disadvantages of newer therapeutic modalities in the treatment of retinoblastoma and choroidal melanoma are stressed.

## CHOROIDAL MELANOMA

There are a number of unresolved issues regarding the definition, natural history and therapy for choroidal melanomas. Some of these important clinical issues include:

(1) At what stage in the history of a small choroidal melanoma does it develop the capacity to metastasize? Is there a recognizable clinical or histological correlate of this event?
(2) At what stage in the natural history of this tumor must intervention occur to avoid metastatic disease?
(3) What is the relative efficacy of various treatment modalities?

Until prospective, randomized treatment trials are performed therapeutic decisions will be based more upon a philosophical opinion than on a secure data base. Although results of multicenter clinical prospective trials are unavailable, clinicians must diagnose and manage patients with pigmented choroidal lesions, and this review provides an empiric approach to the treatment of this neoplasm.

What constitutes a choroidal melanoma is unclear; for the purposes of this chapter we define it as a lesion which has metastatic potential, in contradistinction to a nevus which does not.

## Diagnosis

In patients with clear media, choroidal melanomas greater than 3 mm in elevation can be differentiated from simulating lesions in more than 90% of cases when examined by experienced observers using indirect ophthalmoscopy (Char, 1978*a*). On ophthalmoscopic examination the pigmentation of a choroidal melanoma can vary from amelanotic to a dark-brown color. Often there is superficial orange pigmentation and surrounding subretinal fluid. In larger melanomas which have broken through Bruch's membrane, a 'collar-button' configuration is present which is almost pathognomonic for a melanoma. In contrast to primary choroidal melanomas, metastatic tumors to the choroid are almost always located at the posterior pole, frequently occur as multiple lesions, are usually amelanotic and relatively flat.

The two lesions most difficult to ophthalmoscopically differentiate from small choroidal melanomas are choroidal nevi and hemangiomas. Choroidal nevi are generally slate grey in color, less than 2.0 mm in elevation, and often have overlying drusen. It is unusual to observe subretinal fluid contiguous to a choroidal nevus. Ophthalmoscopically it is almost impossible to differentiate a small melanoma which is less than 2.0 mm in thickness from a choroidal nevus. The presence of orange pigmentation is suggestive of a melanoma, but it is not an absolute sign. Choroidal hemangiomas are often orange or pinkish in color although we have observed a few hemangiomas which could not be distinguished from melanomas either by ophthalmoscopic or fluorescein criteria.

In a number of ocular oncology centers, using non-invasive techniques, the diagnostic accuracy in the differentiation of choroidal melanomas from simulating lesions approaches 98% (Char *et al.*, 1980; Robertson and Campbell, 1979). In lesions greater than 2.5 mm in thickness the diagnostic accuracy, namely, sensitivity and specificity, of a combination of quantitative echography and B-scan ultrasonography is greater than 95% (Ossoinig, 1975; Coleman, 1976). For choroidal mass lesions less than 2 mm in thickness the diagnostic validity of ancillary tests is not sufficiently sensitive.

At the Ocular Oncology Unit, University of California, San Francisco and at other centers a number of false-positive and false negative P-32 tests have been observed in patients with small choroidal lesions (McLean, Zimmerman and Evans, 1978; Shammas, Burton and Weingeist, 1977; Williams *et al.*, 1978; Zakov, Smith and Albert, 1978). While this test has greater than 95% accuracy in large choroidal melanomas, often in those tumors in which there is diagnostic uncertainty the test is unreliable. We therefore do not routinely use this test in the evaluation of patients with choroidal melanomas. Goldmann perimetry, fluorescein angiography, and scleral transillumination are also part of the diagnostic armamentarium; however, we have observed a significant number of false-positive and false-negative results with these assays.

Since the correct diagnosis of choroidal mass lesions less than 2.5 mm in elevation can be difficult, a combination of all non-invasive diagnostic modalities should be used to differentiate choroidal melanomas from simulating lesions. Many choridal melanomas have a typical appearance; they are elevated, pigmented, have surface orange pigmentation, and a small amount of subretinal fluid. Goldmann perimetry demonstrates an absolute scotoma. Fluorescein angiography shows leakage, intrinsic tumor vessels, and 'hot spots'. On ultrasound these lesions have a low-to-medium reflectivity, hard consistency, vascularity, relatively strong sound attenuation, choroidal excavation, and orbital shadowing.

The choice and timing of therapy is based upon the history, clinical findings and laboratory tests. In many patients with small choroidal mass lesions it is impossible to state categorically that the lesion is a melanoma with a potential to metastasize. We therefore follow a number of patients with choroidal mass lesions less than 3 mm in thickness without making a definitive diagnosis.

## Management

A number of investigators have questioned the efficacy of enucleation and have suggested alternative treatment modalities (McLean, Foster and Zimmerman, 1980*a* and *b*; Newman *et al.*, 1970; Stallard, 1966; Vogel and Meyer-Schwickerath, 1978). While these issues can only be resolved with prospective randomized trials, retrospective studies have increased our understanding of the natural history of choroidal melanomas. While it is unclear at what stage a choroidal melanoma develops the capacity to metastasize, lesions of less than 3 mm in thickness appear to have a very low metastatic potential when either serially evaluated without intervention or treated by any modality. Patients with small choroidal melanomas, less than 3 mm in thickness and less than 10 mm in diameter, have less than 10% 5-year tumor-related mortality (Barr, Sipperley and Nicholson, 1978; Char and Hogan, 1977; Curtin and Cavender, 1974; Gass, 1977, 1980; Rubenstein and Myska, 1974; Thomas *et al.*, 1979).

### Serial examination without intervention

In a number of clinical settings serial examination without therapeutic intervention is appropriate. Patients with lesions less than 10 mm in diameter and 3 mm in elevation with an uncertain diagnosis should be followed. It appears reasonable to manage patients with small choroidal melanomas or indeterminant pigmented lesions without therapeutic intervention if the following conditions are met:

(1) the visual acuity in the involved eye is good;
(2) the lesion is less than 3 mm in thickness and 10 mm in diameter;
(3) there is no growth on serial examination with ophthalmoscopy, fundus photography, and ultrasonography.

Patients should initially be followed at 3-month intervals with indirect ophthalmoscopy, Goldmann perimetry, fundus photography, fluorescein angiography and both A- and B-scan ultrasonography. While experienced clinicians can accurately estimate the diameter of a lesion, echography is the most sensitive method to detect an increase in tumor thickness, and photography is the most accurate means to determine if the lesion has changed in horizontal dimension (Char *et al.*, 1980). After each visit, the patient's fundus drawings, serial photographs and ultrasonography are projected on to a large screen and compared to see if horizontal or vertical growth has occurred.

Documentation of growth by clinical evaluation or laboratory tests may indicate that a tumor has increased in its metastatic potential; at that time direct therapeutic intervention is advisable. Unfortunately, at present the only clinical findings which appear to have a good correlation with prognosis are related to tumor diameter and thickness (McLean, Foster and Zimmerman, 1977; Shammas and Blodi, 1977*a*). In our experience, small melanomas usually expand rapidly once they enter their growth phase. Because of this we believe that once there is evidence that a tumor is in its growth phase it may have a greater potential for metastases and should be treated.

At least 200 patients with the diagnosis of small choroidal melanomas have been serially examined without intervention until growth is documented; 5-year tumor mortality has been less than 10%. We have previously reported 20 patients followed with small choroidal melanomas, enucleated only when growth was documented (Char and Hogan, 1977). Of the nine patients who subsequently underwent enucleation, most retained useful binocular vision for 7 years prior to surgery, with a range of 1–19 years, and none have developed metastatic disease during an average follow-up of 4.5 years, with a range of 1.5–9.5 years, since enucleation. Nine additional patients in this group who are still being followed have shown relatively little change in tumor size or visual field defect.

Rubinstein and Myska (1974) and Curtin and Cavender (1974) have also followed a small number of patients with choroidal melanomas and found a similar mortality. Gass (1977) reported on 20 patients with relatively small choroidal tumors examined over periods from 4 months to 11 years. Twelve of these patients had their eyes removed after growth was documented, with a mean of 2.3 years and a range from 4 months to 5 years. Except for one tumor death, these patients have been followed for an average of 3.8 years after enucleation, ranging from 8 months to 11 years, without development of metastatic disease. Seven patients in this group had little or no detectable tumor growth during follow-up.

Among 21 eyes examined pathologically after enucleation following evidence of growth, 20 contained spindle cell melanomas. It is our impression that patients whose tumors do not demonstrate growth on the first few return visits have biologically less active tumors, and can be safely followed without an increase in tumor mortality. These patients can retain useful vision in the affected eye until increased tumor activity is documented by growth. Gass (1977) has suggested that cystic degeneration of the retina, drusen formation, orange pigmentation, and choroidal neovascularization are prognostically important clinical findings suggestive of inactivity in small pigmented choroidal mass lesions. Unfortunately, while we agree that choroidal tumors with these findings are more likely to remain stationary in size, we have noted a number of exceptions. We therefore follow all patients with small choroidal melanomas at frequent intervals since we have found no reliable method of delineating those lesions which are more likely to exhibit serial growth from those which do not.

The choice of therapy in patients with small choroidal melanomas is based on the risk–benefit ratio. We believe that in patients with good visual acuities, management by serial examination without intervention allows them to retain useful binocular vision for prolonged lengths of time without significant increase in tumor-related mortality. When growth is documented treatment is recommended; it is our clinical impression that this event heralds a phase of rapid tumor growth and this may correlate with a poorer prognosis.

## Alternative modes of active intervention

The proper role of alternative modes of therapy including photocoagulation, radiotherapy (radioactive plaques and charged particle irradiation), and either choroidectomy or eyewall resection in the management of choroidal melanoma is unclear. Recent controversy regarding the efficacy of enucleation in preventing metastases has increased the use of alternative therapies. We are convinced that all these modalities can destroy tumors. In patients with small choroidal melanomas without evidence of tumor growth we believe serial examination without intervention incurs less ocular morbidity and is not associated with an increase in tumor-related mortality. We consider alternative therapeutic modalities in the following circumstances:

(1) there is a growing melanoma in a patient's only functional eye;
(2) a small choroidal melanoma less than 10 mm in diameter and less than 3 mm in thickness in an eye with good vision and documented tumor growth;
(3) a medium (10–15 mm in diameter and greater than 5 mm in thickness) or large (greater than 15 mm in diameter or greater than 5 mm in thickness) melanoma in an eye with good vision located at least 3 mm from the optic nerve or fovea;
(4) a choroidal melanoma in a patient who refused enucleation.

In patients in whom active therapeutic intervention is being considered, radioactive phosphorus uptake tests are often performed in many centers. Because the P-32 test is an invasive procedure of questionable sensitivity in patients with small choroidal melanomas, it should only be used when active intervention is contemplated if a positive result is obtained. Some patients with small choroidal melanomas have been noted to have extraocular extension which has not been detectable by either clinical examination, computed tomography or ultrasonography (Duffin *et al.*, 1981). If a radioactive phosphorus uptake test is performed the sclera should be examined for extraocular extension which would require a different form of therapy. As outlined in a number of articles, the P-32 test should be performed in as atraumatic a manner as possible, since a number of complications, including retinal hemorrhage, vitreous hemorrhage and central artery occlusion have been observed with this test. There is also at least a theoretical possibility of tumor spread (Burton, 1976; Char and Hogan, 1977).

We have obtained negative P-32 results in some patients with growing small choroidal melanomas. In such cases, when all of the other diagnostic studies are positive, we proceed with therapy and disregard the negative P-32 results.

## Photocoagulation

Photocoagulation is an alternative therapy which may be used in the treatment of some small choroidal melanomas. The criteria for the use of photocoagulation which have been enumerated by Vogel (1972*a*) only apply to 5–10% of choroidal melanoma patients. The main disadvantage of photocoagulation is its limited applicability. We believe that a choroidal melanoma should be treated by photocoagulation only if in addition to meeting Vogel's criteria one of the following conditions is met:

(1) A patient has decreased vision due to subretinal fluid in the fovea secondary to a small choroidal melanoma superior to the macula.
(2) A patient has a relatively small growing posterior pole choroidal melanoma, less than 4 mm in elevation, and wishes therapy other than radiation or enucleation.

Approximately 50% of cases initially treated with photocoagulation have required enucleation either because of continued tumor growth or complications of photocoagulation (Vogel and Meyer-Schwickerath, 1978). Significant complications associated with photocoagulation include retinal and vitreous hemorrhage, chorioretinal neovascularization, macular folds, retinal exudates, retinal detachment and failure to eradicate the tumor. Visual acuity after photocoagulation depends mainly upon the location of the tumor and the occurrence of complications. Less than a third of patients treated by photocoagulation have had visual acuity better than 20/100.

Patients treated with photocoagulation need frequent serial examination for the rest of their lives. Meyer-Schwickerath *et al.* (1978), François (1974) and our group have all observed tumor recurrences up to 8 years after photocoagulation. In a number of institutions a substantial percentage of eyes treated with photocoagulation eventually require enucleation; on histologic examination there are often numerous areas of active tumor cell proliferation (Duvall and Lucas, 1981; Vogel, 1972*b*). We have found this therapeutic modality useful mainly in patients with relatively flat choroidal melanomas who have visual symptoms due to subretinal fluid leaking from the lesion into the macula. In my experience, lesions over 3 mm in thickness must be treated with xenon photocoagulation, in contradistinction to argon photocoagulation, to destroy a tumor.

The relative efficacy of photocoagulation versus irradiation, using charged particles or plaques, in the management of small choroidal melanomas is unclear. In a relatively thin melanoma where the major symptoms are due to subretinal fluid leaking into the macula, photocoagulation can probably be performed with equal or less morbidity and is more widely available than irradiation. As discussed below, in order to localize a tumor for either plaques or external beam charged particle irradiation a surgical procedure is necessary. In a patient who has lost central vision secondary to a relatively thin, less than 4 mm thick, choroidal melanoma which involves the fovea or is in a peripapillary location, if enucleation is refused, either photocoagulation or irradiation may be used to destroy the tumor.

## Radiation therapy

Radiation therapy has been used in the treatment of choroidal melanoma since 1929. Approximately 500 eyes have been reported after treatment with this modality (Bedford, 1973; Char, Lonn and Margolis, 1977; Lommatzsch, 1974; Moore, 1930; Shields *et al.*, 1982; Stallard, 1961, 1966). In 60% of patients, most of whom had small choroidal melanomas, the tumors have been destroyed obviating the need for enucleation. The 5-year mortality is reported as averaging 11%. As with alternative modes of therapy, the number of patients followed for longer than 5 years after treatment has been small. There are a number of disadvantages with radioactive plaque therapy. Ocular morbidity is a substantial problem in that almost 40% of eyes with choroidal melanomas treated with plaques have required enucleation either because of treatment complications or continued growth. In many patients with posterior pole choroidal melanomas treated with cobalt plaques, visually destructive radiation retinopathy develops (Bedford, Bedetto and MacFaul, 1970; Char, Lonn and Margolis, 1977; Stallard, 1966). Usually the onset of radiation retinopathy is delayed, with a mean of 2 years and a range of 1 month–15 years. Radiation retinopathy has been probably underestimated in those series with relatively short follow-up periods (Davidorf, Makley and Lang, 1976). We have observed the development of radiation retinopathy with markedly decreased visual acuity in over 60% of patients treated with cobalt plaques for melanomas at or behind the equator. In reports by Lommatzsch (1974), Stallard (1966) and others, less than 36% of patients treated with radioactive plaques have had a post-treatment visual acuity of better than 20/60. Because of significant complications associated with the use of radioactive plaques in the treatment of posterior pole melanomas, we believe that plaques should only be considered in the treatment of a small growing choroidal melanoma anterior to the equator. While the potential for visually destructive radiation retinopathy is less with $I^{125}$ or $Ru^{106}$ $Rh^{106}$ plaques, especially if relatively thin tumors are treated, charged particle beam irradiation such as helium ions or protons will probably have a lower incidence of visually destructive complications (Char and Castro, 1982; Lommatzsch, 1979; Packer and Rotman, 1980).

Patients treated with radioactive plaques require frequent serial follow-up examinations since some lesions continue to grow. The radioactive phosphorus uptake test is not useful in the serial follow-up of such patients. Since P-32 is a β-emitting isotope with a tissue penetration of less than 2 mm, viable tumor cells at the apex of a choroidal melanoma will not be detected using this diagnostic assay (Goldberg, Kara and Previte, 1980).

### CHARGED PARTICLE RADIATION (HELIUM IONS OR PROTONS)

Our indications for consideration of charged particle irradiation are the same as for other alternative therapies. Charged particle irradiation, using either helium ions or protons, may be the most effective form of alternative therapy in the management of choroidal melanoma. All charged particles have a characteristic Bragg peak effect that deposits the maximum dose of radiation at the end of the particle range. This and a sharp lateral dose decrement allow irradiation to be localized at the tumor-containing portion of the eye, resulting in a lower potential for radiation retinopathy in areas distant from the tumor. A second advantage of charged particle irradiation is that a uniform tumor dosage is given, which is not possible with radioactive plaques. At the University of California, San Francisco and at Harvard University approximately 200 patients have been treated with charged particle irradiation over the last 5 years (Char *et al.*, 1980, 1982; Gragoudas *et al.*, 1980). At both institutions approximately 90% of patients treated have had large or medium-sized choroidal melanomas. In order to consider charged particle irradiation, a diagnosis of a choroidal melanoma is made using both non-invasive and invasive diagnostic techniques; 2 mm tantalum scleral marker rings are either sutured or glued to the sclera approximately 2 mm outside the tumor's circumference. Radiation treatment planning is performed using a computer program based on polar fundus diagrams, ultrasound, computed tomography and orthogonal roentgenographic localization.

At our institution patients are irradiated using a 460 cm syncyclotron with a 1.5 cm spread Bragg peak of helium ions ranging from 14 to 27 mm. The treatment volume is designed to encompass the entire tumor plus a minimum margin of 2 mm surrounding normal tissue. Patients receive a total of 70 or 80 Grey (7000–8000 cobalt red equivalents) in five outpatient daily fractions over an 8–11 day period. Patient immobilization is facilitated by the use of individually fabricated polystyrene head masks in conjunction with an isocentric positioner. Eye fixation on a red light is verified throughout treatment using a video monitoring system after radiographs confirmed port alignment on the scleral marker rings.

The results of treatment in both institutions using charged particle irradiation are quite similar (Char *et al.*, 1982; Gragoudas *et al.*, 1980). Over 90% of patients who have been treated with helium ion or proton beam irradiation have had evidence of tumor stability or regression when followed for longer than 1 year after therapy. The treated choroidal melanomas have ranged in size from 6 × 4.5 × 3 mm to 20 × 20 × 12 mm in diameter. In an early paper from our institution 17 out of 18 patients followed for at least 1 year after therapy demonstrated tumor regression on ultrasonographic, clinical and photographic evaluation. The mean tumor regression, as measured by the maximum tumor height on quantitative echography before therapy versus the last examination after therapy, was approximately 40% with a range between 17% and 76%. The mean interval between therapy and the onset of detectable shrinkage was 6 months with a range of 1–23 months. Subretinal fluid resorption is often the first sign of tumor regression. The fluid usually reabsorbs within 6 months after therapy with a range of 1–13 months. In most patients who demonstrate tumor shrinkage there are alterations on A-scan ultrasound with a loss of the characteristic homogeneity observed with choroidal melanomas. There are also vascular changes on fluorescein angiography as well as clinically apparent retinal pigmented epithelial, retinal and choroidal surface changes demonstrable on either fundus photography or ophthalmoscopy.

The choice of radiation dose in the treatment of melanomas remains empiric. We have not observed significant differences in the regression or response rates in patients treated with 70 versus 80 Grey nor have we observed differences in those patients with large, medium or small melanomas.

The visual acuity in patients treated with helium ions and followed for more than 1 year has been better than 20/30 in 11 out of 19 patients. Patients who had a visual acuity of less than 20/30 had enucleations, one died within 5 months of treatment from esophageal carcinoma, three had tumors in or adjacent to the optic nerve with secondary radiation retinopathy, and two patients had normal retinal function with cataracts.

Complications associated with charged particle irradiation include continued tumor growth, lid epitheliitis, radiation retinopathy in the field of treatment, cataract, transient extraocular muscle paresis, transient initial increase in subretinal fluid, vitreous hemorrhage during the performance of the P-32 test and clip placement, and neovascular glaucoma.

Approximately 75 patients have been treated with helium ions at the University of California, San Francisco, and none have developed metastatic disease. In the total series both at UCSF and Harvard, only six out of 200 patients have developed metastases. This is less than would be expected on the basis of retrospective controls.

We have not observed radiation retinopathy in areas of the eye outside the radiation field using charged particle beam irradiation. The Bragg peak, which is characteristic of charged particle beam irradiation, potentially allows treatment of a lesion at least 3 mm from the optic nerve or fovea without substantially irradiating either of these structures vital to vision.

There are a number of unresolved issues regarding the use of charged particle irradiation in the management of choroidal melanoma. The effect of this treatment on mortality because of choroidal melanomas is unclear. Current fractionation and dose schedules used are empiric. The length of follow-up with either of the two charged particle therapies is too short to determine the complete incidence and number of complications which may occur in the future. Methods of tumor localization are currently invasive and it is conceivable that the surgical procedures needed to localize these tumors may result in tumor dissemination; however, the low incidence of metastatic disease to date makes this unlikely.

On the basis of current data, it would appear that charged particle irradiation may be more applicable and have less ocular morbidity than either radioactive plaques or photocoagulation and that tumors more than 3 mm from the fovea or optic nerve can be potentially destroyed without the development of visually destructive radiation retinopathy. Tumors closer to the nerve or fovea can also be treated but visually destructive radiation retinopathy will develop.

## Eyewall resection and posterior choroidectomy

We have not performed either full thickness eye resection or posterior choroidectomy for choroidal melanoma in our institution. If indications for these procedures exist, we believe that they are extremely rare. In 16 patients reported by Peyman, Sanders and May (1977) only five had post-treatment visual acuities of 20/100 or better. At the present time, we believe that this mode of therapy is indicated only in a patient who has had markedly elevated anterior choroidal melanoma in their only eye which has not responded to helium ion irradiation.

## Cryotherapy

The results with cryotherapy in the treatment of choroidal melanomas have historically been disappointing (Lincoff, McLean and Long, 1967). We have examined a few patients at our Ocular Oncology Unit who had been previously treated for small peripheral choroidal melanomas with cryotherapy with good results. The role of this therapeutic modality is uncertain.

## Enucleation

A number of investigators have questioned the effect of enucleation on tumor-related mortality (Stallard, 1966; McLean, Foster and Zimmerman, 1980*a*). Using retrospective data, Zimmerman and co-workers have observed a peak in the prevalence of metastases during the first two years after diagnosis and enucleation (Zimmerman, McLean and Foster, 1980; McLean *et al.*, 1980). They hypothesized that this peak could occur as a result of tumor cells being shed into the systemic circulation at the time of surgery. Several other hypotheses have been proposed to explain these retrospective data; it is possible that many high-risk choroidal melanomas may have already developed clinically undetectable micrometastases at the time of enucleation (Siegel *et al.*, 1979; Manschot and van Peperzeel, 1980). A prospective randomized treatment trial is necessary to determine the proper role of enucleation and adjunct therapy in choroidal melanoma management (Char and Phillips, 1982).

The relative indications for enucleation in the management of choroidal melanoma remain unclear. In the following situations, enucleation is a reasonable therapeutic option:

(1) a choroidal melanoma which has destroyed central vision;
(2) a choroidal melanoma of any size in a patient who, after informed consent, wishes to have the eye removed;
(3) a patient in whom alternative therapy has failed;
(4) a medium or large choroidal melanoma in which the shape of the tumor or physical location makes it unlikely that alternative therapy can result in tumor destruction with maintenance of useful vision.

Prior to performing an enucleation for choroidal melanoma, a metastatic evaluation should be done. A patient with metastatic choroidal melanoma has a life-expectancy of less than 1 year and therefore enucleation is not justified in such a case unless the eye is painful (Char, 1978*b*). When primary choroidal melanomas metastasize, approximately 60% of patients develop liver metastases as the initial manifestation of widespread disease. Other common presentations of metastatic disease include the development of subcutaneous nodules, bone pain, often with spinal cord compression, and pleural-pulmonary disease. All patients should have a complete physical examination. Metastases to the lung should be ruled out with plain chest roentgenograms. In numerous studies of systemic melanoma, chest tomography in the presence of a negative chest X-ray has not been efficacious (Char, 1978). Patients with choroidal melanoma metastatic to the liver usually have an elevation of serum alkaline phosphatase, serum lactic dehydrogenase (LDH), and serum glutamyl transpeptidase (GTP). In a large series of patients with metastatic melanoma to the liver, less than 2% had a normal serum LDH, although serum LDH was observed to be 'falsely elevated' in as many as 46% of patients. We routinely obtained these liver chemistries prior to enucleation; if these tests are normal, we do not do further testing of liver function. The sensitivity and specificity of liver spleen scans is probably less than 80%. If abnormal liver function tests are obtained, we perform an abdominal CT scan with fine-needle biopsy if a suspicious area is observed.

In patients with large (greater than 15 mm in diameter or greater than 5 mm in thickness) choroidal melanomas, five-year tumor-related mortality approaches 50%. The use of adjunct radiation either before or shortly after the surgical removal of malignant neoplasms has been advocated for a number of systemic tumors (Char and Phillips, 1982). In a number of carcinomas including rectal, head, neck and bladder, the use of perioperative irradiation has been demonstrated to decrease local recurrence, metastasis to regional nodes, and mortality. While investigators early in the twentieth century believed that melanoma was a radioresistant tumor, recent data indicate responses similar to carcinomas or sarcomas for most melanomas.

The role of preoperative irradiation in the management of choroidal melanomas is unresolved. The results of a number of studies suggest that a prospective randomized treatment trial of perioperative irradiation would be reasonable in high-risk cases. In previous retrospective studies, it appeared that perioperative irradiation of choroidal melanomas might be useful and there was limited morbidity.

Approximately 4 years ago we attempted to determine the feasibility of using 2000 rads of preoperative irradiation in patients with high-risk choroidal melanomas prior to a national prospective randomized study to determine whether preoperative irradiation in this dose and fractionation schedule would decrease the prevalence of metastatic disease. While there are a number of limitations to this approach, we believe that such a study would be useful to test the efficacy of preoperative irradiation as well as to determine the effect of enucleation on the dissemination of tumor cells at the time of surgery. We have observed no untoward side-effects with this therapy and we believe it is a reasonable option in the treatment of poor-prognosis melanoma.

Enucleation should be performed with minimal trauma to lessen the possibility of tumor spread. While some investigators have advocated a 'no touch technique' using a cryoprobe to freeze the tumor, at present we are not convinced that this is a significant improvement over a minimal trauma technique (Wilson and Fraunfelder, 1978). At the time of enucleation, the globe should be carefully examined for extraocular extension; if visible tumor is noted on the bulbar surface, we have routinely performed a limited sector tenonectomy. If no tumor is present, we inject 0.75% marcain into the quadrants and place an orbital implant.

The efficacy of exenteration, sector tenonectomy, or postoperative irradiation for extrascleral extension in the prevention of metastatic disease is under evaluation (Shammas and Blodi, 1977*b*; Starr and Zimmerman, 1962; Wolter, 1971).

While a retrospective study by Shammas and Blodi (1977*b*) which suggested that exenterated patients had a better prognosis than patients treated with chemotherapy or patients followed without further treatment, other investigators have not had similar findings. On an empirical basis we perform a standard enucleation unless there is extraocular extension. If there is a small discrete encapsulated extrascleral nodule a sector tenonectomy is performed. If diffuse extraocular extension is present the patient is offered the option of exenteration and postoperative irradiation with 6000 rads of 4 MeV photons.

Patients who have had an enucleation for a choroidal melanoma are examined every 3 months. Metastatic lesions usually develop between 1 and 4 years after enucleation. However, we have observed that approximately 2% of patients have simultaneous choroidal tumors and metastatic disease, and in some patients delayed metastases have been seen as long as up to 30 years after enucleation.

## Conclusions

A number of issues remain unresolved and only by doing prospective studies in a randomized manner, when ethically feasible, can we better understand the natural history of choroidal melanomas and the effect of different therapeutic modalities on the incidence of metastases. At this time the only clinical signs which correlate with prognosis are tumor diameter and thickness. It appears from the evaluation of limited data that patients with small choroidal melanomas, whether treated by serial evaluation until growth is documented, immediate enucleation or alternative therapies, have a tumor-related 5-year mortality of less than 10%. Because there is currently no evidence that any therapeutic modality significantly alters the incidence of metastatic disease it seems reasonable to attempt to preserve vision in eyes with good visual acuity. We therefore follow patients with small choroidal melanomas until growth is documented.

In patients with larger choroidal melanomas at least 3 mm from the fovea or the optic nerve, early evidence suggests that treatment with charged particle beam irradiation such as helium ions or protons has less morbidity and is more effective than radioactive plaques; charged particle irradiation also has greater applicability than photocoagulation. While the follow-up after treatment with these modalities is at present of short duration the incidence of metastatic disease appears to be no more, and perhaps slightly less, than that historically observed with enucleation.

# RETINOBLASTOMA

Retinoblastoma is the most frequent malignant eye tumor of childhood. It can occur as a result of a germinal (hereditable) or somatic (non-hereditable) mutation; the inheritance pattern is an autosomal dominant with marked penetrance. The incidence of retinoblastoma in the United States is approximately 1:18 000 live births (200 cases per year) (Devesa, 1975; Pendergrass and Davis, 1980). The frequencies of unilateral versus bilateral, familial versus non-familial, and hereditable versus non-hereditable retinoblastoma are inexact as most studies come from referral centers with inherently biased populations. Approximately 6% of all retinoblastoma patients have a positive family history. Bilateral cases have a positive family history of between 10–24% (François, De Bie and Matton-Van Leuven, 1979). Bilateral involvement is observed in 20–35% of retinoblastomas, and in as many as one-fourth of these patients the tumor is initially detected in one eye only (Carlson *et al.*, 1979; Ellsworth, 1969).

## Diagnosis

The most important diagnostic tool in the evaluation of a patient suspected of having retinoblastoma is indirect ophthalmoscopy with 360° scleral depression. The majority of patients present with leukocoria, strabismus or ocular inflammation. Making the correct diagnosis, even in an eye with clear media, can be difficult. The diagnostic error rate of eyes enucleated because of presumed retinoblastoma varies between 6–16% with a greater number of errors in unilateral lesions (Howard, 1969; Robertson and Campbell, 1977). When retinoblastoma occurs in an eye with opaque media or has an unusual presentation there are a number of ancillary tests which may be useful.

In patients with leukocoria or a large mass lesion we have found that thin section high resolution computerized tomography (CT) is the most useful ancillary diagnostic test. All large retinoblastomas (greater than 10 mm in diameter and greater than 5 mm in elevation) examined at our institution have shown calcification on CT. An eye with a lesion of this size, or an eye with leukocoria which does not show calcification on CT suggests an alternative diagnosis. In addition, in a patient with a large retinoblastoma in which the optic nerve cannot be visualized, the CT scan is useful in detecting gross optic nerve invasion, orbital or pineal involvement, or contiguous spread to the central nervous system (Char, 1980; Goldberg and Danziger, 1977; Hedges *et al.*, 1982; Judisch and Patil, 1981). Patients in whom the differential diagnosis of toxocariasis is considered a serum ELISA test for toxocara antigens may be useful (Pollard *et al.*, 1979; Shields, Feldberg and Federman, 1979). This test appears to have a specificity of approximately 91% and a sensitivity of 77%.

Patients with possible retinoblastoma should undergo the following evaluation:

(1) A careful family history, past medical history, and review of systems. Emphasis is placed upon a history of enucleation or death of relatives during infancy, neonatal exposure to oxygen, patient's exposure to cats and dogs, and symptoms consistent with developmental delay or dysmorphic features.
(2) A slit-lamp and fundus examination of the awake infant is performed. If retinoblastoma cannot be definitively excluded, examination under anaesthesia is scheduled. If retinoblastoma is likely, and a large lesion is present, a CT scan, bone scan, liver functions tests, lumbar puncture for cerebrospinal fluid cytology, and bone marrow aspirate and biopsy for histologic examination are scheduled to be performed at the time of examination under anesthesia.

(3) Retinal examination of both parents is performed to detect signs of (or lesions denoting) spontaneous regression of retinoblastoma.
(4) An examination under anesthesia is performed, including measurement of corneal diameter, anterior segment examination using an operative microscope, measurement of intraocular pressures, and indirect ophthalmoscopy with 360° scleral depression of both eyes. The fundi are drawn and composite photographs are made. If a retinoblastoma is diagnosed, bone marrow aspirate and biopsy are performed along with lumbar puncture for cytological examination of the cerebrospinal fluid.
(5) If retinoblastoma is deemed unlikely, other ancillary diagnostic studies are performed depending on the differential diagnosis.

## Therapy

The aim of therapy is to destroy the tumor and retain useful vision, without endangering life.Significantly better results have been obtained in ocular oncology centers than in ophthalmic centers with little experience in retinoblastoma management (Lennox, Draper and Sanders, 1975).

*Table 10.1* Modified Reese–Ellsworth classification of the ocular lesions in retinoblastoma

| | | |
|---|---|---|
| I | a. | Solitary tumor less than 4 DD at or behind the equator |
| | b. | Multiple tumors less than 4 DD at or behind the equator |
| II | a. | Solitary tumor 4–10 DD at or behind the equator |
| | b. | Multiple tumors 4–10 DD at or behind the equator |
| III | a. | Any lesion anterior to the equator |
| | b. | Solitary lesion greater than 10 DD behind the equator |
| IV | a. | Multiple tumors greater than 10 DD |
| | b. | Tumor at the ora serrata |
| V | a. | Massive tumors |
| | b. | Vitreous seeding |

DD: disc diameter

Since there has been little or no observed mortality in stage I–III (*Table 10.1*) lesions treated in ocular oncology centers in the United States, we do not enucleate if the tumor size and location possibly allows the retention of useful vision. Unfortunately, most retinoblastomas are large at the time of presentation. At Columbia, only 19% of unilateral retinoblastoma patients and only 6% of those with bilateral tumors had the largest tumor in stage I–III (Ellsworth, 1977).

### Unilateral retinoblastoma

Controversy exists regarding the criteria for enucleation versus alternative therapy. Some enucleate only if the tumor involves the optic nerve (Bedford, 1977). Since all ocular oncologists have observed tumors growth after radiation, we do not believe this is a reasonable form of management of unilateral cases, especially if the eye has limited or no potential for vision. In unilateral retinoblastomas whose size or location preclude the development of useful vision, we perform an enucleation. As has been stressed by many others, since retinoblastoma often spreads along the optic nerve every attempt should be made to obtain at least 10 mm of nerve at the time of enucleation (Rootman *et al.*, 1976).

We have treated small retinoblastomas with either cryotherapy or photocoagulation if they do not involve the optic nerve or macular regions. Unfortunately, most unilateral retinoblastomas are not amenable to alternate therapy since more than 80% are relatively large at the time of diagnosis. In a recent series from Indiana University, only one of 16 unilateral tumors was felt to be suitable for alternate therapy and treatment was unsuccessful in that case (Shidnia *et al.*, 1977). In those rare unilateral retinoblastomas in the posterior fundus that are at least 3 mm away from the disc and outside the central arcade, we treat with xenon photocoagulation if the lesion is less than 6 mm in diameter and 3 mm in elevation. Similar-sized lesions anterior to the equator are treated with triple freeze–thaw cryotherapy, with freezing into the vitreous on each application.

We have had no experience of treating unilateral retinoblastomas with either radioactive plaques or external beam such as 4 MeV linear accelerator irradiation. After our adverse experience with cobalt plaques in choroidal melanomas, and recent data demonstrating good results with other types of radioactive plaques, we would be inclined to treat a medium-sized retinoblastoma, less than 10 mm in diameter and 4 mm in elevation at the mid-periphery, with either a $^{125}I$ or a $^{106}Ru$ $^{106}Rh$ plaque (Char, Lonn and Margolis, 1977; Lommatzsch, 1977). The radiation dosimetry with these forms of local irradiation may allow tumor destruction with a lower incidence of visually destructive radiation retinopathy than has been observed with cobalt plaques. Lommatzsch has treated 33 patients with $^{106}Ru$ $^{106}Rh$ plaques and noted a good response in 28 cases (84%). Unfortunately, in neither his publications nor those of Hopping and Schmidt (1977), is it possible to distinguish the percentage of cures in unilateral versus bilateral cases. Lommatzsch believes that tumors in stages I, II and IV which are less than 5 mm in elevation and greater than 3 mm from either the fovea or the optic nerve can be treated with this form of local irradiation.

## Bilateral retinoblastoma

The management of retinoblastoma depends to a large measure on the extent of ocular involvement. Four patterns are commonly seen:

(1) a stage V tumor involving one eye and small peripheral lesions in the second eye;
(2) tumors involving the optic nerve and/or fovea bilaterally;
(3) large symmetric tumors in both eyes;
(4) tumor initially involving one eye (20% of bilateral retinoblastomas initially present with unilateral involvement).

We have tended to treat both eyes in poor prognosis bilateral retinoblastomas if at least one-third of the retina is uninvolved (even if it is detached). In those eyes in which the size of the tumor precludes useful vision enucleation is performed. Our success in treating very large retinoblastomas and retaining useful vision has been quite limited; we only consider treating an eye with a stage V tumor if there is symmetrical involvement.

Since hereditary retinoblastoma patients are at increased risk of developing another malignancy and may have a non-demonstrable DNA repair defect, we try to avoid irradiation or other potentially carcinogenic agents whenever possible (Cleaver *et al.*, 1982). In patients with a large tumor in one eye and a small peripheral tumor in the second eye, we enucleate the non-seeing eye and use cryotherapy to treat the second eye. Cryotherapy of small peripheral tumors is often successful. Total eradication of tumor usually occurs within 4 weeks. Unlike irradiation which usually results in tumor regression with some residual mass, if the tumor is not totally obliterated with either photocoagulation or cryotherapy the retinoblastoma is still active and requires further treatment.

If there is asymmetric involvement with a very large tumor in one eye and only posterior tumors outside the central arcade and away from the disc of the second eye, we treat the second eye with photocoagulation. Our criteria for photocoagulation and cryotherapy in bilateral and unilateral retinoblastomas are the same.

In larger tumors (6–10 mm in diameter and 3–5 mm in elevation) external beam irradiation or radioactive plaque therapy is indicated. A number of investigators have reported good results with plaque therapy in tumors of this size; approximately 85% of these patients can be successfully treated (Hopping and Schmidt, 1977; Lommatzsch, 1977). In addition to use for a solitary tumor in the mid-periphery, radioactive plaques are useful if choroidal extension is present or for a tumor recurrence too large for treatment with photocoagulation and cryotherapy.

In patients with bilateral symmetrical large tumors with at least one-third of the retina involved by tumor in each eye, or in those patients with tumor involving the macula or within 3 mm of the disc, external beam irradiation is indicated. Most American institutions have used lateral port irradiation with a 4 MeV linear acceleration source of external beam irradiation, the advantage being a lower incidence of cataracts; however, lesions at or near the ora serrata often need to be treated with either cryotherapy or photocoagulation (Bedford, 1975; Egbert *et al.*, 1978; Ellsworth, 1977). At our institution we have not used a head stabilization device but have had closed circuit monitoring of patients under ketamine anesthesia. Patients generally receive between 3500–4500 rads over a period of 6 weeks. While there are disadvantages to lateral port irradiation, notably the lack of tumoricidal dose to the retina near the ora, it has a much lower incidence of cataract development than anterior port irradiation.

The success of external beam radiation depends on the size of the tumor. Generally between 80 and 90% of stage I–III lesions can be cured, whereas only 29% of stage IV–V lesions are successfully treated (Egbert *et al.*, 1978; Ellsworth, 1977; Freeman *et al.*, 1980). Complications of irradiation include radiation retinopathy, cataracts, and possibly radiation-induced neoplasia. In a series reported from Stanford, 25/38 eyes (66%) developed cataracts and seven developed vitreous hemorrhages. In a large series from New York, only 39% of patients receiving external beam irradiation developed radiation side-effects. As has been repeatedly stressed, a second course of external beam radiation is fraught with complications as most cases develop visually destructive radiation retinopathy, and there is probably a greater chance for the development of a radiation-induced neoplasia. If additional therapy is needed because of recurrence after external beam irradiation, cryotherapy, or photocoagulation, or experimental forms of dye therapy coupled with photocoagulation can be used (Dougherty *et al.*, 1978; Murphree *et al.*, 1981).

In patients with recurrent tumors too large to treat with either photocoagulation or cryotherapy, treatment with a localized plaque, or a potentially more sharply focusable form of radiation such as helium ion or proton beam, should be considered to attempt to destroy the tumor without inducing radiation retinopathy. Because these newer forms of heavy ion irradiation, such as helium ions or protons, can be delivered more selectively to the retina involving the tumor, there is a lower potential for complications.

There are three types of post-irradiation regression patterns:

(1) 'cottage-cheese' regression pattern;
(2) differentiated regression pattern;
(3) mixed regression pattern (a combination of (1) and (2)).

Patients undergoing a 'cottage-cheese' regression pattern are relatively easy to follow; however, in those with either a mixed or differentiated regression pattern it can be difficult to differentiate active from regressed tumors. Generally, a successfully treated tumor is grey and on serial examination shows no growth, whereas an active tumor is pinkish. We routinely make montages of fundus photographs to follow the patient's progress. If there is no growth 6 months after treatment, the tumor is usually arrested; however, growth can occur within 3 years.

## Serial evaluation

Following enucleation the orbit and the other eye are re-examined with 360° scleral depression at 6 weeks, then examinations under anesthesia are performed every 3 months for the first year. If the lesion was a stage IV or V tumor, we obtain bone scans, liver function tests, CT scans of the orbit, bone marrow biopsy/aspirates, and cerebrospinal fluid at 6-month intervals. If no new tumors are observed, during the 2nd year the patient is examined every 4 months and in the 3rd year every 6 months, and annually thereafter.

Patients treated with alternative therapy such as irradiation, photocoagulation or cryotherapy are examined 1 month after the completion of therapy, and again in 6 weeks. If no new or recurrent tumors are observed, then the patients are followed temporally as discussed above. If chemotherapy is not undertaken (*see below*), metastatic evaluation is performed as outlined in the preceding paragraph. Fundus drawings are made, and composite photographs are taken during each examination under anesthesia.

## Chemotherapy

Chemotherapy may be useful in the management of retinoblastoma in two clinical situations:

(1) Microscopic or gross disease outside the eye.
(2) Far advanced bilateral retinoblastoma in combination with external beam irradiation.

The value of adjunctive chemotherapy in retinoblastoma has yet to be determined. There is significant morbidity associated with the use of chemotherapeutic agents, and the prognosis for patients with unilateral stage IV–V tumors without involvement of the optic nerve behind the lamina is probably greater than 85% survival (Rootman *et al.*, 1976). In patients with microscopic or gross tumor outside the eye, the prognosis is from 0 to 35% survival at 5 years (Stannard *et al.*, 1979). There is increasing evidence to suggest that these patients may do much better with chemotherapy (Carbajal, 1959, Freeman *et al.*, 1980; Judisch, Apple and Fratkin, 1980). In patients with far-advanced ocular retinoblastoma, either symmetric bilateral disease or advanced tumor in an only eye, chemotherapy may act synergistically with radiation and increase the chance of local tumor control. The data are limited for this latter point at present. Recent work with a nude mouse *in vivo* culture system for retinoblastoma cells may increase our ability to develop better chemotherapeutic agents (Gallie *et al.*, 1977).

## Prognosis

Overall there is approximately a 15–19% mortality associated with retinoblastoma. In major ocular oncology centers mortality is observed almost exclusively in patients with stage IV–V disease (Jensen and Miller, 1971). Histological criteria are the most accurate prognostic predictors. A number of parameters do not appear to correlate consistently with prognosis. These include endophytic versus exophytic tumor growth pattern, unilateral or bilateral tumor, and degree of tumor differentiation (Stannard *et al.*, 1979; Mashiah and Barishak, 1977). While some investigators believe that photocoagulation may be detrimental by allowing choroidal invasion, review of the initial data does not substantiate this hypothesis (Ellsworth, 1977). Massive choroidal involvement, in contrast to minimal involvement, does adversely affect prognosis (Mashiah and Barishak, 1977). The most important histological parameter is involvement of the optic nerve. When tumor is at the cut end of the optic nerve, the mortality approaches 65%; in most series, tumor beyond the lamina but not involving the cut end of the nerve has a significant but lesser mortality (Reese, 1976). Immunological studies are not sufficiently reliable to be used clinically in the evaluation of prognosis.

Death due to extraocular spread of retinoblastoma almost always occurs within 4 years of the diagnosis (Gaitan-Yanguas, 1978; Redler and Ellsworth, 1973). Approximately 60% of metastases occur by hematogenous spread and 50% involve the central nervous system via contiguous spread along the optic nerve. Extraocular retinoblastoma outside the central nervous system often involves the skeletal system, namely the skull, vertebral column, ribs and long bones, or the orbit. Other areas of involvement include the liver, kidney and adrenal glands (Gaitan-Yanguas, 1978; Lennox, Draper and Sanders, 1975; Reese, 1976).

As discussed under chemotherapy, microscopic or gross extraocular disease should be treated with chemotherapy. In orbital and skeletal involvement local irradiation is useful as a palliative measure.

In a review of a large series of retinoblastoma deaths, approximately 80% were due to extraocular spread and 20% were caused by the development of another malignancy. In patients with germinal hereditable retinoblastoma death is more often due to a second tumor than to metastases of retinoblastoma.

## Genetic counseling

An important component in retinoblastoma management is to acquaint the patient's family with the relative risk of retinoblastoma development in other potential offspring of the parents or the affected patient.

A counseling scheme for the risk of developing retinoblastoma is shown in *Table 10.2* (Char, 1980). Generally, if a germinal mutation is inherited, the risk of developing this autosomal dominant tumor with marked penetrance is approximately 40–50%. If the patient has had only a somatic mutation, the risk of retinoblastoma in the rest of his pedigree is minimal. The reason that his risk, or the risk for children of normal siblings in a germinal mutation retinoblastoma patient, is not zero is due to the possibility that the patient may be a phenotypically non-expressed germinal mutation carrier.

*Table 10.2* Retinoblastoma genetic counseling

| | *Risk of retinoblastoma in future children* |
|---|---|
| Negative family history | |
| Parents with one affected child | 2–5% |
| Parents with unilateral disease | 5% |
| Parents with bilateral disease | 40% |
| Positive family history | |
| Patients | 40% |
| Healthy siblings | 2–6% |
| Healthy offspring | 2–6% |

## Conclusions

Multidisciplinary management is the most effective approach in retinoblastoma diagnosis and therapy. The combined efforts of ocular oncologists, radiotherapists and pediatric oncologists yield the highest percentage of correct diagnoses and cures. Six cardinal points are paramount in the management of retinoblastoma patients:

(1) Patients presenting to the ophthalmologist with a possible retinoblastoma in eyes with potential vision can be correctly diagnosed in greater than 95% of cases.
(2) Significantly better results are obtained in ocular oncology centers than in ophthalmic centers with little experience in retinoblastoma management.
(3) There has been almost no mortality associated with relatively small (stage I–III) retinoblastoma treated in ocular oncology centers in the United States.
(4) Hereditary retinoblastoma patients are at increased risk of developing other malignancies, and treatment modalities other than radiation, because of its potentially greater carcinogenic effects, are preferable when feasible.
(5) In bilateral retinoblastoma patients with a poor prognosis in whom irradiation is necessary, it is difficult to predict which eye will respond better to therapy. Enucleation of the 'worse eye' should usually be postponed until the effect of radiation can be determined.
(6) Adjunct chemotherapy may be useful in the management of patients with orbital, central nervous system or metastatic disease.

## References

Barr, C., Sipperley, J. O. and Nicholson, D. H. (1978) Small melanoma of the choroid. *Archives of Ophthalmology*, **96,** 1580–1582

Bedford, M. A., Bedotto, C. and MacFaul, P. A. (1970) Radiation retinopathy after the application of a cobalt plaque. *British Journal of Ophthalmology*, **54,** 505–509

Bedford, M. A. (1973) The use and abuse of cobalt plaques in the treatment of choroidal malignant melanoma. *Transactions of the Ophthalmological Society of the United Kingdom*, **93,** 139–143

Bedford, M. A. (1975) Treatment of retinoblastoma. *Advances in Ophthalmology*, **13,** 1–2

Bedford, M. A. (1977) Management of retinoblastoma. *Modern Problems in Ophthalmology*, **18,** 101

Burton, T. C. (1976) Iatrogenic breaks in Bruch's membrane in choroidal melanoma. *Transactions of the American Academy of Ophthalmology and Otolaryngology*, **81,** 841–848

Carbajal, U. M. (1959) Metastasis in retinoblastoma. *American Journal of Ophthalmology*, **48,** 47

Carlson, E. A., Letson, R. D., Ramsay, N. K. C. and Desnick, R. J. (1979) Factors for improved genetic counseling for retinoblastoma based on a survey of 55 families. *American Journal of Ophthalmology*, **87,** 449

Char, D. H. and Hogan, M. J. (1977) The management of small elevated pigmented choroidal lesions. *British Journal of Ophthalmology*, **61,** 54–58

Char, D. H., Lonn, L. and Margolis, L. (1977) Complications of cobalt plaque therapy for small choroidal melanomas. *American Journal of Ophthalmology*, **84,** 536–541

Char, D. H. (1978a) Management of small choroidal melanomas. *Survey of Ophthalmology*, **22,** 377–386

Char, D. H. (1978b) Metastatic choroidal melanoma. *American Journal of Ophthalmology*, **86,** 70–80

Char, D. H. (1980) Current concepts in retinoblastoma. *Annals of Ophthalmology*, **12,** 792–804

Char, D. H., Stone, R. D., Irvine, A. R., Crawford, J. B., Hilton, G. F., Lonn, L. I. and Schwartz, A. (1980) Diagnostic modalities in choroidal melanoma: sensitivity, specificity and reproducibility. *American Journal of Ophthalmology*, **89,** 223–230

Char, D. H. *et al.* (1980) Helium ion charged particle therapy for choroidal melanoma. *Ophthalmology*, **87,** 565–570

Char, D. H. and Castro, J. R. (1982) Helium ion therapy for choroidal melanoma. *Archives of Ophthalmology*, **100,** 935–938

Char, D. H. and Phillips, T. L. (1982) The potential for adjuvant radiotherapy in choroidal melanoma. *Archives of Ophthalmology*, **100,** 247–248

Char, D. H., Crawford, J. B., Woodruff, K. H. and Stone, R. D. Failure of choroidal melanoma to respond to helium ion therapy. *Archives of Ophthalmology* (in press)

Cleaver, J. E., Char, D. H., Charles, W. C. and Rand, H. (1982) Repair and replication of DNA in hereditary (bilateral) retinoblastoma cells after X-irradiation. *Cancer Research*, **42,** 1343–1347

Coleman, D. J. (1976) Ultrasonic evaluation of ocular and orbital tumors. In *Tumors of the Eye*, edited by A. B. Reese, 332–342. Hagerstown: Harper and Row

Curtin, T. V. and Cavendar, J. C. (1974) Natural course of selected malignant melanomas of the choroid and ciliary body. *Modern Problems in Ophthalmology*, **12,** 523–527

Davidorf, F. H., Makley, T. A. and Lang, J. R. (1976) Radiotherapy of malignant melanoma of the choroid. *Transactions of the American Academy of Ophthalmology and Otolaryngology*, **81,** 849–861

Devesa, S. S. (1975) The incidence of retinoblastoma. *American Journal of Ophthalmology*, **80,** 263

Dougherty, T. J., Kaufman, J. E., Goldfarb, A., Weishaupt, K. R., Boyle, D. and Mittleman, A. (1978) Photoradiation therapy for the treatment of malignant tumors. *Cancer Research*, **38,** 2628–2635

Duffin, R. M., Straatsma, B. R., Foos, R. Y. and Kerman, B. M. (1981) Small malignant melanoma of the choroid with extraocular extension. *Archives of Ophthalmology*, **99,** 1827–1830

Duvall, J. and Lucas, D. R. (1981) Argon laser and xenon arc coagulation of malignant choroidal melanomata: histological findings in 6 cases. *British Journal of Ophthalmology*, **65,** 464–468

Egbert, P. R., Donaldson, S. S., Moazed, K. and Rosenthal, A. R. (1978) Visual results and ocular complications following radiotherapy for retinoblastoma. *Archives of Ophthalmology*, **96,** 1826

Ellsworth, R. M. (1969) The practical management of retinoblastoma. *Transactions of the American Ophthalmological Society*, **67,** 462

Ellsworth, R. M. (1977) Retinoblastoma. *Modern Problems in Ophthalmology*, **18,** 94

François, J. (1974) Treatment of malignant melanoma of the choroid by light coagulation. *Modern Problems in Ophthalmology*, **12,** 550–555

Francois, J., De Bie, S. and Matton-Van Leuven, M. T. (1979) The Costenbader Memorial Lecture: genesis and genetics of retinoblastoma. *Journal of Pediatric Ophthalmology*, **16,** 85

Freeman, C. R., Esseltine, D. L., Whitehead, V. M., Chevalier, L. and Little J. M. (1980) Retinoblastoma: the case for radiotherapy and for adjunct chemotherapy. *Cancer*, **46,** 1913–1910

Gaitan-Yanguas, M. (1978) Retinoblastoma: analysis of 235 cases. *International Journal of Radiation Oncology and Biological Physics*, **4,** 359

Gallie, B. L., Albert, D. M., Wong, J. J. Y., Buyukmihci, N. and Puliafito, C. A. (1977) Heterotransplantation of retinoblastoma into the athymic 'nude' mouse. *Investigative Ophthalmology and Visual Science*, **16,** 256

Gass, J. D. M. (1977) Problems in the differential diagnosis of choroidal nevi and malignant melanomas. *Transactions of the American Academy of Ophthalmology and Otolaryngology*, **83,** 19–48

Gass, J. D. M. (1980) Observation of suspected choroidal and ciliary body melanomas for evidence of growth prior to enucleation. *Ophthalmology*, **87,** 523–528

Goldberg, B., Kara, G. B. and Previte, L. R. (1980) The use of radioactive phosphorus $^{32}P$ in the diagnosis of ocular tumors. *American Journal of Ophthalmology*, **90,** 817–827

Goldberg, L. and Danziger, A. (1977) Computed tomographic scanning in the management of retinoblastoma. *American Journal of Ophthalmology*, **84,** 380

Gragoudas, E. S., Goitein, M., Verhey, L. *et al.* (1980) Proton beam irradiation. *Ophthalmology*, **87,** 565–570

Hedges, T. R. III, Pozzi-Mucelli, R., Char, D. H. and Newton, T. H. (1982) Computed tomographic demonstration of ocular calcification: correlations with clinical and pathological findings. *Neuroradiology*, **23,** 15–21

Hopping, W. and Schmidt, G. (1977) The treatment of retinoblastoma. *Modern Problems in Ophthalmology*, **18,** 106

Howard, G. M. (1969) Erroneous clinical diagnoses of retinoblastoma and uveal melanoma. *Transactions of the American Academy of Ophthalmology and Otolaryngology*, **73,** 199

Jensen, R. D. and Miller, R. W. (1971) Retinoblastoma: epidemiologic characteristics. *New England Journal of Medicine*, **285,** 307

Judisch, G. F. and Patil, S. R. (1981) Concurrent hereditable retinoblastoma, pinealoma, and trisomy X. *Archives of Ophthalmology*, **99,** 1767–1769

Judisch, G. F., Apple, D. J. and Fratkia, J. D. (1980) Retinoblastoma: a survivor 12 years after treatment for metastatic disease. *Archives of Ophthalmology*, **98,** 711–713

Lennox, E. L., Draper, C. J. and Sanders, B. M. (1975) Retinoblastoma: a study of natural history and prognosis of 268 cases. *British Medical Journal*, **3,** 731

Lincoff, H., McLean, J. and Long, R. (1967) The cryosurgical treatment of intraocular tumors. *American Journal of Ophthalmology*, **63,** 389–399

Lommatzsch, P. (1974) Treatment of choroidal melanomas with $^{106}$Ru/$^{106}$Rh β-ray applicators. *Survey of Ophthalmology*, **19,** 85–100

Lommatzsch, R. K. (1977) Experience with β-irradiation [$^{106}$Ru/$^{106}$Rh] of patients suffering from retinoblastoma. *Japanese Journal of Ophthalmology*, **2,** 424

Lommatzsch, R. K. (1979) Radiotherapy der intraokularen Tumoren, insbesondere bei Aderhautmelanom. *Klinische Monatsblatter für Augenheilkunde*, **174,** 948–958

Manschot, W. A. and van Peperzeel, H. A. (1980) Choroidal melanoma. *Archives of Ophthalmology*, **98,** 1301–1303

Mashiah, M. and Barishak, Y. R. (1977) Photoreceptor differentiation in retinoblastomas and its significance in prognosis. *British Journal of Ophthalmology*, **61,** 417–422

McLean, I. W., Foster, W. D. and Zimmerman, L. E. (1977) Prognostic factors in small malignant melanomas of the choroid and ciliary body. *Archives of Ophthalmology*, **95,** 48–58

McLean, I. W., Zimmerman, L. E. and Evans, R. M. (1978) Reappraisal of Callender's spindle A type of malignant melanoma of the choroid and ciliary body. *American Journal of Ophthalmology*, **86,** 557–564

McLean, I. W., Foster, W. D. and Zimmerman, L. E. (1980a) Choroidal melanoma. *Archives of Ophthalmology*, **98,** 1298–1301

McLean, I. W., Foster,W. D., Zimmerman, L. E. *et al.* (1980b) Inferred natural history of uveal melanoma. *Investigative Ophthalmology and Visual Science*, **19,** 760–770

Moore, R. F. (1930) Choroidal sarcoma treated by the intraocular insertion of radon seeds. *British Journal of Ophthalmology*, **14,** 145–152

Murphree, A. L., Benedict, W. F., Lingua, R. W., Doiron, D. R. and Gomer, C. J. (1981) *ARVO Abstracts*, p. 162

Newman, G. H., Davidorf, F. H., Havener, W. H. *et al.* (1970) Conservative management of malignant melanoma. *Archives of Ophthalmology*, **83,** 21–26

Ossoinig, K. C., Bigar, F. and Kaefring, S. L. (1975) Malignant melanoma of the choroid and ciliary body. A differential diagnosis by clinical echography. *Bibliotheca Ophthalmologica*, **83,** 141–154

Packer, S. and Rotman, M. (1980) Radiotherapy of choroidal melanoma with iodine-125. *Ophthalmology*, **87,** 582–590

Pendergrass, T. W. and Davis, S. (1980) Incidence of retinoblastoma in the United States. *Archives of Ophthalmology*, **98,** 1204–1210

Peyman, G. A., Sanders, D. R. and May, D. R. (1977) Local excision of malignant melanoma of the choroid. In *Intraocular Tumors*, edited by G. A. Peyman, D. J. Apple and D. R. Sanders, 167–188. New York: Appleton-Century-Crofts

Pollard, Z. F., Jarrett, W. H., Hagler, H. S., Allain, D. S. and Schantz, P. M. (1979) ELISA for diagnosis of ocular toxocariasis. *Ophthalmology*, **86,** 743

Redler, L. D. and Ellsworth, R. M. (1973) Prognostic importance of choroidal invasion in retinoblastoma. *Archives of Ophthalmology*, **90,** 294

Reese, A. B. (1976) *Tumors of the Eye,* 3rd edition, Hagerstown: Harper and Row

Robertson, D. M. and Campbell, R. J. (1977) Analysis of misdiagnosed retinoblastoma in a series of 726 enucleated eyes. *Modern Problems in Ophthalmology*, **18,** 156

Robertson, D. M. and Campbell, R. J. (1979) Errors in the diagnosis of malignant melanoma of the choroid. *American Journal of Ophthalmology*, **87,** 269

Rootman, J., Hofbauer, J., Ellsworth, R. M. and Kitchen, D. (1976) Invasion of the optic nerve by retinoblastoma: a clinicopathological study. *Cancer Journal of Ophthalmology*, **11,** 106

Rubinstein, K. and Myska, V. (1974) Life cycle of choroidal melanoma. *Modern Problems in Ophthalmology*, **12,** 517–522

Shammas, H. F. and Blodi, F. C. (1977*a*) Prognostic factors in choroidal ciliary body melanomas. *Archives of Ophthalmology*, **95,** 63–69

Shammas, H. F. and Blodi, F. C. (1977*b*) Orbital extension of choroidal and ciliary body melanomas. *Archives of Ophthalmology*, **95,** 2002–2005

Shammas, H. F., Burton, T. c. and Weingeist, T. A. (1977) False-positive results with the radioactive phosphorous test. *Archives of Ophthalmology*, **95,** 2190 –2192

Shidnia, H., Hornback, N. B., Helveston, E. M., Gettlefinger, T. and Biglan, A. W. (1977) Treatment results of retinoblastoma at Indiana University Hospital. *Cancer*, **40,** 2917

Shields, J. A., Augsburger, J. J., Brady, L. W. and Day, J. L. Cobalt plaque therapy of posterior uveal melanomas. *Ophthalmology* (in press)

Shields, J. A., Feldberg, N. T. and Federman, J. L. (1979) Discussion. *Ophthalmology*, **86,** 750

Siegel, D., Myers, M., Ferris, F. L. III, *et al.* (1979) Survival rates after enucleation of eyes from malignant melanoma. *American Journal of Ophthalmology*, **87,** 761–765

Stallard, H. B. (1966) Radiotherapy for malignant melanoma of the choroid. *British Journal of Ophthalmology*, **50,** 147–155

Stallard, H. B. (1961) Malignant melanoma of the choroid treated with radioactive applicators. *Annals of the Royal College of Surgeons of England*, **29,** 170–182

Stannard, C., Lipper, S., Sealy, R. and Sevel, D. (1979) Retinoblastoma: correlation of invasion of the optic nerve in choroid with prognosis and metastases. *British Journal of Ophthalmology*, **63,** 560–570

Starr, H. J. and Zimmerman, L. E. (1962) Extra scleral extension and orbital recurrence of malignant melanomas of the choroid and ciliary body. *International Ophthalmology Clinics*, **2,** 369–385

Thomas, J. V., Green, W. R. and Maumenee, A. E. (1979) Small choroidal melanomas: a long-term follow-up study. *Archives of Ophthalmology*, **97,** 861–864

Vogel, M. H. (1972a) Treatment of malignant melanomas with photocoagulation. *American Journal of Ophthalmology*, **74,** 1–11

Vogel, M. H. (1972b) Histopathologic observations of photocoagulated malignant melanomas of the choroid. *American Journal of Ophthalmology*, **74,** 466–474

Vogel, M. and Meyer-Schwickerath, G. (1978) Results of photocoagulation treatment of malignant melanoma of the choroid. In *Ocular and Adnexal Tumors*, edited by F. A. Jakobiec, 71–75. Birmingham: Aesculapius Publishing Co.

Williams, A. T., Font, R. L., Van Dyk, H. J. L. and Riekhof, T. (1978) Osseous choristoma of the choroid simulating a choroidal melanoma. *Archives of Ophthalmology*, **96,** 1874–1877

Wilson, R. S. and Fraunfelder, F. T. (1978) 'No-touch' cryosurgical enucleation: a minimal trauma technique for eyes harboring intraocular malignancy. *Ophthalmology*, **85,** 1170–1175

Wolter, J. R. (1971) Tenonectomy. *Archives of Ophthalmology*, **86,** 529–533

Zakov, Z. N., Smith, T. R. and Albert, D. M. (1978) False-positive P-32 uptake test. *Archives of Ophthalmology*, **96,** 2240–2243

Zimmerman, L. E., McLean, I. W. and Foster, W. D. (1980) Statistical analysis of follow-up data concerning uveal melanomas and the influence of enucleation. *Ophthalmology*, **87,** 557–564

# 11
# Instrumentation for closed intraocular microsurgery

Robert J. Cooling

## INTRODUCTION

Instrumentation for closed intraocular microsurgery has undergone a period of remarkable development since the introduction of the vitreous infusion suction cutter (VISC) in 1971 (Machemer *et al.*, 1971). With continued refinement of basic instruments and the advent of a wealth of specialized devices, the techniques have become increasingly sophisticated. During this period of rapid development, important changes have occurred in the concepts of instrumentation. In the early 1970s, several instruments were designed based upon the original concept of a single instrument with combined facilities for suction-cutting, infusion and illumination (full-function probes). The introduction of two-instrument techniques (Machemer, 1974) extended the capabilities of pars plana vitrectomy and prompted the development of accessory instruments. Subsequently, functions originally assigned to one vitrectomy probe have become divided among instruments of standard shaft diameter accommodated within multiple pars plana incisions of less than 1 mm in diameter (*Figure 11.1*). This common-gauge principle, conceived by Connor O'Malley (O'Malley and Heintz, 1975), has become a feature of most commercially produced systems, endowing considerable flexibility and fostering the development of a wide range of complementary instrumentation which has assumed an ever-increasing role in vitreous surgery.

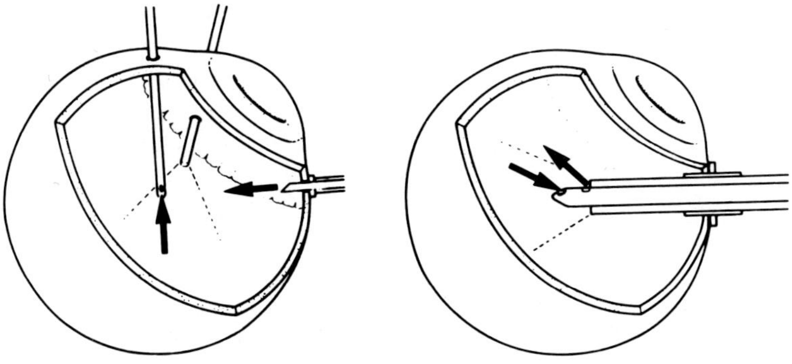

(*a*) (*b*)

*Figure 11.1* (*a*) Common gauge instrumentation versus (*b*) full-function vitrectomy probe

## SUCTION CUTTERS

In the past few years, full-function probes have increasingly given way to smaller gauge cutters used in conjunction with an independent infusion system and separate fibreoptic endoillumination. Presently, several instruments of this type are marketed, the choice of which will depend upon a variety of considerations including the overall cost, availability, and frequently the preference of the surgeon. In general, these instruments are simpler in construction and more readily assembled than previous designs and, with few exceptions, can be steam autoclaved to allow rapid recycling.

In principle, material for excision must first be engaged by suction force within a bevelled port and subsequently cut by a shearing action produced by movement of an inner blade housed within a stationary outer tube. Fragmented tissue and fluid is then conducted from the cutting port to the collection bottle by the aspiration system. The hollowed inner blade may rotate or oscillate about its long axis or undergo a linear reciprocating guillotine movement. Oscillatory cutters may be fitted with a springloaded inner blade to increase the cutting efficiency and to provide a degree of self-sharpening. However, when reduced in efficiency rotary, and to a lesser extent oscillatory cutters, may result in spooling of tissue around the inner blade to produce exaggerated vitreoretinal traction. Guillotine cutters, which do not induce this effect, are generally preferred and depend upon precision manufacture and a sharpened blade for efficient cutting. However, in all suction cutters various factors exist which militate against continued sharpness of the cutting surfaces, necessitating periodic resharpening or replacement of the cutting tip. Movement of the inner blade may be powered by a DC micromotor or electromagnet contained within the handpiece, or by pneumatic drive from a vacuum pump, so reducing the overall dimensions of the handpiece (*Figure 11.2*). The instrument must be capable of a rapid and variable cutting speed, although in

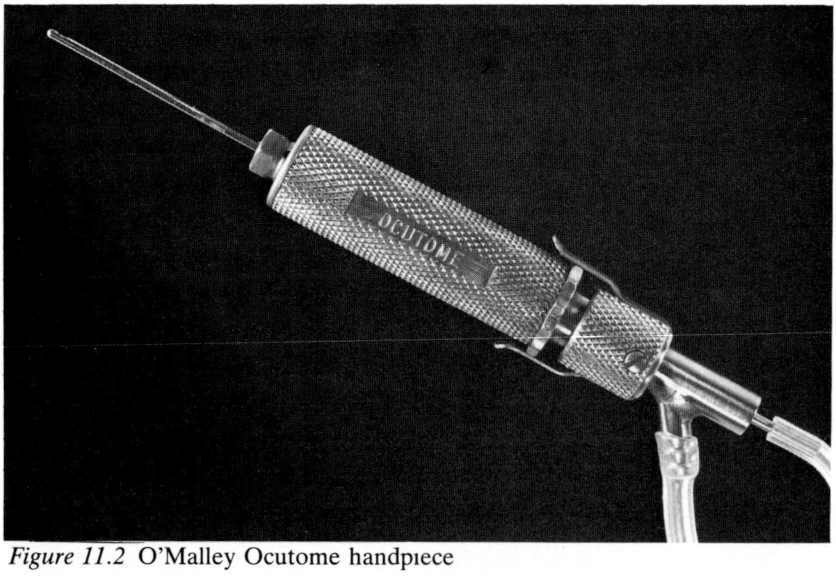


*Figure 11.2* O'Malley Ocutome handpiece

general the maximum frequency is used to ensure safer and more effective removal of vitreous gel.

The aspiration port is most commonly located on the side of the outer stationary tube at a distance from the tip which varies between different instruments (*Figure 11.3*). In the Klöti vitreous stripper, the port is located on the inner shaft which is

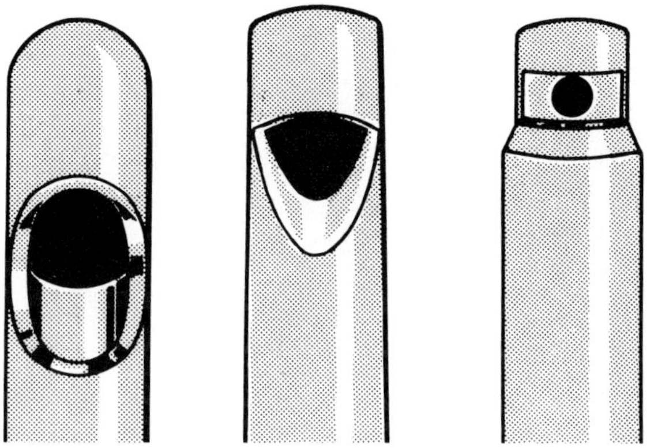

(*a*) (*b*) (*c*)

*Figure 11.3* Intraocular tips of 20-gauge guillotine suction cutters: (*a*) O'Malley Ocutome, (*b*) Peyman disposable vitrophage, (*c*) Klöti vitreous stripper

retracted against the sharpened terminal edge of the outer blade, providing an extremely fast and efficient cutting mechanism. The aperture of the cutting port may be adjustable (for example, O'Malley Ocutome) or of a wide-angled configuration (for example, Peyman disposable vitrophage), facilitating the impaction of less deformable tissues. A reduced aperture increases cutting efficiency and permits the use of lower levels of suction force.

In recent years the aspiration system has undergone increasing sophistication. Suction force, originally produced by a syringe operated by the assistant, is now generated by an automated unit using a vacuum or peristaltic pump. Suction may be activated by closure of a venting port (such as the Peyman vitrophage) or compression of a hollow bypass ring as in the Federman SITE located on the handpiece. This open system affords some control over the level of suction, but, despite venting of the aspiration system to atmospheric pressure, tissue may continue to be engaged within the cutting port by a pressure gradient maintained by the infusion system. In a closed system, the level of vacuum is selected on the console and activated by a foot-switch controlled suction valve with instant cessation of fluid outflow. With the necessity for constant and wide variation in suction levels, several systems now employ a linear suction control (*Figure 11.4*) allowing continuous regulation of suction force up to a preselected maximum by variable depression of a foot pedal (Charles, 1981*a*). This refinement is seen as a significant advance, allowing the application of minimal suction force and the avoidance of undue vitreoretinal traction.

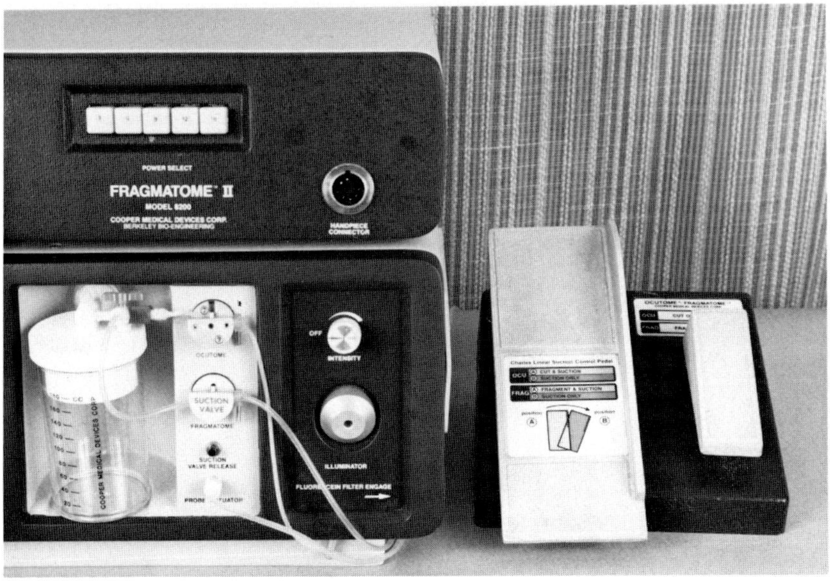


*Figure 11.4* Ocutome and Fragmatome 8000 consoles with linear suction control pedal

The aspiration system must be of sufficient dimensions to prevent tissue clogging and be completely filled with fluid prior to use to prevent air locking and decreased flow. The system also provides a reflux facility to disengage tissue from the cutting port by simply reversing the direction of flow with a syringe connected to the aspiration tubing.

## ULTRASONIC LENS FRAGMENTERS

In many instances suction cutting probes are inappropriate for lensectomy with frequent obstruction of the aspiration system by lens material and unnecessary lengthening of the procedure. Consequently, most systems now include an ultrasonic module for fragmentation of the lens nucleus using a specially designed handpiece (*Figure 11.5*). Ultrasonic phakoemulsification has also replaced mechanical lens fragmenters which were designed for use with full-function probes (Peyman, Huamonte and Goldberg, 1975; Douvas, 1976). The ultrasonic needle

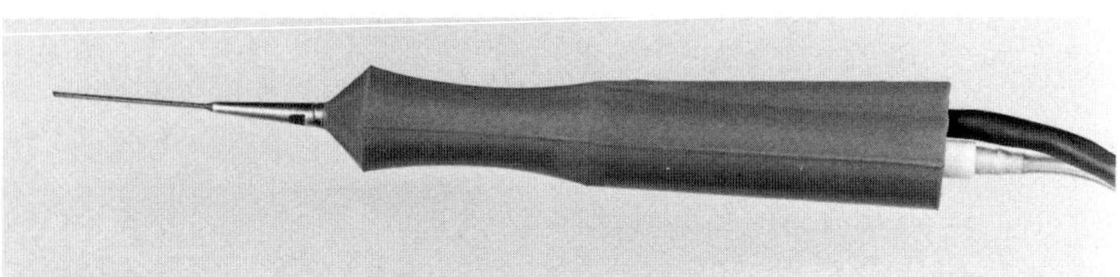

*Figure 11.5* Fragmatome handpiece with 20-gauge ultrasonic needle

can be accommodated within the same sclerotomy as the vitreous cutter and continuous sonification and aspiration (at high levels) are used to allow efficient fragmentation. Uninterrupted flow is vital to ensure internal cooling of the needle and avoidance of thermal damage to the sclera.

## INFUSION SYSTEMS

The use of an infusion system independent of the cutter presents a number of important advantages and has gained widespread acceptance. An indwelling 20-gauge cannula (*Figure 11.6*), introduced through a pars plana sclerotomy and secured by a mattress suture, ensures adequate infusion of replacement fluid to maintain intraocular pressure in spite of wide fluctuations in the rate of outflow.

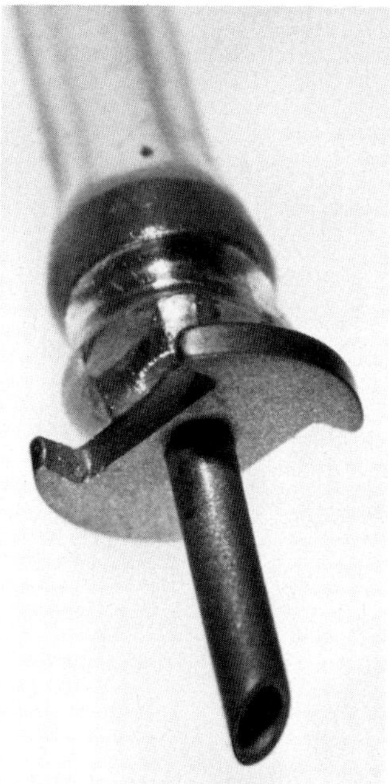

*Figure 11.6* Indwelling 4 mm infusion cannula

Intraocular pressure can also be controlled following the removal of other intraocular instruments combined with temporary occlusion of the sclerotomies by stainless steel plugs (O'Malley and Tripp, 1977). In addition, a separate infusion system reduces the dispersion of cellular and particulate debris throughout the vitreous cavity and decreases total fluid exchange. Extrusion techniques are facilitated and, in the presence of a retinal break, reduced accumulation of subretinal fluid may occur during vitrectomy, in contrast to that seen using full-function probes. Before commencing infusion, it is essential to confirm complete penetration of the pars plana by the tip of the infusion cannula to avoid progressive ciliochoroidal detachment by infusion into the suprachoroidal space. Dense opacities within the media may prevent visualization of the tip of the cannula and require the use of a long-reach cannula (4 or 6 mm) or preliminary infusion with an alternative device.

Infusion is most commonly gravity-dependent, the maximum intraocular pressure being determined by the height of the fluid reservoir above the eye. Infusion pressure may be raised to control capillary bleeding or lowered to allow peripheral indentation (collapsing technique). To regulate intraocular pressure below a selected maximum, automated infusion systems have been developed which utilize a compressor or modified peristaltic pump and pressure transducers. Recently, a motorized injector has also become available for the non-pulsatile insufflation of gas (Charles, 1981*a*).

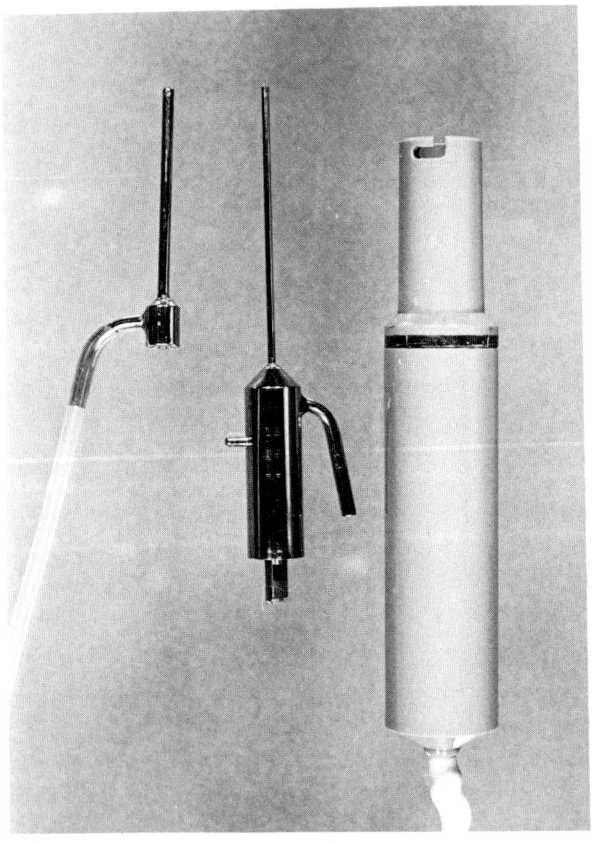

*Figure 11.7* SITE-TXR handpiece with end-cutting tip and universal infusion sleeve

Alternative facilities for infusion, largely employed for anterior segment procedures, include a universal infusion sleeve placed over the tip of the suction cutter (*Figure 11.7*) and an angulated blunt-ended needle (20-gauge) introduced via the limbus or pars plana for two-instrument techniques (May, 1981).

**ILLUMINATION**

In contrast to extraocular light sources, fibreoptic endoillumination eliminates reflexes from various optical interfaces and provides an adequate level of illumination for detailed resolution of the operative field even under high magnification.

Initially, endoillumination was provided by sleeved fibreoptics around the vitrectomy probe. This system presented a number of inherent limitations and carried a significant risk of entry site tears during introduction of the blunt end of the sleeve. With standard two-instrument techniques, a separate fibreoptic probe is used to provide focal, diffuse or dark-field illumination and permits variable positioning of illumination with respect to other intraocular instruments. A continuous fibreoptic cable and integral illuminator is now routinely used and substantially increases the intensity of intraocular illumination compared with the standard bayonet-fitted probe (*Figure 11.8*). Dual-purpose endoilluminators may

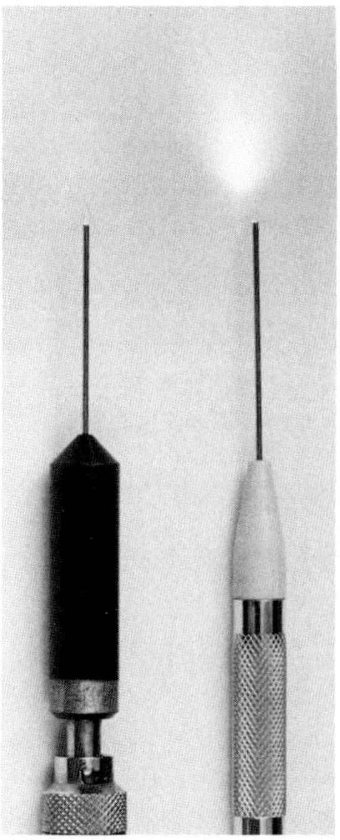

*Figure 11.8* Fibreoptic endoilluminators showing high intensity output of continuous-fibre probe

also be used in which illumination is combined with a dissector (O'Malley, 1977) or infusing device (Poole and Sudarsky, 1979). An indwelling fibreoptic light source for diffuse illumination, designed in the manner of the infusion terminal, has also been developed but experience has not revealed any significant advantage over existing endoilluminator probes.

Several years ago, experimental studies raised the possibility of permanent damage to the photoreceptors and pigment epithelium in the human eye from exposure to intraocular light sources (Fuller, Machemer and Knighton, 1978). With the advent of more intense endoilluminators, the risk of cumulative light toxicity has increased (Meyers and Bonner, 1982) and is of particular concern with the use of prolonged focal illumination for epiretinal dissection. However, insufficient attention has been paid to the use of filtered light sources and the elimination of damaging short wavelength light (Sliney and Wolbarsht, 1980).

## VISUALIZATION

The use of an operating microscope with coaxial illumination and incorporating motorized focusing, zoom magnification and XY coupling with foot-switch controls is essential. A beam splitter with binocular side-tube attachment provides coaxial but non-stereoscopic viewing for the assistant. In addition, the use of a beam-splitter provides facilities for photography or television recording. To reduce the working distance, a short-bodied microscope with inclinable eyepieces is preferred, and the unit should be ceiling-mounted to release valuable floor space within the vicinity of the operating table.

To allow observation of deeper structures, a neutralizing fundus contact lens is used. It may be self-retaining or flanged to allow fixation to the globe but these designs have largely been replaced by infusing plano-concave lenses rigidly mounted or gimballed to a curved handle held by an assistant, affording improved central and peripheral visualization (*Figure 11.9*). Constructed of scratch-resistant

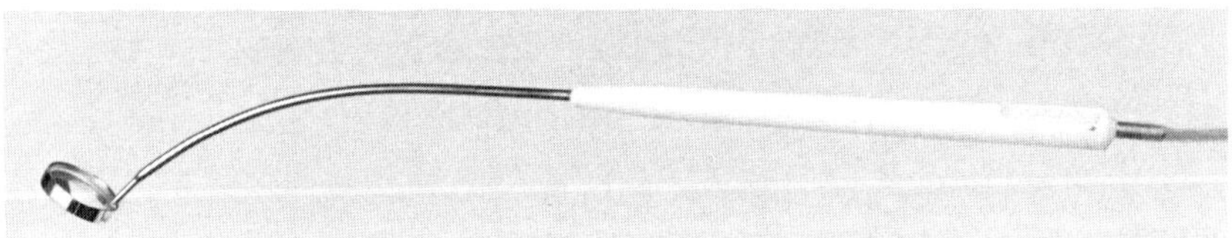

*Figure 11.9* Irrigating quartz fundus contact lens designed by Parel and Machemer

material, the lens is lightly held on the cornea and maintained coaxial with the objective lens of the microscope during ocular rotation (Parel and Machemer, 1981). Continuous irrigation of physiological fluid eliminates air or blood from beneath the lens and a reduced flow rate minimizes hydration of the corneal epithelium. High powered biconcave lenses are also now available to enable peripheral viewing with reduced rotation of the globe (Sebestyen, 1982) and for observation of the posterior fundus in the gas-containing phakic eye (Landers, Stefansson and Wolbarsht, 1981).

## INTRAOCULAR DISSECTORS AND MICROFORCEPS

Microsurgical dissection of various tissue planes within the posterior segment now forms an essential part of many pars plana vitrectomy procedures and for which a wide range of instruments of varying complexity has been developed.

The angulated tip of a disposable 20-gauge hypodermic needle fitted to a tuberculin syringe or infusing handle serves as a suitable dissector for most non-vascularized epimacular membranes. The edge of the membrane is engaged with the tip of the needle and gently peeled from the surface of the retina to relieve tangential traction. To facilitate edge dissection, Michels and co-workers (1979) have designed a series of special membrane picks with differing tip and edge configurations. In the absence of a discrete edge, the membrane is initially incised with an exquisitely sharp knife such as the microvitreoretinal blade, customarily used to create pars plana sclerotomies. Similarly, the blade may be used to fenestrate a thickened posterior hyaloid interface or pupillary membrane so as to facilitate subsequent engagement within the port of the cutter.

Various designs of manually operated intraocular microscissors are available, principally used for the segmentation or resection of more intimately adherent epiretinal membranes. Right-angled 20-gauge scissors (*Figure 11.10*) in which axial movement of the proximal or distal blade is activated by compression of the handle, allow membrane division perpendicular to the retinal surface. For the resection or

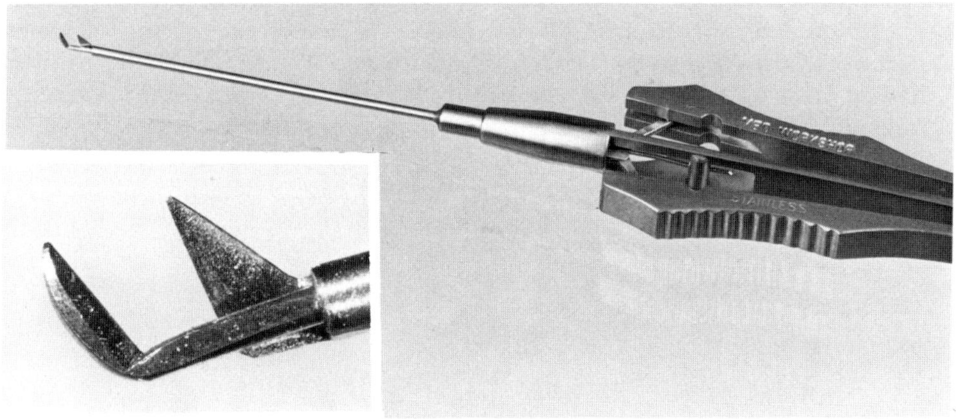

*Figure 11.10* Right-angled 20-gauge intraocular scissors

delamination of epiretinal membranes, scissors described by Sutherland (*Figure 11.11*) are used in which the cutting blades are orientated at an oblique angle to the shaft to allow cutting parallel to the surface of the retina. These scissors are activated by depressing a lever against the tension of a light spring, and turning a knurled ring on the handpiece allows complete rotation of the blades around the instrument shaft (Heinze, 1978). Irrespective of the design, intraocular microscissors pose a significant risk of entry site tears and therefore require careful introduction in a closed position through an enlarged sclerotomy.

Remotely activated intravitreal scissors were developed many years ago to reduce the risk of retinal damage from inadvertent deflection of the blades during manual activation (Couvillion, Freeman and Schepens, 1970). Recently, several designs of automated intraocular microscissors have become commercially available, and although not yet fully evaluated offer more controlled and efficient

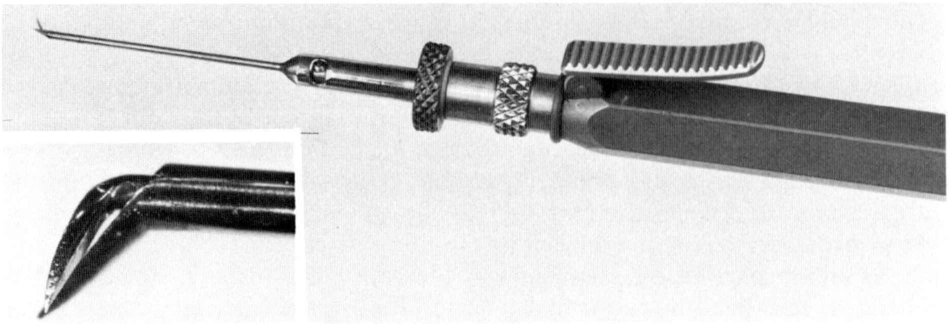

*Figure 11.11* Sutherland 20-gauge rotatable intraocular scissors

cutting (Machemer *et al.*, 1981; Charles and Wang, 1981). The membrane peeler cutter, developed by Machemer and co-workers, is constructed on a guillotine principle with 90° parallel-edged blades and powered by a micromotor within the handpiece. The fixed distal blade is used as a dissector and the rate of movement of the upper blade is electronically controlled by a foot-switch. Pneumatically driven 20-gauge microscissors which interface with the handpiece of the O'Malley Ocutome probe have also been designed (Charles and Wang, 1981).

A wide range of intraocular microforceps has been developed for the extraction of retained foreign material. Selection of the most appropriate instrument is dictated by the dimensions, attitude and location of the foreign body. The 20-gauge forceps with serrated jaws have, in the author's experience, proved the most satisfactory design (*Figure 11.12*). To reduce the risk of displacement of the foreign

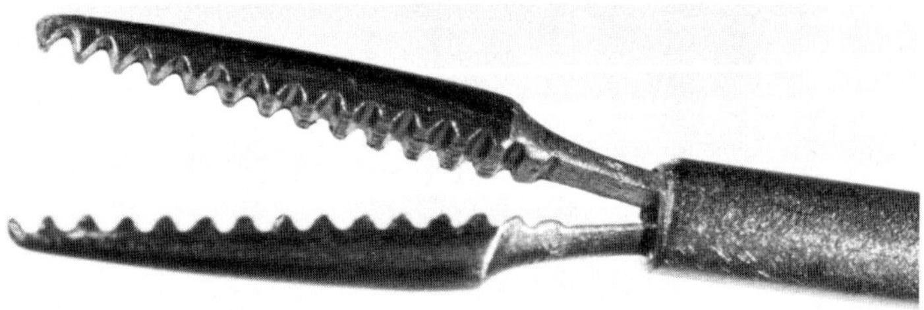

*Figure 11.12* 20-gauge intraocular microforceps with serrated jaws

body during delivery, the blades may be covered by silastic tubing (Hutton, 1977) or be diamond-coated (Hickingbotham, Parel and Machemer, 1981). The 20-gauge microforceps have also proved useful as an accessory in epimacular membrane peeling and for intraocular tissue biopsy.

## EXTRUSION DEVICES

Several instruments can be used to undertake a number of important and commonly employed procedures collectively described as extrusion techniques. These techniques include 'vacuum cleaning' of sedimented debris from the surface of the retina, internal drainage of the subretinal space via a retinal break, and simultaneous exchange of intraocular fluid for gas or other fluid substitutes. The extruding force is principally provided by the infusion system and the device may be vented to the atmosphere or linked to a closed outflow system.

The Charles flute needle consists of a blunt-ended 20-gauge needle connected to a handle with an internal channel and recessed side-opening exit port. The flow of fluid or gas is controlled by the forefinger placed over the exit port. Several modified handles (*Figure 11.13*) have been devised including siting of the exit port on a mount to allow more precise control of fluid outflow (McLeod and Leaver, 1981) and the use of a disposable syringe with a perforated barrel providing a reflux facility (Escoffery and Grand, 1980).

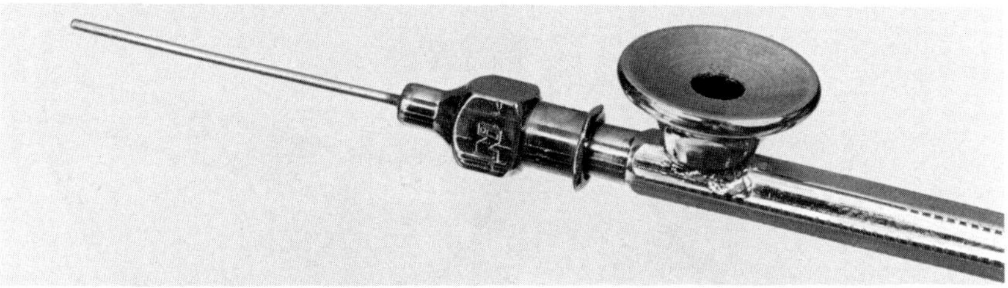

*Figure 11.13* Modified Charles flute needle

An improved extrusion system is currently used in which the vacuum-cleaning needle is attached to a short handpiece connected by the debris line to an automated suction unit with foot-switch control (*Figure 11.14*). Recently a further modification has been introduced with replacement of the vacuum-cleaning needle

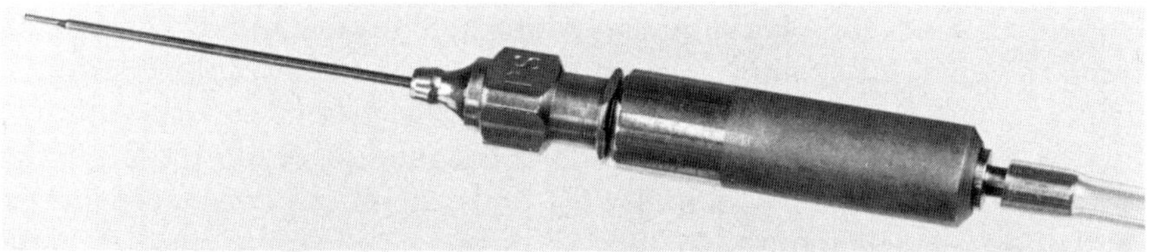

*Figure 11.14* Tapered linear extrusion needle and handpiece

by a tapered extrusion needle (19/20–26 gauge). When used with linear suction control, this system offers a substantially improved method of internal subretinal fluid drainage especially via small pre-existing or 'created' posterior retinal breaks, reducing the risks of tear enlargement or inadvertent retinal incarceration (Yarian and Parel, 1981).

## INTRAOCULAR TISSUE COAGULATION

### Endodiathermy

Intraocular diathermy, originally employed for the treatment of posterior retinal breaks (Mamoli, 1937), is principally used to directly coagulate potential or actual bleeding sites within vascularized epiretinal tissue.

Although a number of insulated unipolar and coaxial bipolar endodiathermy probes have been developed (Shea, 1972; Tate *et al.*, 1975, Klöti, 1976; Parel, O'Grady and Machemer, 1981) intraocular diathermy is most conveniently and safely applied, using a bimanual bipolar technique (*Figure 11.15*). The electrical

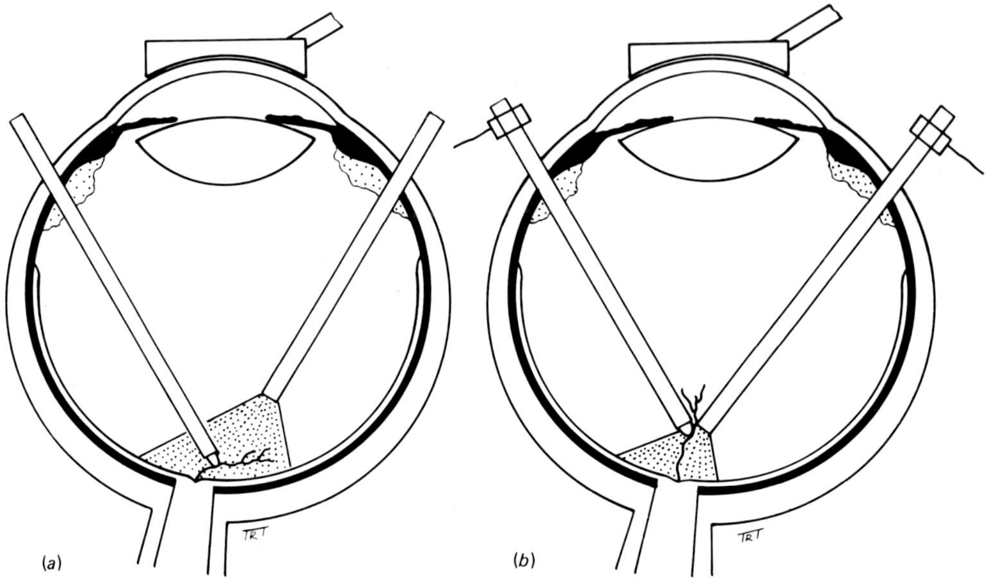


*Figure 11.15* (*a*) Unimanual bipolar endodiathermy probe; (*b*) bimanual bipolar endodiathermy

leads of a low-frequency bipolar unit are connected by microclips to separate intraocular instruments; for example, the endoilluminator and a second instrument such as scissors, suction cutter or extrusion device. The flow of current within an elliptical field between the instrument tips allows coagulation of interposed tissues and, in contrast to radiofrequency unipolar methods, significantly reduces the risk of electrical damage to neighbouring tissues, in particular the optic nerve (Charles *et al.*, 1976).

## Intraocular cryotherapy

Improved designs of intraocular cryoprobe (including 20-gauge diameter) have become available since the introduction of transvitreal cryotherapy by Cibis in 1965 (Machemer and Aaberg, 1979; Woldoff, 1980; Bradbury and Fung, 1980). The cryotherapy unit must be capable of rapid defrosting and the iceball confined to the tip of the probe (features equally desirable for extraocular cryoprobes). This technique has been used for focal treatment of retinal breaks situated in the vicinity of the optic nerve or macula, softening of the lens nucleus prior to ultrasonic emulsification (Shock, 1974) and the open-sky removal of a dislocated lens or selected intraocular foreign body. As a method of direct retinal coagulation, the technique has largely fallen into disuse with the difficulty of determining the end-point, and risks of choroidal haemorrhage or tearing of the retina with premature retraction of the probe from the retinal surface.

## Endophotocoagulation

A method of endophotocoagulation has been devised by Charles (1981*b*) using a specialized 20-gauge fibreoptic probe coupled to a portable xenon arc photocoagulator (*Figure 11.16*). In the absence of a focusing system the tip of the probe must

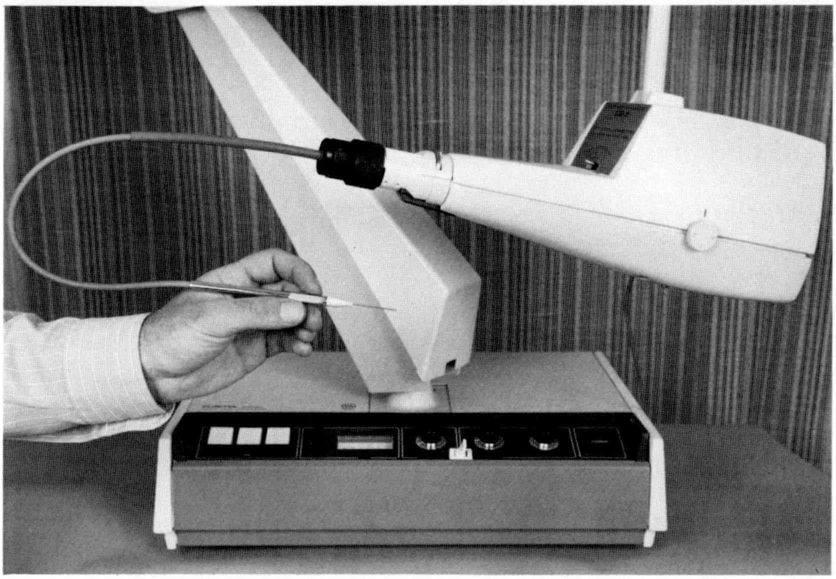

*Figure 11.16* Charles endophotocoagulator probe and log 3 xenon light coagulator

be stationed within 0.5 mm of the attached retina to produce 800–1000 μ burns. This method has proved to be of value in the treatment of posterior retinal breaks and for panretinal ablation in the management of preoperative iris neovascularization. Diffuse illumination is usually provided by a separate endoilluminator but the endophotocoagulator probe emits sufficient light between applications to permit simultaneous use of an extrusion device. During prolonged treatment sessions, the use of a barrier filter advanced beneath the objective lens of the microscope has been recommended to improve the comfort and protection of the surgeon and assistant from the reflection of attenuated light (Carroll and Peyman, 1981). Unfortunately, the probe cannot be fired in air, gas or silicone fluid without damage to the tip and, despite careful handling, the lifespan of the probe has often proved disappointingly short.

Recently, systems for the delivery of argon laser photocoagulation using remotely located sources and low energy-loss fibreoptics have been developed

(Fleischman, Swartz and Dixon, 1981; Peyman, Salzano and Green, 1981). A number of advantages are offered over existing techniques of xenon endophotocoagulation, and preliminary experiences have been encouraging. With reduced divergence of the light beam, the endolaser probe can be used at a distance of 3 mm or more from the retinal surface and may also be fired from within a gas bubble. In addition, a rapid firing sequence can be achieved providing a more efficient method of panretinal endophotocoagulation. With the rapid development of laser technology, it is likely that intraoperative delivery systems will undergo considerable improvement and that intraocular laser dissectors using various sources will be developed in the near future.

## MISCELLANEOUS

There are a number of additional items of equipment which have come to be regarded as important if not essential for the undertaking of modern vitreoretinal surgery.

A freestanding instrument carriage, of which several designs are commercially available, is required to accommodate the large number of consoles and ancillary power sources. The trolley may straddle the operating table (Hilton and Avins, 1979) or be placed to one side to allow the surgeon an unobstructed view of instrument gauges. The prototype stand, illustrated in *Figure 11.17*, is of sturdy and lightweight construction with sufficient shelf-space to accommodate basic instrument consoles, a back-up vitrectomy system and various gas cylinders. A detachable tray fitted to the front of the trolley provides a suitable working surface for

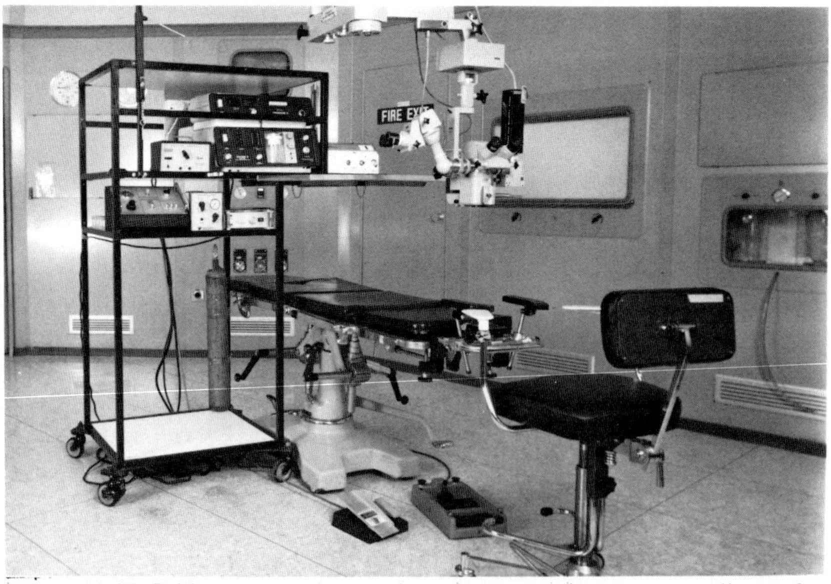

*Figure 11.17* Ceiling-mounted operating microscope, instrument trolley and operating chair

instrument assembly and for the orderly placement of conducting tubes and instrument leads during surgery. A bank of electrical sockets is located to the rear of the consoles and a single cable is connected to a wall socket. With completion of the intraocular part of the procedure, the trolley may be wheeled from the operating table to allow dismantling of equipment. The trolley also provides safe and convenient storage of equipment following surgery.

To ensure stability and appropriate positioning of the patient's head during surgery, a suitable headrest is used and may be fitted with side arms to form part of a draining trough for fluid overflow from the irrigating contact lens.

During prolonged procedures, a comfortable operating stool or chair of adjustable height is required and may include arm rests providing support for the surgeon's elbows.

Finally, despite the complexity of modern instrumentation, familiarity with the capabilities, limitations and workings of each individual instrument is essential. Many of the instruments described are delicately constructed and for optimal performance appropriate care and handling must be constantly exercised. Particular attention should be paid to guarding the intraocular tips of various cutting instruments and the avoidance of kinking of fibreoptic light probes. Whilst the care of instrumentation is ultimately the responsibility of the surgeon, the services of a dedicated technician as a member of the vitreoretinal surgical team are regarded as indispensable in any busy vitrectomy programme.

## Acknowledgements

The author wishes to thank Miss Fehmida Latif for preparation of the manuscript, Messrs T. R. Tarrant and A. Chopping for the illustrations and Dr Jay L. Federman for kindly supplying *Figure 11.7*.

## References

Bradbury, M. J. and Fung, W. E. (1980) A new 20-gauge intravitreal cryoprobe. *American Journal of Ophthalmology*, **90,** 424–425

Carroll, C. P. and Peyman, G. A. (1981) A microscope filter for endophotocoagulation. *Archives of Ophthalmology*, **99,** 327

Charles, S. (1981a) *Vitreous Microsurgery*, 26–28. Baltimore: Williams and Wilkins

Charles, S. (1981b) Endophotocoagulation. *Retina*, **1,** 117–120

Charles, S. and Wang, C. (1981) Pneumatic intraocular microscissors. *Archives of Ophthalmology*, **99,** 1251

Charles, S., White, J., Dennison, C. and Eichenbaum, D. (1976) Bipolar, bimanual intraocular diathermy. *American Journal of Ophthalmology*, **81,** 101–102

Couvillion, G. C., Freeman, H. M. and Schepens, C. L. (1970) Vitreous surgery. V. Modification of the vitreous scissors. *Archives of Ophthalmology*, **83,** 722–723

Douvas, N. G. (1976) Vitrectomy instrumentation, roto-extractor indications, and techniques and results. In *Current Concepts of the Vitreous including Vitrectomy*, edited by K. A. Gitter, 159–161. St Louis: C. V. Mosby

Escoffery, R. F. and Grand, M. G. (1980) A flute syringe for vitreous surgery. *Archives of Ophthalmology*, **98,** 2059

Fleischman, J. A., Swartz, M. and Dixon, J. A. (1981) Argon laser endophotocoagulation – an intraoperative trans-pars plana technique. *Archives of Ophthalmology*, **99,** 1610–1612

Fuller, D., Machemer, R. and Knighton, R. W. (1978) Retinal damage produced by intraocular fibreoptic light. *American Journal of Ophthalmology*, **85,** 519–537

Heinze, J. (1978) Sutherland rotatable microsurgery instruments. *Transactions of the Ophthalmological Society of New Zealand*, **33,** 112–115

Hickingbotham, D., Parel, J. M. and Machemer, R. (1981) Diamond-coated all-purpose foreign-body forceps. *American Journal of Ophthalmology*, **91,** 267–268

Hilton, G. F. and Avins, L. R. (1979) Instrument tables for pars plana vitrectomy. *American Journal of Ophthalmology*, **88,** 773–774

Hutton, W. L. (1977) Vitreous foreign body forceps. *American Journal of Ophthalmology*, **84,** 430

Klöti, R. (1976) Vitrectomy via the pars plana ciliaris with the vitreous stripper. In *Advances in Vitreous Surgery*, edited by A. R. Irvine and C. O'Malley, 243–257. Springfield, Illinois: C. C. Thomas

Landers, M. B., Stefansson, E. and Wolbarsht, M. L. (1981) The optics of vitreous surgery. *American Journal of Ophthalmology*, **91,** 611–614

Machemer, R. (1974) A new concept for vitreous surgery. 7. Two-instrument techniques in pars plana vitrectomy. *Archives of Ophthalmology*, **92,** 407–412

Machemer, R. and Aaberg,T. M. (1979) *Vitrectomy,* 2nd Edition, 119–124. New York: Grune and Stratton

Machemer, R., Buettner, H., Norton, E. W. D. and Parel, J-M. (1971) Vitrectomy, a pars plana approach. *Transactions of the American Academy of Ophthalmology and Otolaryngology*, **75,** 813–820

Machemer, R., Parel, J. M., Hickingbotham, D. and Nose, I. (1981) Membrane peeler cutter. *Archives of Ophthalmology*, **99,** 152–153

Mamoli, L. (1937) A case of retinal detachment with macular hole: tentative treatment with trans-bulbar diathermy. *Annales d'Oculistique (Paris)*, **174,** 309–312

May, D. R. (1981) An anterior segment 30° bent infusion needle. *Archives of Ophthalmology*, **99,** 1288

McLeod, D. and Leaver, P. K. (1981) Modified Charles flute needle. *British Journal of Ophthalmology*, **65,** 69

Meyers, S. M. and Bonner, R. S. (1982) Retinal irradiance from vitrectomy endoilluminators. *American Journal of Ophthalmology*, **94,** 26–29

Michels, R. G., Rice, T. A. and Ober, R. R. (1979) Vitreoretinal dissection instruments. *American Journal of Ophthalmology*, **87,** 836–837

O'Malley, C. (1977) Viewing and illumination during intraocular surgery. In *Vitreous Surgery and Advances in Fundus Diagnosis and Treatment*, edited by

H. M. Freeman, T. Hirose and C. L. Schepens, pp. 159–162. New York: Appleton-Century-Crofts

O'Malley, C. and Heintz, R. M. (1975) Vitrectomy with an alternative instrument system. *Annals of Ophthalmology*, **7,** 585–594

O'Malley, C. and Tripp, R. M. (1977) Plugs and stiletto: entry incisions for a 20-gauge instrument system. *Ophthalmic Surgery*, **8,** 76

Parel, J-M. and Machemer, R. (1981) Steam-sterilizable fundus contact lenses. *Archives of Ophthalmology*, **99,** 151

Parel, J-M., O'Grady, G. E. and Machemer, R. (1981) A bipolar coaxial microprobe for safe transvitreal diathermy. *Archives of Ophthalmology*, **99,** 494–497

Peyman, G. A., Huamonte, F. and Goldberg, M. F. (1975) Management of cataract in patients undergoing vitrectomy. *American Journal of Ophthalmology*, **80,** 30–36

Peyman, G. A., Salzano, T. C. and Green, J. L. (1981) Argon endolaser. *Archives of Ophthalmology*, **99,** 2037–2038

Poole, T. A. and Sudarsky, R. K. (1979) A 20-gauge illumination and irrigation instrument for pars plana vitrectomy. *American Journal of Ophthalmology*, **88,** 1093–1095

Sebestyen, J. G. (1982) An improved contact lens for trans-pars plana vitreous surgery. *American Journal of Ophthalmology*, **93,** 122–124

Shea, M. (1972) Intravitreal electrocoagulation of retinal vessels. *Canadian Journal of Ophthalmology*, **7,** 268–270

Shock, J. P. (1974) Phacocryolysis combined with phacofragmentation and irrigation for removal of cataracts. *American Journal of Ophthalmology*, **77,** 860–864

Sliney, D. H. and Wolborsht, M. L. (1980) Safety standards and measurement techniques for high intensity light sources. *Vision Research*, **20,** 1133–1141

Tate, G. W., Hutton, W. L., Vaiser, A. and Snyder, W. B. (1975) A coaxial electrode for intraocular diathermy. *American Journal of Ophthalmology*, **79,** 691–693

Woldoff, H. S. (1980) A 20-gauge intravitreal cryoprobe. *American Journal of Ophthalmology*, **90,** 262

Yarian, D. and Parel, J. M. (1981) *The Ocutome Newsletter*, **6,** 3–4

# 12
# Silicone oil injection in retinal detachment surgery

R. H. B. Grey

## INTRODUCTION

In 1962 Cibis *et al.* first published reports of silicone oil injection into the vitreous cavity for treatment of retinal detachment. At that time conventional surgical techniques were less reliable than those used today and a search for alternative methods led to a variety of vitreous substitutes being tried but discovered to be of limited or temporary benefit. Following injection into the vitreous cavity in laboratory animals, silicone oil was found to be inert and to remain optically clear (Stone, 1958). It was used, therefore, in cases of recalcitrant retinal detachment in man in an attempt to tamponade the retina against the pigment epithelium (Cibis *et al.*, 1962).

The early workers in this field found silicone oil to be useful for reattaching the retina, but with a high risk of complications (Dufour, 1964; Kanski and Daniel, 1973; Okun, 1968; Rosengren, 1966; Watzke, 1967). However, while the latter finding, together with a gradual improvement in standard surgical techniques producing better results, led to the abandonment of silicone oil injection in all but a few centres, certain complicated retinal detachments still failed to respond to scleral buckling procedures, and Scott (1972; 1973; 1974) championed the use of liquid silicone for such cases. More recently there has been a reawakening of interest in the use of silicone oil injection for complicated retinal detachments and currently it is the most successful method of producing long-term reattachment and maintenance of useful vision (Grey and Leaver, 1977; 1979).

## INDICATIONS FOR USE OF SILICONE OIL

### Massive periretinal proliferation (MPP)

Retinal detachments with good retinal mobility should be treated by standard scleral buckling procedures, and in cases where localized immobility is associated with star folds scleral buckling should be attempted initially. This may be combined with division of preretinal membranes and temporary internal tamponade with air or air–gas mixtures to improve the chances of success. However, in cases where extensive formation of fibrous epiretinal membranes greatly reduces retinal mobility (massive periretinal proliferation) and prevents closure of retinal breaks with buckling procedures, silicone oil injection is one method of freeing the retina of membranes, re-establishing retinal mobility and closing the breaks. Anatomical reattachment of the retina can be achieved and useful vision restored by this method in more than 50 per cent of such cases in experienced hands (*Figure 12.1*).

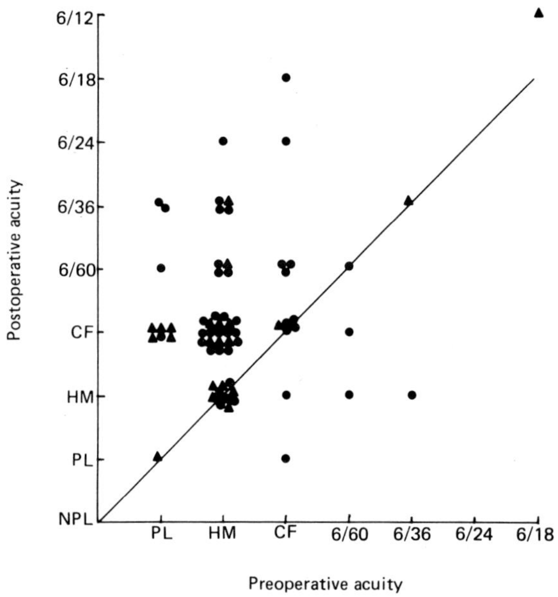


*Figure 12.1* Scattergram showing the visual results of silicone oil injection in the treatment of massive periretinal proliferation. Points above the diagonal line show an improvement in vision, points on the line no change, and those below a deterioration following surgery. (●) Phakic; (▲) aphakic. (From Grey and Leaver (1979), courtesy of the Editor and Publishers, *British Journal of Ophthalmology*)

Once the retina has been replaced, further periretinal proliferation is commonly of no serious significance because the incompressibility of the oil globule prevents the retina reseparating from the pigment epithelium. Redetachment following successful silicone oil injection in cases of massive periretinal proliferation occurs in less than 10 per cent of cases.

Alternative methods of treatment involving pars plana vitrectomy and division of preretinal membranes together with insufflation of sulphur hexafluoride gas and air into the vitreous cavity produce similar initial results to those obtained with silicone oil injection. However, owing to the temporary nature of the tamponade combined with further membrane proliferation the long-term success rate is no better than 30 per cent.

## Giant retinal tears

In eyes with retinal detachment caused by giant tears, redetachment due to massive periretinal proliferation is extremely high even following an initially successful buckling procedure. The use of silicone oil combined with limited buckling and vitrectomy has greatly improved the long-term results in these eyes (*Figure 12.2*) (Lean *et al.*, 1982; Leaver and Lean, 1981).

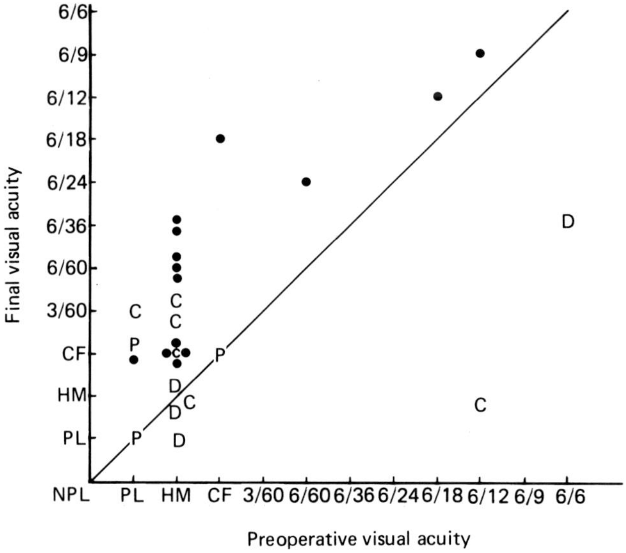


*Figure 12.2* Scattergram showing the visual results of vitrectomy and silicone oil injection in the treatment of giant retinal tears. Points above the diagonal line show an improvement in vision, points on the line no change, and those below it a deterioration following surgery. (C) cataract; (D) retina detached; (P) macular pucker

## Posterior retinal breaks

Silicone oil has a role in the treatment of certain other complex retinal detachments associated with breaks and traction in the posterior retina. Such breaks can be very difficult to close by explants and, when surface or anteroposterior traction is present, their closure by internal tamponade with air or sulphur hexafluoride gas may be only temporary. In these cases silicone oil is a useful alternative and the greater the degree of retinal immobility the greater the indication for its use. Thus detachments associated with posterior breaks in penetrating trauma, myopic staphylomata and proliferative diabetic retinopathy (PDR) or in conjunction with choroidal colobomata, often respond better to silicone oil injection than to internal gas tamponade.

## TECHNIQUES OF SILICONE OIL INJECTION

The principle of successful oil injection is the complete exchange of the fluid in the preretinal space with oil. In the absence of vitrectomy, it is important to remove as much retrohyaloid fluid and subretinal fluid as possible in order to achieve a maximum-size oil globule, and therefore a correspondingly minimum volume of residual fluid. If large volumes of retrohyaloid fluid remain, residual peripheral retinal traction elevates retinal breaks and the fluid becomes redistributed in the subretinal space, causing redetachment of the retina (*Figure 12.3*). Small quantities

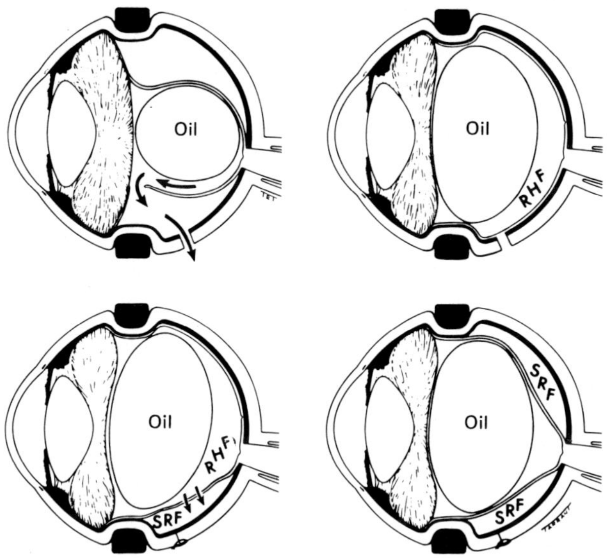


*Figure 12.3* Diagrams showing successful reattachment of the shortened retina by silicone oil initially followed by redistribution of residual retrohyaloid fluid (RHF) to the subretinal space (SRF) postoperatively

of subretinal fluid remaining at the end of surgery will absorb provided the retinal breaks are sealed. However, continuing peripheral circumferential traction tends to hold the retina elevated inferiorly if fluid remains at the end of the operation and occasionally the inferior retina re-elevates in spite of complete subretinal fluid drainage.

Because silicone oil has a lower specific gravity than water the oil globule tends to fill the superior vitreous cavity when fluid replacement is incomplete so that the oil tamponades the superior more than the inferior retina. Provided the macular area is attached the functional result reflects anatomical reapposition of the superior and central retina; the permanent nature of silicone oil tamponade prevents redetachment in the large majority of cases, so that persistence of subretinal fluid inferiorly is of no clinical importance. Unlike conventional surgery where persistence of subretinal fluid indicates an open retinal break, it does not have the same significance after oil injection.

When injecting silicone oil it may be necessary to buckle large retinal breaks to prevent the oil from passing into the subretinal space. Although the surface properties of the oil tend to maintain the integrity of the single globule, where retinal rigidity and shortening is severe it is sometimes possible for oil to be forced through a large tear, and an encircling buckle enhanced with additional silastic sponges or circumferential solid silicone gutters is used to seal such tears. Small holes similar to those in lattice degeneration do not usually require buckling.

Retrohyaloid fluid can be evacuated with a hollow needle, helped by gentle external ocular pressure. However, problems can be encountered if vitreous gel becomes impacted in the needle tip before it reaches the retrohyaloid space. In order to minimize this it is advisable to use a sharp 20-gauge hypodermic needle rather than a blunt-tipped needle. Once the retrohyaloid fluid has been removed its volume should be replaced with oil, thus restoring the intraocular pressure and assisting in the subsequent drainage of subretinal fluid.

If there is massive periretinal proliferation, it is advisable to perform the sclerotomy in an area of marked retinal immobility as this allows the majority of the fluid to be drained. The retina reattaches first in areas of greatest mobility and, therefore, if a drainage site is chosen in an area of mobile retina, subretinal fluid is likely to become sequestered under the more rigid areas. Once the retina flattens over the draining sclerotomy, a further drain site has to be chosen in order to obtain further retinal flattening. Silicone oil should be injected simultaneously in order to prevent hypotony and to provide drainage by gentle positive pressure applied to the inner retinal surface.

Recently, a more sophisticated method has been developed, particularly useful in the treatment of giant retinal tears, which combines vitrectomy and membranectomy with silicone oil injection (Lean *et al.*, 1982). This technique offers a more complete exchange of fluid for oil in the preretinal space, internal rather than external drainage of subretinal fluid using the operating microscope, and greater control of the oil injection through a sclerotomy cannula (*Figure 12.4*).

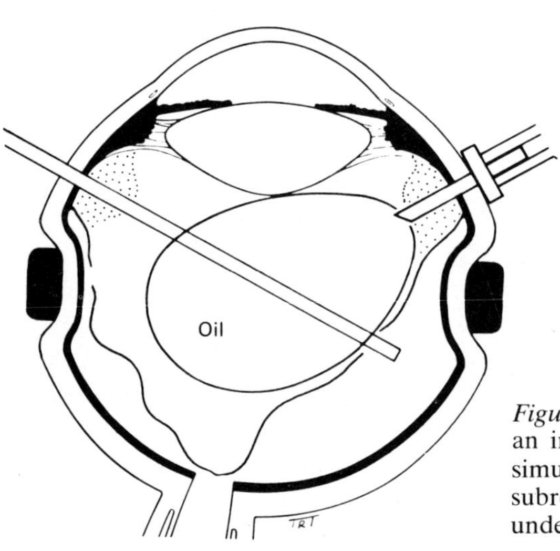


*Figure 12.4* Injection of silicone oil through an infusion cannula in the pars plana with simultaneous drainage of the preretinal and subretinal spaces using a Charles flute needle under microscopic control

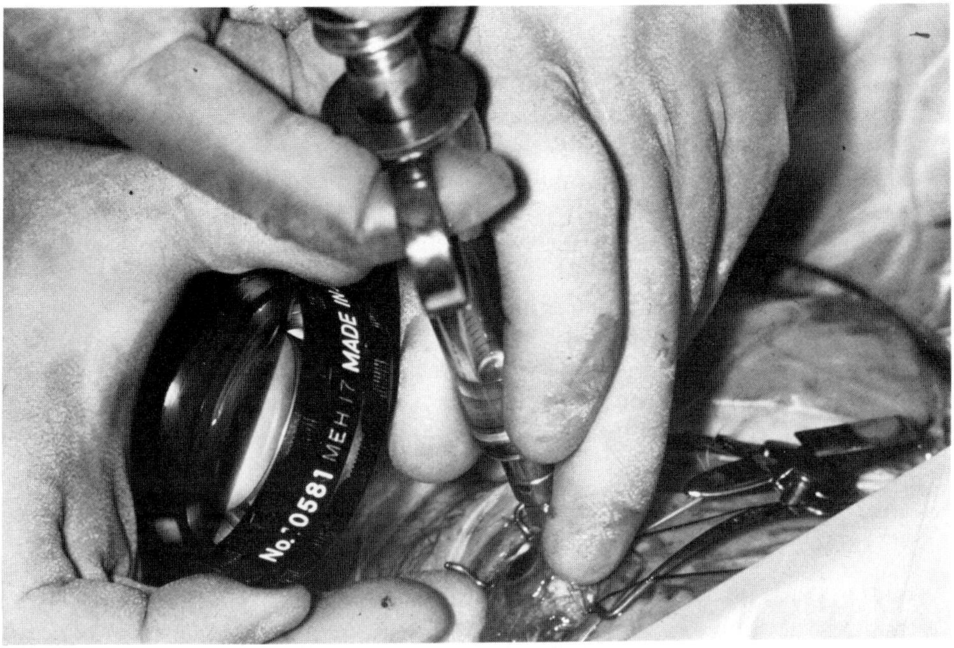


*Figure 12.5* Glass three-ring syringe operated by the assistant under indirect ophthalmoscopic control by the surgeon

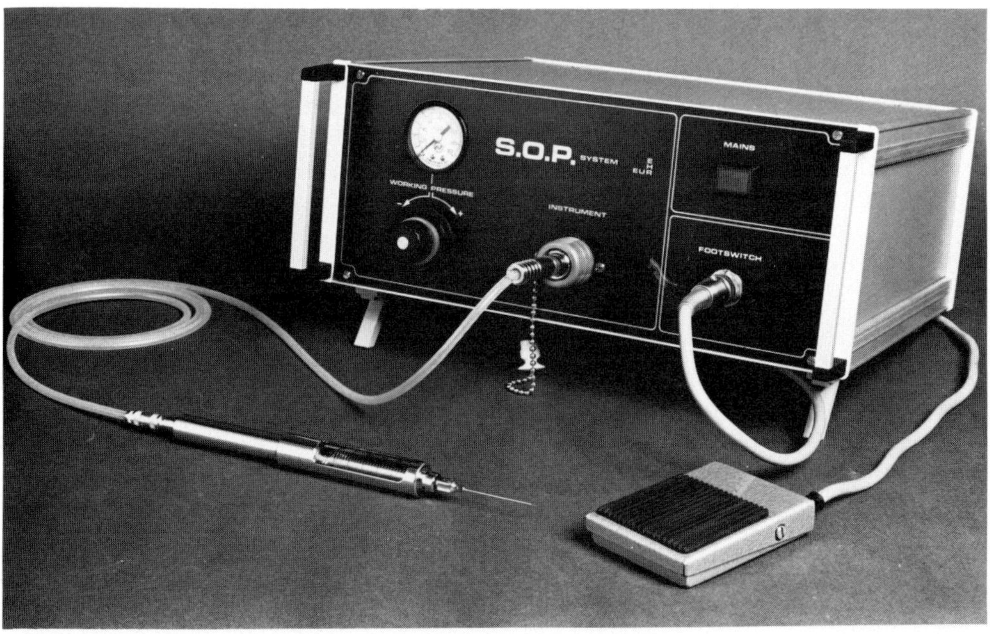


*Figure 12.6* Silicone oil pressure (SOP) unit with syringe powered by compressed air. (Courtesy of Mr G. Vijfvinkel and Medical Workshops Ltd.)

The posterior flap of a giant tear can be unfolded and replaced directly using a bimanual intraocular microsurgical technique, whilst the entire preretinal space is filled with silicone oil under microscopic control. In order to prevent further extension, the ends of the giant tear are supported by explants and a circumferential buckle is used to support the peripheral retina inferiorly. Buckling of the sclera in the bed of the giant tear is normally not indicated as it frequently jeopardizes the success of surgery. Indentation of the sclera produces folding of the retina, preventing its reapposition to the pigment epithelium and permanent adhesion by cryopexy.

The oil may be injected either manually by means of a reinforced glass syringe (*Figure 12.5*) or by a mechanized pressure unit designed for the purpose (*Figure 12.6*). The syringe, manually operated by the assistant, is cumbersome which makes it difficult to control the needle tip in the retrohyaloid space. The purpose-built but more expensive pressure units allow perfect control of injection by the surgeon.

## COMPLICATIONS OF SILICONE OIL INJECTION

### Operative complications

#### Haemorrhage

Silicone oil injection is frequently associated with small retinal haemorrhages which absorb postoperatively and do not produce long-term effects. Severe choroidal haemorrhage may occur during the operation, reducing the potential volume for oil replacement within the eye. Such haemorrhages can be prevented partially by careful attention to the sclerotomy during external drainage and by avoiding hypotony. Sclerotomy is best performed under the microscope, allowing the surgeon to identify large choroidal vessels which may then be cauterized. Hypotony is difficult to avoid throughout the entire procedure, but external pressure on the eye during retrohyaloid fluid removal and simultaneous injection of oil during subretinal fluid drainage is helpful.

#### Tear formation

Silicone oil can enter the subretinal space during the operation due either to failure to close an existing tear or to the development of a new tear in shortened retina during the operation. Fresh tears developing during the operation are usually a sign of gross preretinal retraction and in the majority of such cases the procedure has to be abandoned. When an existing break in shortened retina is not closed subretinal oil can be drained, the tear sealed by an explant and the procedure continued.

#### Entry into anterior chamber

In some aphakic eyes oil enters the anterior chamber during surgery. This unusual occurrence is rarely troublesome as the oil usually passes back into the vitreous cavity and becomes incorporated into the main globule in the early postoperative period.

## Postoperative complications

### Cataract

The major long-term complication of silicone oil injection is the development of cataract. In cases with a successful surgical outcome, approximately 55 per cent of phakic eyes will develop some degree of lens changes from 6 to 18 months after oil injection (Leaver, Grey and Garner, 1979). However, it is only in a minority of cases that the degree of cataract becomes significant. The earliest visible lens change is posterior subcapsular vacuolation (*Figure 12.7*). This sometimes occurs soon after surgery and disappears, but usually progresses to posterior subcapsular opacity and, on some occasions, to dense cataract.

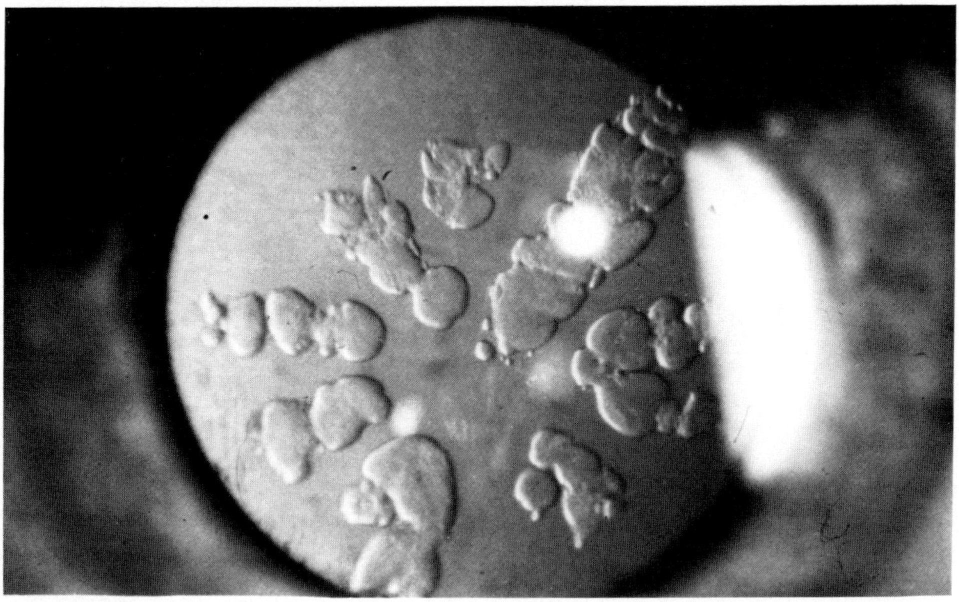

*Figure 12.7* Posterior subcapsular lens vacuoles after silicone oil injection

When the cataract interferes with vision extraction can be undertaken without undue difficulty. The extracapsular approach has been the method of choice until recently, but some surgeons express a preference for a routine intracapsular technique.

### Silicone oil in the anterior chamber

In approximately one-third of patients small oil droplets can be detected in the superior anterior chamber angle on gonioscopy (Leaver, Grey and Garner, 1979). This incidence is not increased by aphakia and the presence of these small droplets is of no serious clinical significance. The droplets may become numerous and circulate in the anterior chamber similar to inflammatory cells in anterior uveitis.

## Glaucoma

Glaucoma develops in some patients following silicone oil injection, and the role of these droplets in its causation has been studied. However, the number of patients with droplets in the anterior chamber greatly exceeds the number of patients with glaucoma. In the author's experience the incidence of glaucoma is 15 per cent but in the majority of cases there is pre-existing chronic simple glaucoma, or a significant degree of chronic angle closure in aphakic eyes. The number of cases in which droplets of oil can be incriminated as the most likely cause of glaucoma is less than 5 per cent. The management of patients with raised intraocular pressure after silicone oil injection is similar to that of other patients with glaucoma. Medical therapy is generally effective but on rare occasions trabeculectomy has been used to good effect, although this carries the risk of oil entering the anterior chamber.

## Keratopathy

A single large globule of oil enters the anterior chamber in 8 per cent of cases. The majority of such eyes are aphakic and the absence of the lens appears to result in

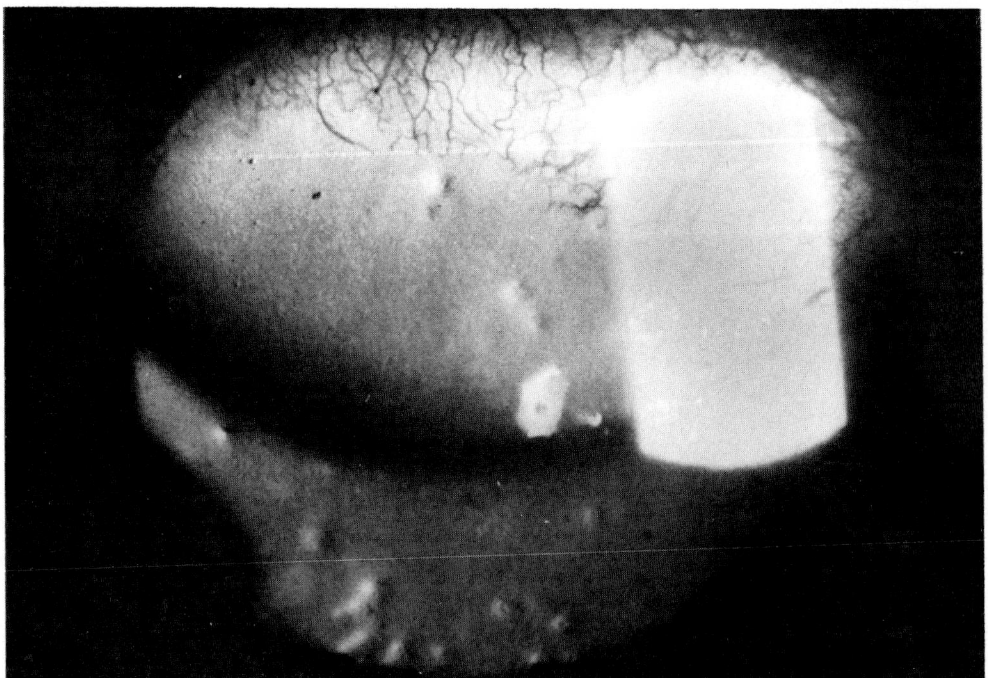

*Figure 12.8* Vascularized keratopathy related to silicone oil in contact with the corneal endothelium superiorly. (From Leaver, Grey and Garner (1979), courtesy of the Editor and Publishers, *British Journal of Ophthalmology*)

loss of a mechanical barrier holding the oil in the vitreous cavity. This complication can lead to the development of band-shaped or vascularized keratopathy. The mechanism of this typical keratopathy is not fully understood but appears to relate to the mechanical pressure of oil against the endothelium. When the oil touches only the upper endothelium, the area of cornea in contact with the oil vascularizes first (*Figure 12.8*). Vessels grow into the superficial stroma from the limbus, producing stromal oedema and such eyes can be extremely painful. Early keratopathy sometimes resolves if the oil is removed from the anterior chamber, but dense opacification or severe pain may have to be treated by keratoplasty.

### Retinal toxicity

In the author's experience there is no evidence that silicone oil is retinotoxic, despite earlier reports (Lee *et al.*, 1969; Mukai *et al.*, 1975; Mukai and Schepens, 1972). Electroretinographic studies have to be interpreted with care as silicone oil is an electrical insulator (Constable, Mohammed and Tan, 1982), but there is mounting experimental and clinical evidence that electrical activity is restored to the retina which has been reattached by silicone oil (Leaver, Grey and Garner, 1979). Histology of the retina has been carried out on severely disorganized eyes which have required enucleation. Droplets of oil can be found in the preretinal fibrous membranes and amongst the Muller cells, but there is no intracellular invasion of the retina by oil and no inflammatory reaction to suggest toxicity.

Although there is a high complication rate after silicone oil injection, the complications usually respond well to conventional treatment. Such complications are acceptable in eyes otherwise blinded by recurrent retinal detachment. Future developments may show that silicone oil injection should be followed by removal of the oil a few months later. Such removal could prevent the long-term complications and allow the retina to remain reattached long enough for active preretinal fibrosis to become quiescent so that removal of the oil would not result in subsequent retinal detachment.

## CONCLUSION

Silicone oil injection is an effective method of reattaching the retina when conventional procedures have either failed or are likely to fail. Owing to the poor state of the macula in many of these cases, recovery of central visual acuity is limited, but a large area of visual field and navigating vision can usually be restored (*Figure 12.9*). Silicone oil injection should be used to treat patients blind from detachment in one eye who develop detachment in their second eye with preretinal fibrosis and shortening. It should also be considered in patients with complicated detachments in whom there is an appreciable risk of detachment in the fellow eye from high myopia or extensive lattice degeneration.

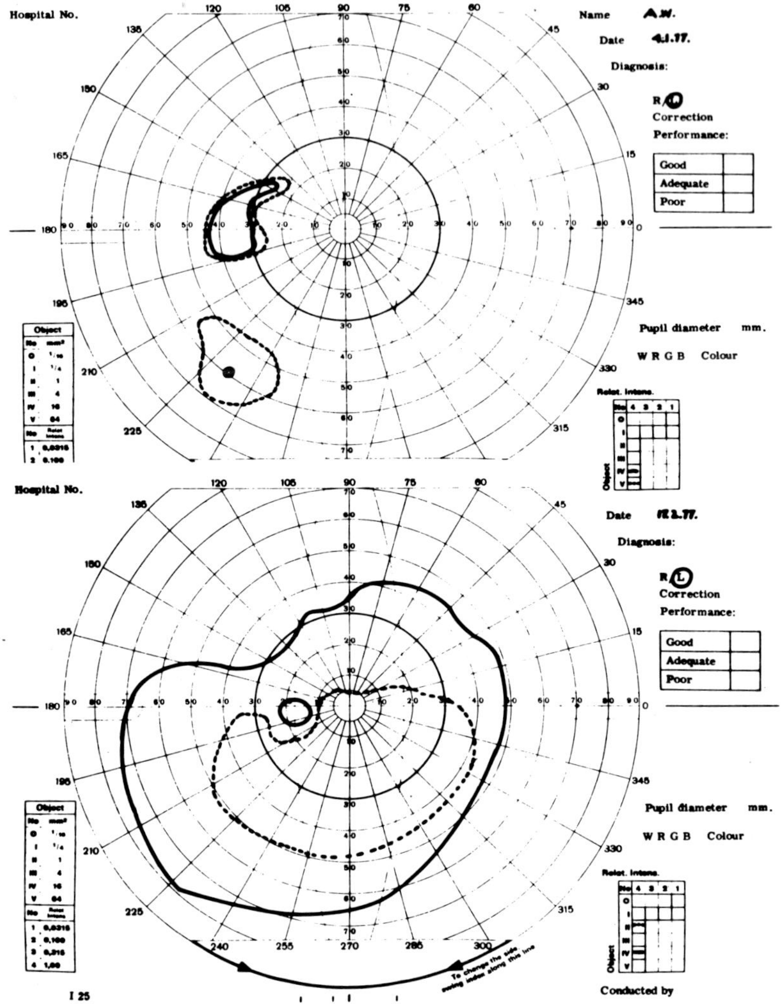


*Figure 12.9* Example of improvement in visual field in a patient with massive periretinal proliferation after reattachment of the retina with silicone oil. (From Grey and Leaver (1977), courtesy of the Editor and Publishers, *Transactions of the Ophthalmological Society of the United Kingdom*)

## References

Cibis, P. A., Becker, B., Okun, E. and Canaan, S. (1962) The use of liquid silicone in retinal detachment surgery. *Archives of Ophthalmology*, **68**, 590–599

Constable, I., Mohammed, S. and Tan, P. L. (1982) Super viscous silicone liquid in retinal surgery. *Australian Journal of Ophthalmology*, **10**, 5–11

Dufour, R. (1964) L'injection intra-vitréene de silicone liquide dans le décollement rétinique déséspéré. *Ophthalmologica (Basel)*, **147**, 160–166

Grey, R. H. B. and Leaver, P. K. (1977) Results of silicone oil injection in massive preretinal retraction. *Transactions of the Ophthalmological Society of the United Kingdom*, **97**, 238–241

Grey, R. H. B. and Leaver, P. K. (1979) Silicone oil in the treatment of massive preretinal retraction. I. Results in 105 eyes. *British Journal of Ophthalmology*, **63**, 355–360

Kanski, J. and Daniel, R. (1973) Intravitreal silicone injection in retinal detachment. *British Journal of Ophthalmology*, **57**, 542–545

Lean, J. S., Leaver, P. K., Cooling, R. J. and McLeod, D. (1982) Management of complex retinal detachments by vitrectomy and fluid/silicone exchange. *Transactions of the Ophthalmological Society of the United Kingdom*, **102**, 203–205

Leaver, P. K., Grey, R. H. B. and Garner, A. (1979) Silicone oil injection in the treatment of massive preretinal retraction. II. Late complications in 93 eyes. *British Journal of Ophthalmology*, **63**, 361–367

Leaver, P. K. and Lean, J. S. (1981) Management of giant retinal tears using vitrectomy/silicone oil/fluid exchange. *Transactions of the Ophthalmological Society of the United Kingdom*, **101**, 189–191

Lee, P. F., Donovan, R. H., Mukai, N., Schepens, C. L. and Freeman, H. M. (1969) Intravitreal injection of silicone oil; an experimental study. I. Clinical picture and histology of the eye. *Annals of Ophthalmology*, **1** (2), 15–25

Mukai, N., Lee, P. F., Oguri, M. and Schepens, C. L. (1975) A long-term evaluation of silicone retinopathy in the monkey. *Canadian Journal of Ophthalmology*, **10**, 391–401

Mukai, N. and Schepens, C. L. (1972) Intravitreous injection of silicone: an experimental study. *Annals of Ophthalmology*, **4**, 273–287

Okun, E. (1968) Intravitreal surgery using liquid silicone. *Transactions of the Pacific Coast Oto-ophthalmological Society*, **49**, 141–159

Rosengren, B. (1966) Intravitreal injection of liquid silicone for retinal detachment. *Acta Ophthalmologica (Kbh.)*, **Suppl. 84**, 975–976

Scott, J. D. (1972) Treatment of the detached immobile retina. *Transactions of the Ophthalmological Society of the United Kingdom*, **92**, 351–357

Scott, J. D. (1973) The treatment of massive vitreous retraction. *Transactions of the Ophthalmological Society of the United Kingdom*, **93**, 417–423

Scott, J. D. (1974) Macular holes and retinal detachment. *Transactions of the Ophthalmological Society of the United Kingdom*, **94**, 319–324

Stone, W. (1958) Alloplasty in surgery of the eye. *New England Journal of Medicine*, **258**, 486–533

Watzke, R. C. (1967) Silicone retinopiesis. *Archives of Ophthalmology*, **77**, 185–196

# 13

# Closed intraocular microsurgery for advanced diabetic eye disease

D. McLeod

## SURGICAL PATHOLOGY

The potentially blinding sequelae of proliferative diabetic retinopathy (PDR), *vitreous haemorrhage and tractional retinal detachment*, provide vitreoretinal surgeons with a substantial part of their workload. A thorough understanding of the pathogenesis and surgical pathology of severe diabetic eye disease is essential for patient management.

### Extraretinal neovascularization

The proliferative phase of diabetic retinopathy is characterized by multiple outgrowths of vascular mesenchyme through the inner limiting lamina of the retina, so-called extraretinal neovascularization. The new vessels usually arise from retinal veins and venules, though a choroidal origin has been demonstrated in some patients with disc neovascularization or after heavy photocoagulation of the retina. The neovascularization appears to be a response to retinal capillary non-perfusion and ischaemia, which in diabetes is characteristically initially located in the midperipheral retina, with later central encroachment (Shimizu, Kobayashi and Muraoka, 1981). There is as yet no clear evidence of an association between extraretinal neovascularization and so-called 'intraretinal neovascularization', which may be looked upon simply as a process of vascular remodelling deep to the inner limiting lamina within areas of capillary non-perfusion. It has been postulated that a 'vasoproliferative factor', produced in ischaemic retina, is responsible for stimulating neovascularization; certainly extracts of the vitreous from eyes with PDR encourage neovascularization experimentally.

Once the vascular mesenchyme has penetrated the inner limiting lamina, 'flat new vessels' proliferate on the retinal surface within the most cortical part of the vitreous gel as vascularized epiretinal membranes. The vessels do not penetrate into the central gel, except occasionally within Cloquet's canal (McMeel, 1971), owing to either inhibitory substances within the gel or the absence of a suitable gel scaffolding. Wherever a vascularized epiretinal membrane proliferates, cortical gel becomes incarcerated within the membrane (Foos, 1974). Since the membrane adheres to the retina at points of laminar dehiscence and tissue outgrowth, an exaggerated attachment develops between the vitreous and retina via such a membrane, and this adhesion resists vitreoretinal separation. The membranes, together with the annular vitreoretinal adhesion at the vitreous base (*Figure 13.1a*), constitute the anchoring zones upon which vitreoretinal traction systems are subsequently founded.

The endothelium of new vessels within an epiretinal membrane has no well-developed tight junctions so that serum transudes into the gel (as demonstrated by fluorescein angiography). In addition to the vascular component of the membrane,

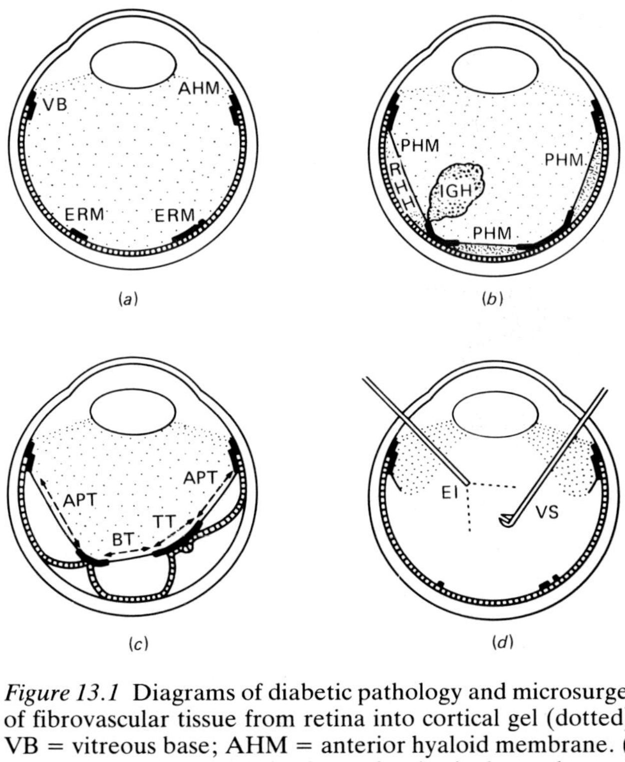


*Figure 13.1* Diagrams of diabetic pathology and microsurgery. (*a*) Two posterior outgrowths of fibrovascular tissue from retina into cortical gel (dotted). ERM = epiretinal membrane; VB = vitreous base; AHM = anterior hyaloid membrane. (*b*) Incomplete posterior vitreous detachment with avulsed edges of epiretinal membranes, 'cone' and 'trampoline' membranes, and haemorrhage. PHM = posterior hyaloid membrane; IGH = intragel haemorrhage; RHH = retrohyaloid haemorrhage. (*c*) Two posterior tractional retinal detachments with apical (*left*) or truncated (*right*) vitreoretinal interfaces. APT = anteroposterior traction; BT = bridging traction; TT = tangential traction. (*d*) Closed intraocular microsurgery via pars plana, with circumcision and segmentation of epiretinal membranes and retinal reattachment. EI = endoilluminator; VS = vitreous scissors

there is a fibroblastic component which, in keeping with other epiretinal membranes, has the potential for contraction (*Figure 13.2*). The ensuing tangential (or surface) retinal traction is mediated by intracellular filaments (Wallow, Greaser and Stevens, 1981), and the fibroblasts are also responsible for collagen synthesis. The collagen fibres consolidate and stabilize tangential traction on the underlying retina exerted by cellular contraction. At an early stage of neovascularization,

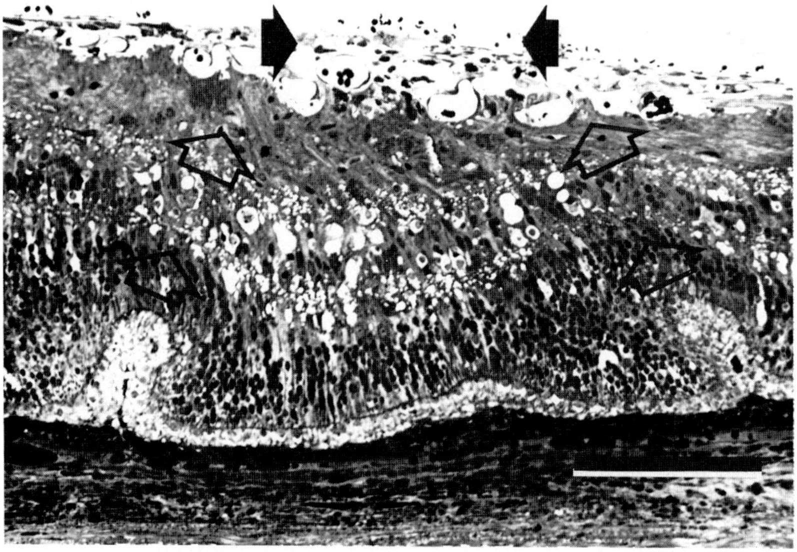

*Figure 13.2* Light micrograph. Fibrovascular epiretinal membrane (closed arrows), with wrinkling of retinal surface; transmission of tangential traction forces through retina (open arrows), with folding of external limiting membrane. (From McLeod, Marshall and Grierson, 1981, courtesy of the Editor and Publishers, *Transactions of the Ophthalmological Societies of the United Kingdom*)

panretinal photocoagulation may arrest or reverse at least the vascular component of the membrane. It also has a favourable influence on the process of fibroblast proliferation and contraction. Once fibroblastic activity is well established, however, photocoagulation is less effective and in some circumstances appears to enhance or accelerate membrane contraction. Argon laser photocoagulation appears to be less dangerous than xenon arc photocoagulation, while trans-scleral panretinal cryotherapy has a particularly sinister reputation in this respect. When the membrane is well established, much larger vessels may be visible in its central part, their size sometimes exceeding that of the underlying intraretinal vasculature. These large vessels may remain visible within the membrane despite spontaneous or photocoagulation-induced arrest of active capillary proliferation at the edge of the membrane.

It should be appreciated that epiretinal vasoproliferation is dependent upon gel–retina contact (McLeod and Restori, 1981). In the absence of gel or after complete posterior vitreous detachment, such proliferation either does not occur or is restricted to localized 'abortive' outgrowths. This peculiar, unexplained and crucial aspect of the biological behaviour of extraretinal neovascularization is evident from examination of diabetic eyes before, during and after vitrectomy (Michels, 1978), and is also demonstrable in cases of retinal branch vein occlusion with extensive capillary closure (Shilling, McLeod and Restori, 1979; Trempe, Takahashi and Topilow, 1981). Thus, complete posterior vitreous detachment not only prevents any possible vitreoretinal tractional consequences of neovascularization (Scott, 1969; Foos, 1974), but also precludes significant extension of new vessels over the retinal surface and any consequent tangential traction. This phenomenon explains many cases of diabetic rubeosis which present with little or no associated PDR. Apparent exceptions, notably the vascularized membranes occasionally discovered during vitrectomy in the posterior pole behind detached gel, can probably be explained by 'delamination' of attenuated cortical vitreous from the underlying membrane owing to eccentric, asymmetrical contraction in a contiguous part of the membrane.

Proliferations originating from multiple fibrovascular outgrowths often coalesce to form widespread sheets of vascularized tissue covering the retinal surface. The membranes are most commonly located at and around the optic disc, nasal to the disc and along the major temporal vascular arcades. However, no part of the retina is immune, and vascularized membranes sometimes develop over the macula, and even peripherally in the immediately post-basal region. The major complications of PDR are vitreous haemorrhage, vitreoretinal traction and retinal break formation, the last two processes resulting in retinal detachment. Each of these complications tends to be associated with detachment of the vitreous (Davis, 1965), though there are exceptions. Whether posterior vitreous detachment in diabetic eyes is stimulated by retinal ischaemia, by changes in the gel from protein insudation, or by a distant effect of tangential traction exerted by epiretinal membranes is still unclear. When vitreous detachment occurs, it is *incomplete* owing to exaggerated vitreoretinal adhesions at each site of vasoproliferation (except in those rare instances where a vascularized membrane avulses completely from the retinal surface and comes to lie as a 'ghost membrane' on the detached posterior hyaloid face). Usually, however, only the *edges* of epiretinal membranes become avulsed, and these spring forward in the plane of the detached posterior hyaloid membrane as 'forward new vessels' (*see Figure 13.1b*).

Once the vitreous has detached as far as the vitreoretinal adhesions allow, no further surface vasoproliferation occurs. Nevertheless, forward new vessels, in continuity with vascularized epiretinal membranes at their base and the original vascular outgrowths from the retina, may proliferate anteriorly along the detached posterior hyaloid interface. The vessels may be observed to 'sway' in concert with gel movements after ocular saccades; alternatively, marked contraction and collagen synthesis in a frond of forward vessels may result in an immobile 'stalk' connecting the gel to the retina or disc. Further anteriorly, non-vascular proliferation of cells and collagen synthesis may also occur, resulting in a taut 'fibrocellular' membrane connecting the vitreous base anteriorly with the edges of the vascularized tissue posteriorly (*Figure 13.3a*). Machemer has coined the term 'trampoline membrane' to describe a similar structure bridging the macula between vascular-

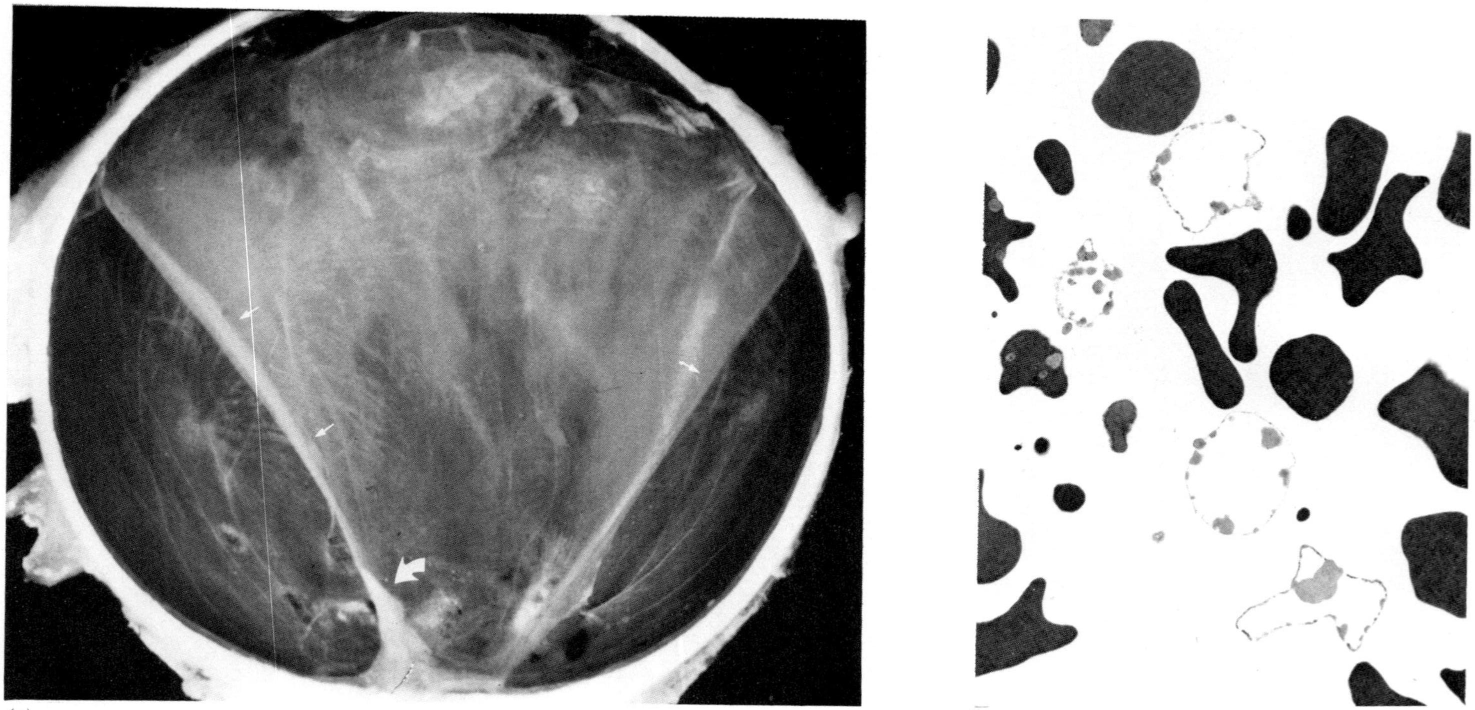

(a) (b)

*Figure 13.3* (*a*) Hemisected globe with incomplete posterior vitreous detachment and ischaemic retina; fibrocellular (small arrows) and fibrovascular (curved arrow) components of posterior hyaloid cone; focal (*right*) and wide (*centre*) vitreoretinal adhesions. (*b*) Electronmicrograph of vitreous haemorrhage; erythrocytes and erythroclasts. (Courtesy of Dr G. Glover and Dr I. Grierson)

ized membranes along the superior and inferior temporal vascular arcades (*see Figure 13.1b*). Immobilization of the vitreous results purely from the contraction process along its boundaries. Unless invaded by haemorrhage, with ensuing syneresis, the gel itself has a normal consistency and should not be thought of as having actively contracted, though the volume occupied by gel is undoubtedly diminished.

## Vitreous haemorrhage

Intravitreal bleeding is frequently associated with vitreous detachment and avulsion of the edge of a fibrovascular membrane (*see Figure 13.1b*). It arises either from capillaries within the membrane or from stem vessels growing out of the retina. However, other factors, such as hypoglycaemia and hypotony, may also predispose to bleeding and it is generally believed that new vessels on the disc are more prone to haemorrhage than those in the periphery. Bleeding may occur into the vitreous gel itself (intragel haemorrhage) or, more frequently, into the retrohyaloid compartment (*Figures 13.1b* and *13.4a*). Nevertheless, retrohyaloid haemorrhage may penetrate into the vitreous gel through dehiscences in the continuity of the detached vitreous, for example via a hiatus in the cortical gel frequently present in the macular area (Davis, 1965). The blood initially clots, but in the subsequent few days undergoes fibrinolysis. Within the gel this results in diffuse blood-staining, while red blood cells loculated in the retrohyaloid compartment often sediment out from the defibrinated plasma to form a red carpet over the retina. The interface between plasma and red cells produces a fluid level on B-scan ultrasound examination (*Figure 13.4d*) which flows or 'creeps' over the retina in response to gravitational forces (McLeod and Restori, 1979).

In addition to fibrinolysis, the red cells undergo a form of haemolysis (Forrester, Grierson and Lee, 1978), with release of pigmented haemoglobin breakdown products and transformation of the biconcave erythrocytes into spheroidal erythroclasts (*see Figure 13.3b*). The blood-stained gel may take on an ochre-yellow, grey or white colour, with erythroclasts clogging the cortical gel to form an 'ochre membrane' (Smith, Van Heuven and Streeten, 1976) tethered by a fibrovascular adhesion to the retina or disc (*Figure 13.4b*). The retrohyaloid space may be similarly silted up with free erythroclasts.

The mechanism of spontaneous clearing of vitreous haemorrhage is uncertain, though macrophages undoubtedly play a part: however, erythroclasts appear to be less digestible than erythrocytes. Retrohyaloid haemorrhage tends to clear more quickly than intragel haemorrhage. Some red cells seem to escape via the anterior chamber and trabecular meshwork (especially in aphakic eyes), and blood pigments may diffuse anteriorly to stain the iris stroma, causing haemosiderosis iridis. However, to what extent blood pigments truly stain (and irreversibly damage) the *retina* during persistence of vitreous haemorrhage is unclear. In clinical practice, this seldom appears to be of importance.

Although the presence of haemorrhage has been implicated as a stimulus to fibrosis *after trauma*, it is not known whether vitreous haemorrhage influences the

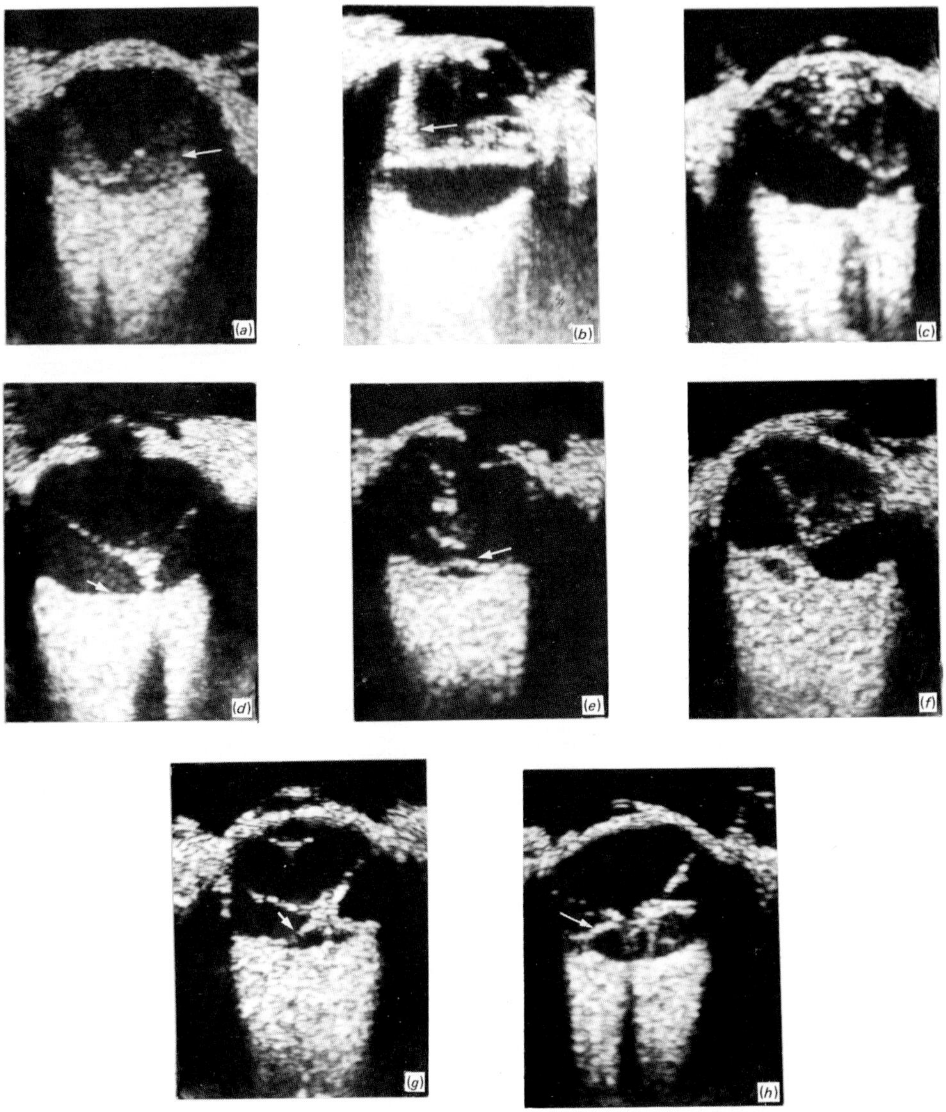


*Figure 13.4* Horizontal B-scan ultrasound sections. (*a*) Retrohyaloid haemorrhage (arrow) and echo-free gel; vitreopapillary adhesion. (*b*) Eye deviated right; intragel haemorrhage and ochre membrane (arrow) with focal attachment to retina posteriorly. (*c*) Intragel haemorrhage tethering to wide zone of epiretinal fibrosis nasal to the disc; clear retrohyaloid compartment. (*d*) Retrohyaloid haemorrhage with fluid level over macula (arrow); stalk-like vitreopapillary attachment of posterior hyaloid cone. (*e*) Intragel haemorrhage and localized traction retinal detachment in posterior pole (arrow). (*f*) Intragel haemorrhage and 'apical' attachment (in this plane) to traction retinal detachment. (*g*) Truncated vitreoretinal attachment with retinal surface showing anterior concavity (arrow). (*h*) 'Table-top' retinal detachment with retinal surface showing anterior convexity (arrow), implying a rhegmatogenous component. (From McLeod, Leaver and Feretis, 1980, courtesy of the Editor and Publishers, *Transactions of the Ophthalmological Societies of the United Kingdom*)

fibroblastic component of *diabetic* vascularized membranes. Intragel haemorrhage is a potent stimulus to posterior vitreous detachment, and as such paradoxically protects the retina from further epiretinal vasoproliferation. The use of the term *organization* of the vitreous in the context of diabetes is inappropriate; this term has a specific meaning in pathology, namely 'invasion of a haematoma by macrophages, capillaries and fibroblasts, with ultimate replacement of the haematoma by a fibrous scar'. In diabetic eye disease the central gel is not so invaded, and neovascularization is the *cause*, not the result, of vitreous haemorrhage.

## Retinal detachment

Diabetic retinal detachment seldom occurs in the absence of tangential traction on the underlying neuroepithelium by contracting epiretinal membranes. The greater the extent of epiretinal vasoproliferation, the greater the tendency to tractional detachment. Initially, the surface layers, i.e. the inner limiting lamina and the nerve-fibre layer, become wrinkled (*see Figure 13.2*), the intraretinal vasculature is distorted and retinal landmarks are displaced, for example ectopia of the macula (*Figure 13.5a*). Transmission of strong surface traction forces through the retina thereafter causes full thickness folding and detachment of the retina (*Figures 13.5b and c*). Other factors, however, may also be involved in causing retinal detachment. Traction may occur from contraction of fibroblastic elements along the detached posterior hyaloid interface (or cone) between the vitreous base anteriorly and the edges of the vitreoretinal adhesions posteriorly (anteroposterior traction). Traction also occurs between individual sites of posterior vasoproliferation (bridging traction) for example, via a premacular trampoline membrane (*see Figure 13.1c*). The detached (and possibly schitic) retina assumes an angular configuration with an anterior concavity of its surface (*see Figures 13.1c and 13.4e, f and g*). Where the epiretinal elements have a focal distribution, and anteroposterior tractional elements predominate, the apex of the posterior hyaloid cone inserts into the summit of the retinal elevation (*Figures 13.1c and 13.4f*). Where the epiretinal contraction is more widespread, the apex of the detachment is replaced by a plane surface or plateau, the apex of the posterior hyaloid cone being similarly truncated (*see Figures 13.1c, 13.4g and 13.5c*). Such truncation is most evident in the so-called 'table-top' configuration of detachment, which results from contraction of widespread coalescent membranes covering the postequatorial retina (*Figure 13.6; see also Figures 13.4g and h*).

Retinal breaks may also contribute to retinal elevation (*Figure 13.5d*). Indeed, formation of a break sometimes causes the retina to detach when no such complication would otherwise arise. Retinal breaks in PDR are characteristically small and oval, are located postequatorially adjacent to the avulsed edge of a vascularized epiretinal membrane (Davis, 1965) and are tractional rather than trophic in origin. Occasionally, however, huge breaks occur in atrophic retina, or peripheral tears may develop in relation to postbasal vitreoretinal adhesions associated with lattice degeneration. Full thickness macular holes are also occasionally seen.

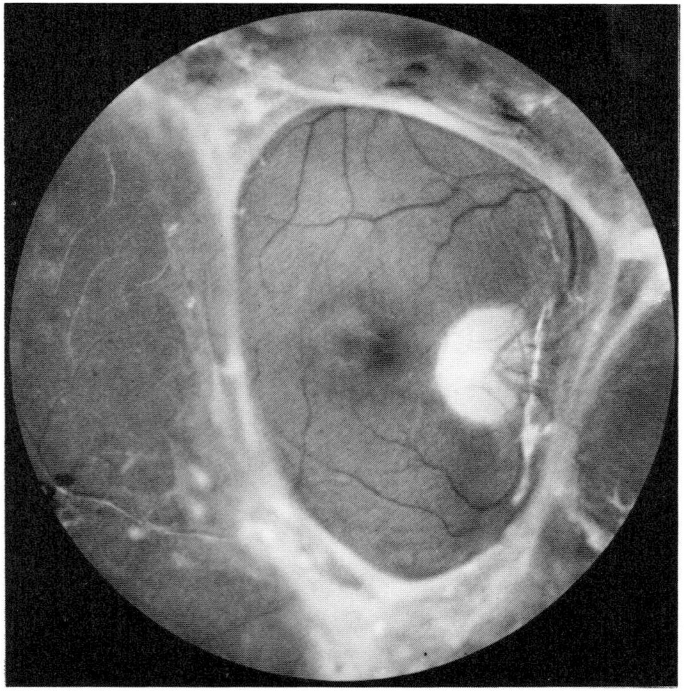

(a)

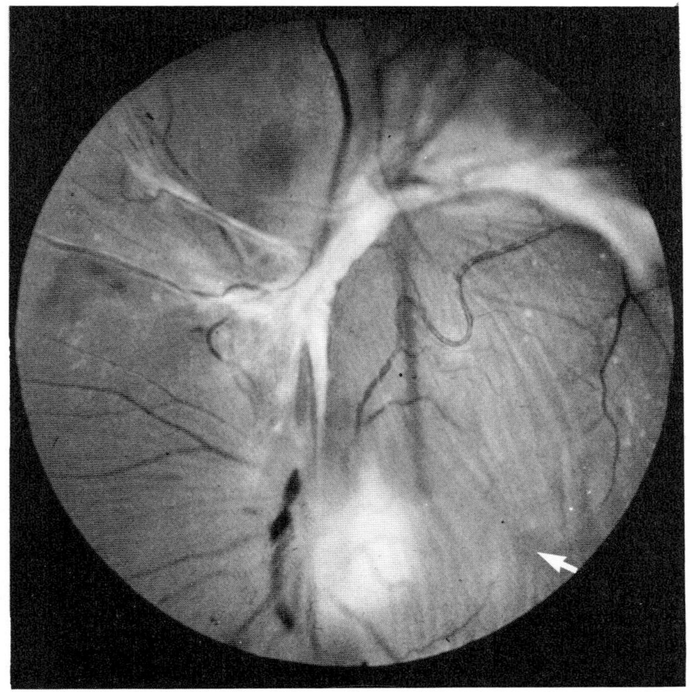

(b)

*Figure 13.5* Fundus photographs of diabetic detachments. (*a*) Ring of fibrovascular proliferation; shallow traction detachment peripheral to major vascular arcades; hiatus in central cortical gel reveals attached central retina, but nasal ectopia of macula including subfoveal pigment epithelium (acuity 6/9). (*b*) Surface wrinkling and detachment of posterior retina with fovea dragged nasally (arrow); narrow arch of contracted fibrovascular tissue along major superotemporal vein

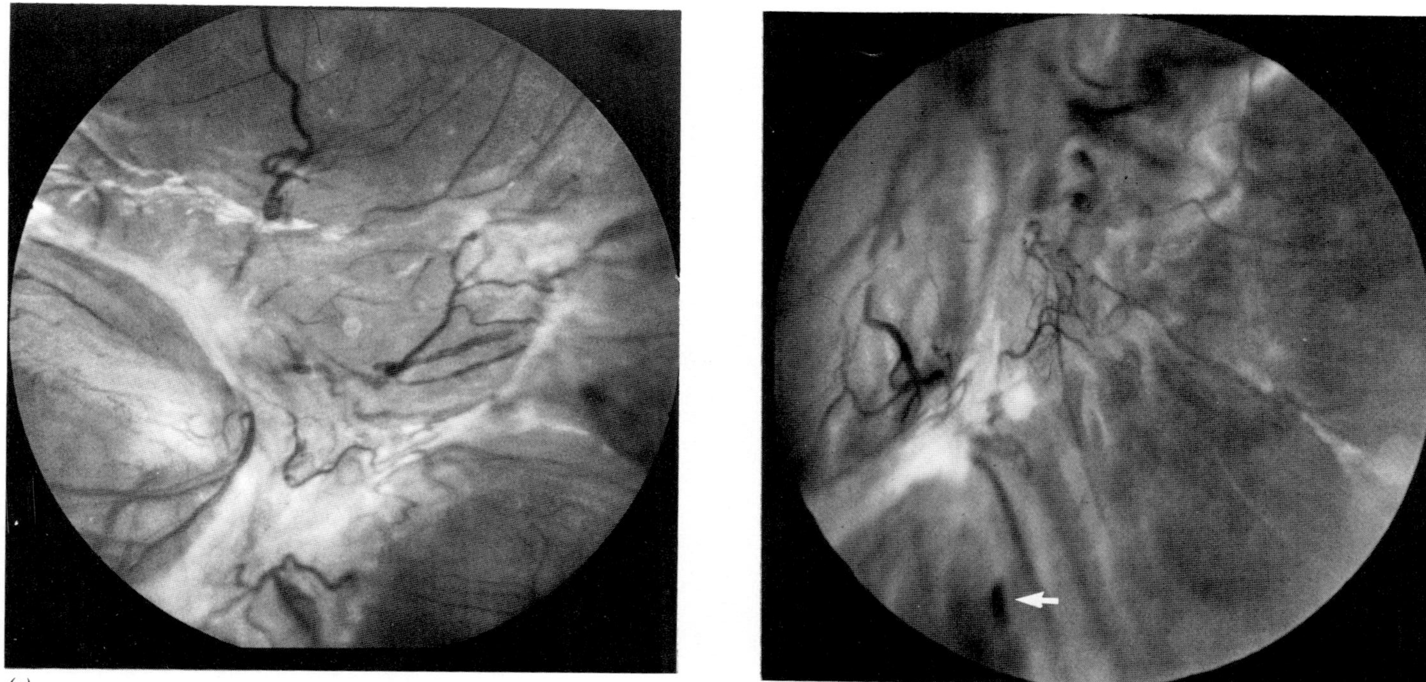

(c) (d)

*Figure 13.5* (*c*) Wide sheets of coalescent fibrovascular proliferation over detached peripapillary retina. (*d*) Bullous retinal detachment along inferior major vascular arcade, with oval break (arrow) just peripheral to contracted fibrovascular tissue. ((*b*) and (*c*) from Barrie *et al*., 1982, courtesy of the Editor and Publishers, *British Journal of Ophthalmology*)

A retinal break allows transfer of fluid from the retrohyaloid space into the subretinal space, and the retinal detachment usually (but not necessarily) becomes more extensive and has a bullous configuration (*see Figure 13.4h*). Anterior extension of detachment to the ora serrata is much more likely in such rhegmatogenous detachments than in pure traction detachments. If the retrohyaloid space contains haemorrhage at the time of break formation, the subretinal fluid may become blood-stained, and not infrequently such progression to a combined rhegmatogenous and traction retinal detachment accelerates clearance of haemorrhage from the eye. Thus, a patient presenting initially with a vitreous haemorrhage may subsequently have a clear vitreous and a detached retina. Because fluid in the retrohyaloid compartment empties into the subretinal space via the break, anteroposterior elements of traction may be less evident than previously; indeed, relaxation of the posterior hyaloid membrane may allow it to come into renewed contact with the retinal surface over a wide area.

Some diabetic retinal detachments are rapidly progressive whether due to formation of retinal breaks or overwhelming traction. Others, even rhegmatogenous detachments, are very stable, remaining unchanged in extent and elevation for months or years, with development of high-water marks and retinal atrophy (Davis, 1965). Because the macula is usually free of vasoproliferation, the

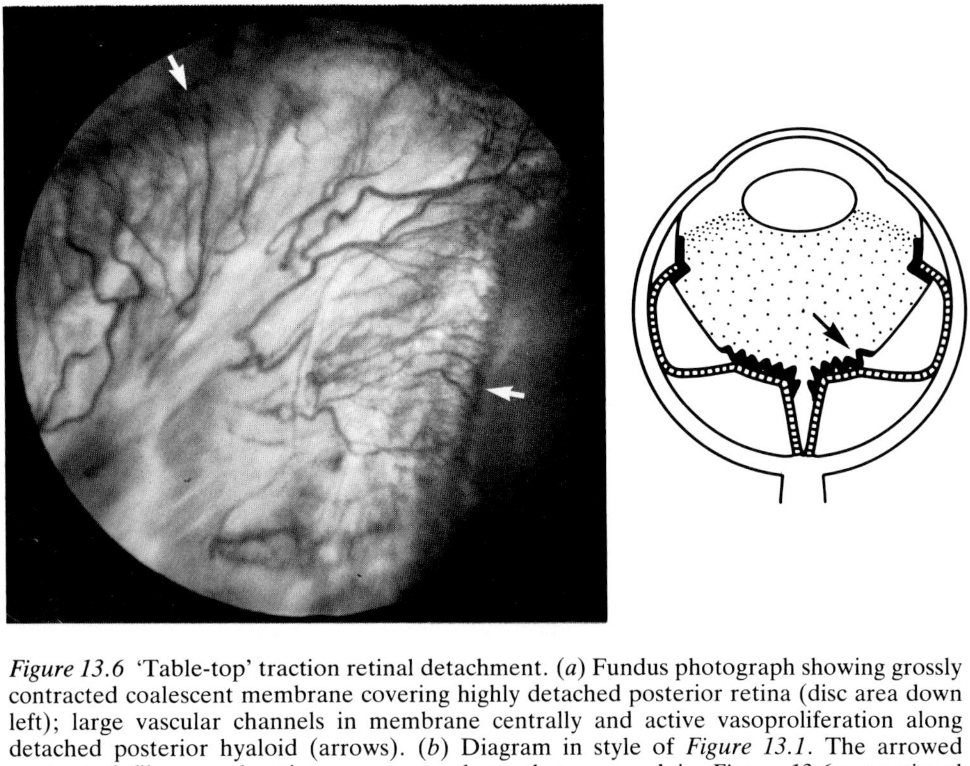

*Figure 13.6* 'Table-top' traction retinal detachment. (*a*) Fundus photograph showing grossly contracted coalescent membrane covering highly detached posterior retina (disc area down left); large vascular channels in membrane centrally and active vasoproliferation along detached posterior hyaloid (arrows). (*b*) Diagram in style of *Figure 13.1*. The arrowed contracted fibrovascular tissue corresponds to that arrowed in *Figure 13.6a*; tractional detachment in vitreous base region

fovea is often the last part of the posterior retina to become detached. Some detachments undergo spontaneous reattachment (Davis, 1965; McMeel, 1971; Tasman, 1972; Cohen, McMeel and Franks, 1979). This usually reflects further avulsion of fibrovascular epiretinal membranes from the retina so the area of surface traction and truncation is reduced. However, there is usually no functional recovery owing to atrophic changes in the reapposed retina and pigmented epithelium following prolonged detachment.

There are two circumstances in which retinal detachment is unlikely. Firstly, when the vitreous is attached posteriorly only at the optic disc (McMeel, 1971), and, secondly, when focal vitreous attachments over large veins cause the vessels to be drawn forwards into the vitreous cavity as 'vascular loops'. In all eyes with a mobile detached gel, however, dynamic traction may result in tearing of the retina along any irregularity of the posterior border of the vitreous base. Furthermore, static anteroposterior traction in an immobile cone may produce a traction detachment involving the oral retina (*see Figure 13.6b*). Such pathology increases the risk of entry site complications during pars plana microsurgery.

### Non-vascularized epiretinal proliferation

In addition to vascularized epiretinal proliferation, non-vascularized fibrocellular membranes may proliferate on the retinal surface (Lee, 1968; McMeel, 1971). Their development appears to be *independent* of gel–retina contact, as fibrocellular membranes proliferate both within attached cortical gel and posterior to a detached vitreous cortex. Epimacular membranes frequently occur in eyes in which the macula is surrounded by vascularized proliferations from the disc and temporal vascular arcades. The fibrocellular membranes appear to have less propensity to contract than fibrovascular membranes (McMeel, 1971).

Surprisingly, isolated macular pucker is relatively unusual in PDR, even though simple, non-contracting, glial epiretinal membranes and surface-wrinkling retinopathy are common features of the autopsied diabetic eye (Foos, 1974). Furthermore, proliferation of extensive non-vascularized epiretinal membranes producing a picture similar to that seen in massive periretinal proliferation (MPP) is extremely rare, even in eyes with combined rhegmatogenous and tractional detachment. However, a type of non-vascularized epiretinal proliferation – 'reparative fibrosis' – is an important complication of surgical dissection of diabetic epiretinal membranes (*see below*), and may produce an MPP-like configuration of immobile detachment postoperatively.

## PRESURGICAL ASSESSMENT

Patients being considered for vitreoretinal surgery should give details of ocular symptoms and undergo a complete ophthalmic examination so that the indications for intervention and the likely prognosis can be determined.

## History

Particular attention should be paid to the onset, nature and duration of visual loss, and an attempt made to distinguish impaired vision due to haemorrhage from that due to retinal detachment. A record of the visual acuity prior to vitreous haemorrhage or macular detachment is of great value. Details of previous ocular treatment, for example photocoagulation, should be obtained.

## Visual function

The visual acuity in each eye is recorded, with careful assessment of those degrees of visual loss between 6/60 and finger counting; 3/60 is the least acuity for independent navigation. The swinging flashlight test comparing central function between eyes is frequently of value. Haemorrhage in the vitreous *scatters* light, rather than absorbing it like a neutral-density filter, and only the very densest of haemorrhages produce a relative afferent pupillary defect *per se*. It must be remembered, however, that an afferent defect is found after panretinal photocoagulation, and that its presence does not necessarily contraindicate surgery, for example if it results from macular detachment.

## Ocular examination

In the anterior segment, particular attention should be paid to the iris and lens. The iris in diabetes undergoes a number of changes in addition to the glycogen deposition in the pigmented epithelium which results in increased transillumination and pigment dispersion during mydriasis. Staining of the iris stroma by blood pigments (haemosiderosis) may complicate long-standing vitreous haemorrhage and its presence is felt by some to be a poor prognostic feature in that it may correlate with retinal toxicity from intravitreal blood. This issue has not been proven. Posterior synechiae from iritis, and miosis and immobility of the iris resulting from neuropathy/myopathy or stray photocoagulation, may result in poor pupillary dilatation. This may cause problems at surgery if the lens is to be spared. Before dilating the pupil, however, it is essential to assess the iris for rubeosis, which is almost certainly a distant response to retinal ischaemia. The small vessels at the pupil margin which constitute the earliest sign of rubeosis may become invisible after pupil dilatation, especially with vasoconstrictors like phenylephrine.

The degree of sclerosis of the lens nucleus is important in respect of difficulties likely to be encountered during phacoemulsification. Most eyes with more than minimal posterior subcapsular lens opacities will require lens removal, especially in preparation for a difficult epiretinal membrane dissection.

The posterior segment is examined by binocular indirect ophthalmoscopy and biomicroscopy using the Goldmann 3-mirror lens in order to determine the extent and distribution of fibrovascular proliferation, and the likelihood and location of retinal breaks. The overall configuration of tractional elements operating along the posterior hyaloid membrane and on the retinal surface is determined. It is important to appreciate that diabetic vitreoretinal pathology is *planar*, seldom showing discrete traction bands. Apparent bands and strands comprise denser areas, for example from fibrovascular (as opposed to fibrocellular) proliferation on the retinal surface and detached hyaloid (*see Figure 13.3a*), or from collagen condensation in relation, for example, to a premacular hiatus in a trampoline membrane (*see Figure 13.5a*). In eyes with retrohyaloid haemorrhage, it is still possible to determine the overall vitreous configuration, since areas of fibrovascular membrane delineate and loculate the retrohyaloid space.

The most important function of ophthalmoscopy of eyes with clear media is to determine the state of the macula, in particular whether or not the macular neuroepithelium is elevated from the pigmented epithelium. This is sometimes very difficult to define with certainty. The macula is also examined for evidence of ischaemic or exudative maculopathy. These are the essential determinants of the surgical decision-making process, since microsurgery is usually only indicated if the macula is detached and if an improvement in visual function can be anticipated after reattachment.

## Ocular investigations

### Ultrasound

Real-time grey-scale B-scan ultrasound is an essential investigation in patients with cloudy media from cataract or vitreous haemorrhage (McLeod and Restori, 1979, 1981); A-scan is of limited value in diabetes. The overall anatomical configuration of the vitreous and retina is readily determined (*see Figure 13.4*) and, as with ophthalmoscopy, particular attention should be paid to the posterior retina. Owing to limitations of axial resolution, however, shallow extension of a tractional detachment into the macula may be difficult to recognize.

### Electrical tests

In practice, electrophysiological testing – ERG, EOG and VER – is frequently unrewarding in diabetic eyes. Mass responses are almost invariably diminished (as a result of the associated widespread ischaemia or from previous photocoagulation) and fail to discriminate between impaired macular and general retinal function. Bright-flash ERG testing in eyes with very dense haemorrhage also suffers this serious limitation. Many patients have functioning retina only central to the major temporal vascular arcades and may have excellent acuity postoperatively despite grossly diminished electrical activity. Tests more indicative of macular function (e.g. the VER) fail to distinguish between damage from irreversible macular ischaemia and potentially reversible macular detachment. What is required is a test which indicates potential macular function after clearance of haemorrhage and macular reattachment!

### Fluorescein angiography

Fluorescein angiography has very little place in previtrectomy assessment in diabetes. It may be useful in indicating the extent of macular capillary perfusion in eyes in which the degree of ischaemia is not apparent from ophthalmoscopic examination. Iris angiography may be helpful in the evaluation of early rubeosis, but is not in routine use.

## Systemic examination

General factors regarding anaesthetic risks and life prognosis, for example renal failure, hypertension and ischaemic cardiovascular disease, are determined in co-operation with the patient's diabetic physician. Surgery while diabetic control is unstable should be avoided.

## Indications and contraindications for surgery

Closed intraocular microsurgery is indicated when the likelihood that this will result in significant visual benefit exceeds the risk of potentially irreversible surgically induced deterioration of function. The possibility of spontaneous improvement during the natural course of the disease must also be borne in mind. Stated simply, the principal indications for operation are *persistent vitreous haemorrhage in an only eye*, and *recent extension of retinal detachment to include the macula in any eye*. In practice, a host of readily determined factors, together with many ill-defined influences, must be brought to bear on the problem. Frequently, the ultimate decision to operate can be reached only after careful weighing of conflicting arguments, considering the following criteria.

### Type and duration of pathology

Visual loss from haemorrhage, whatever its duration, is potentially completely reversible after spontaneous clearing or surgery; retinal haemosiderosis appears to be unimportant (Charles, 1981). Nevertheless, concurrent deterioration may occur as the result of progressive diabetic maculopathy or the development of macular detachment. There is no absolutely defined level of acuity above which vitrectomy for haemorrhage is contraindicated. Some patients with persistently annoying mobile opacities and an extremely fleeting 6/9 vision may benefit greatly from surgery.

Visual loss from macular detachment is virtually completely reversible, provided reattachment is achieved within a few days. Thereafter, visual deterioration becomes progressively irreversible the longer the detachment persists because of receptor damage and gross cystoid oedema. The duration of detachment after which no functional recovery can be anticipated is impossible to define. It would appear that a shallow traction detachment can be associated with reversibility for a much longer period than a highly elevated detachment, for example from combined rhegmatogenous and traction detachment, where reattachment after 6 months or so is seldom rewarding. The possibility of spontaneous reattachment of the retina rarely enters the decision-making process. In eyes with very slow progression of macular elevation, however, there is no strictly defined level of acuity at which operation is advised; the decision to operate is based on a variety of additional factors.

The severity of pathology, particularly the extent of epiretinal vasoproliferation, is an important determinant of surgical prognosis in both haemorrhage and detachment cases (Barrie *et al.*, 1982). Table-top traction detachments carry a poor prognosis when compared with eyes with non-coalescent multifocal vasoproliferation. It must be remembered that many diabetic eyes with traction detachment maintain a low level of useful vision for a protracted period (Cohen, McMeel and Franks, 1979), while unsuccessful surgery soon tends to be associated with absence of light perception.

## Activity of neovascularization

The risk of complications, especially rubeosis iridis and rebleeding, is least if neovascularization has arrested spontaneously or has reversed following photocoagulation. The presence of mild rubeosis, recurrent bleeding or active capillary budding along the edges of preretinal membranes is, in itself, a relative contraindication to vitrectomy. Provided these can be influenced by intraoperative photocoagulation, however, surgery can be considered; indeed, the appearance of rubeosis may be an indication for early operation. Whether reattachment of the retina at vitrectomy *per se* can reverse rubeosis is unclear.

## Unilateral/only eye status

Other things being equal, macular detachment is an indication for immediate surgery whatever the status of the other eye. In contrast, surgery for haemorrhage is generally indicated solely for an 'only eye' or if better vision can be anticipated in the treated eye than in the fellow eye, as determined by the swinging flashlight test. Exceptions may have to be made in young patients needing binocular vision, or if previously considered factors, such as development of rubeosis, likelihood of treatable diabetic maculopathy, or the discovery on ultrasound of extensive temporal vitreoretinal adhesions or extramacular traction detachment, indicate a high risk of macular detachment.

## Patient temperament

Patients vary widely in their reactions to blindness and also to the surgeon's statement of prognosis. For example, a predicted 70 per cent success rate may represent a glorious opportunity to one individual, but a dismal prospect for another who demands a virtual guarantee of success before considering operation.

The emotional state and social needs of the patient are frequently the essential determinants of the timing of surgery for haemorrhage in an only eye.

In patients with a poor life prognosis, surgery which has the prospect of only marginal visual improvement cannot be justified, though vitrectomy for uncomplicated haemorrhage in an only eye may be considered even for patients on dialysis for chronic renal failure. The following factors militate strongly against a decision to proceed with surgery.

## Extramacular tractional detachment

Because the risks of visual deterioration after microsurgery for traction detachment are seldom less than 20%, and the chances of progression to macular detachment are only of the order of 14% per year (Charles and Flinn, 1981), operation is not indicated for extramacular detachment except in some eyes with associated cataract, haemorrhage or progressive rubeosis. It is particularly difficult to withstand the temptation to intervene in eyes with good visual acuity, but extensive detachment surrounding the fovea and reducing the visual field to the central 3–5°. In some cases, photocoagulation of attached ischaemic retina may be indicated on the basis of active neovascularization or recurrent haemorrhage, but the risk of inducing progression of fibrous contraction must be recognized.

## Combined rhegmatogenous and traction detachment

Those few detachments with a visible, accessible and closeable retinal tear in which sealing of the break is thought to be sufficient to allow macular reattachment should be treated by scleral buckling and subretinal fluid drainage (Gragoudas and McMeel, 1976).

## Preponderance of irreversible pathology

Surgery is contraindicated if there is evidence of a major irreversible element of visual loss, for example from optic atrophy following ischaemic optic neuropathy, ischaemic maculopathy or post-detachment retinal atrophy following prolonged macular separation. Surgery should not be considered in an eye with a gross afferent pupillary defect if the macula is flat or in an eye known to have had very poor vision prior to the onset of retinal detachment or vitreous haemorrhage.

## Severe rubeosis iridis

Once rubeosis is well established, with peripheral anterior synechiae and secondary glaucoma, vitreous surgery is contraindicated.

## VITREORETINAL SURGERY

Scott (1969) of Cambridge employed an open-sky vitrectomy technique for managing severe diabetic eye disease over a decade ago, while closed vitrectomy via the pars plana was pioneered in the early 1970s by Machemer (1974). The common-gauge system of closed intraocular microsurgery was thereafter popularized by Charles (1981).

### Management objectives

The purpose of surgery is to restore and maintain the maximum possible vision in the operated eye.

#### Removal of opacities

Axial opacities in the lens, vitreous gel and retrohyaloid space must be removed so as to restore transparency of the media.

#### Retinal reattachment

Vitreoretinal tractional elements (anteroposterior, bridging and tangential) must be eliminated and any breaks sealed so that the neuropithelium can be restored to a smooth contour in contact with the pigment epithelium.

#### Stabilization of vision

The above mechanical objectives can be simply stated and frequently achieved, but it must be emphasized that the vitrectomized diabetic eye is highly susceptible to further damage which may militate against a successful outcome in the short or long term. After complete vitrectomy, no new vasoproliferation occurs on the retinal surface (Michels, 1978), but the scaffolding structure of the basal gel cannot be removed and this region may be invaded by fibrovascular tissue of either episcleral or uveal origin (Tardiff and Schepens, 1977). This entry site complication is a feature particularly of ischaemic retinopathies, whether from diabetes or Eales' disease, and is more sinister than the non-vascularized healing process normally associated with vitrectomy procedures, especially in causing rebleeding. While haemorrhage may be localized to certain vitreous compartments preoperatively, postoperative haemorrhage tends to obscure the entire vitreous cavity or the whole eye.

Similarly, while complete gel removal precludes further *epiretinal* neovascularization, it increases the access of vasoproliferative factor to the *iris*, stimulating rubeosis. The risk is greatest after combined lensectomy and vitrectomy procedures

(Michels, 1978). Rubeosis occurs less frequently after vitrectomy alone, provided the diffusion-barrier function of the anterior cortical gel is left intact (Charles, 1981). Both the tendency to rebleeding (whether from fibrovascular ingrowth or residual neovascularization) and the tendency to rubeosis appear to be significantly reduced by panretinal photocoagulation. Thus, vitrectomy in diabetics should never be thought of simply as an alternative to photocoagulation. Iris neovascularization is the most sight-threatening complication of retinal production of vasoproliferative factor, and in this respect the likelihood of irreversible demise of vision is increased rather than decreased by vitrectomy.

Finally, the physical continuity of the neuroepithelium must be maintained after surgery. Unfortunately, the most elegant and complicated of microsurgical dissections can be rendered useless by a tiny unrecognized retinal break causing complete redetachment. Retinal detachment in diabetic eyes appears to cause an increased production of vasoproliferative factor, possibly because of decreased choroidal oxygenation of the retina, and therefore a markedly increased risk of rubeosis.

## Preoperative treatment

Ischaemic retina should be photocoagulated some days prior to surgery in order to reduce the risk of postoperative rebleeding and rubeosis. Equatorial areas around a central haemorrhage or attached retina around a traction detachment can be so treated. The practicality and desirability of trying to reduce iris neovascularization by retinal cryopexy is not established; cryotherapy has a considerable propensity for increasing traction in eyes with widespread fibrovascular proliferation.

Only exceptionally should cataract extraction precede vitrectomy. With modern phacoemulsification capabilities it is best to remove the lens and vitreous during the same procedure. If the lens nucleus is too sclerotic to permit phacoemulsification, a combined intracapsular or extracapsular extraction and vitrectomy can be performed. There is, however, a group of patients with both lens and vitreous opacities in whom cataract extraction alone will facilitate spontaneous clearance of haemorrhage and obviate the need for vitrectomy and its attendant risks, especially rubeosis.

## Preliminary manoeuvres

Most surgeons prefer general to local anaesthesia. The location within the eye of breaks and major fibrovascular proliferations (nasal, temporal, superior or inferior) determines the optimal inclination of the patient's head under the operating microscope. A lateral canthotomy is frequently helpful. Maximal pupillary dilatation should be achieved with drops and subconjunctival mydriatics; topical phenylephrine drops should be avoided in view of possible endothelial toxicity. If an encircling strap is to be used, this can be secured, though not tightened, prior to closed microsurgery. Three pars plana entry sites are prepared in the standard fashion 3 or 4 mm from the limbus (Charles, 1981), infusion is established and surgery carried out in the following sequence.

## Lens removal

Unless the nucleus is densely sclerotic, the lens can be removed by phacoemulsification via the pars plana. After removing the cortex, nucleus, posterior capsule and anterior subcapsular epithelium, some surgeons leave the anterior capsule intact and remove it along with any remaining hydrated equatorial lens cortex towards the end of surgery in order to minimize damage to the corneal endothelium. Lens removal is indicated if there is significant cataract, but removal of a clear lens, though undesirable, may sometimes be necessary in order to facilitate peripheral vitreoretinal dissection or simultaneous fluid–gas exchange.

## Vitrectomy

The 'core' of the vitreous gel is first excised, preferably using a suction cutter with a rapid guillotine action. If the posterior hyaloid interface is opaque, it should be penetrated at a point well clear of the retina, as determined by preoperative ultrasound examination. A taut posterior hyaloid membrane may require to be punctured by a needle or a microvitreoretinal (MVR) blade and the opening extended with vitreous scissors. In eyes with retrohyaloid haemorrhage, lysed blood or a 'sand storm' of erythroclastic debris wells forth through the hyaloid defect; this should not be mistaken for intraoperative bleeding (which forms a fibrinous clot). Provided the central gel is removed first, the retrohyaloid space can be rapidly cleared of blood by vacuum-cleaning with a flute needle or linear suction using an extrusion hand-piece (Charles, 1981). The entire 360° cone of posterior hyaloid membrane should be removed so as to isolate each fibrovascular complex and disconnect the membranes from the vitreous base (*Figure 13.7*); anteroposterior and bridging elements of traction are thereby eliminated and the tendency to rebleeding and redetachment is reduced. Remarkably, the apparent vascularity of posterior fibrovascular proliferations immediately diminishes once the vitreous attachments have been severed (Machemer, 1978). Circumcision of posteriorly located adhesions is readily accomplished, but may prove more difficult if the neovascularization is sited equatorially. New vessels proliferating forward along the posterior hyaloid should be precoagulated by bimanual bipolar diathermy (Charles *et al.*, 1976), care being taken to keep the optic nerve out of the elliptical field of current by coagulating well forward of the disc.

Using scleral indentation, the anterior part of the posterior hyaloid membrane and associated vitreous should be removed so as to leave only a small frill of basal gel. Otherwise erythroclasts may be released from the gel frill postoperatively and contribute to haziness of the media or trabecular obstruction. Furthermore, untoward pathology in the basal and equatorial retina may remain hidden, and possible tractional and haemorrhagic consequences of fibrovascular ingrowth may be increased. Nevertheless, suction cutting close to the vitreous base should be avoided in view of the risk of causing retinal damage.

In phakic eyes, the cortical gel forming the anterior hyaloid membrane should be left intact so as to reduce anterior diffusion of vasoproliferative factor towards the

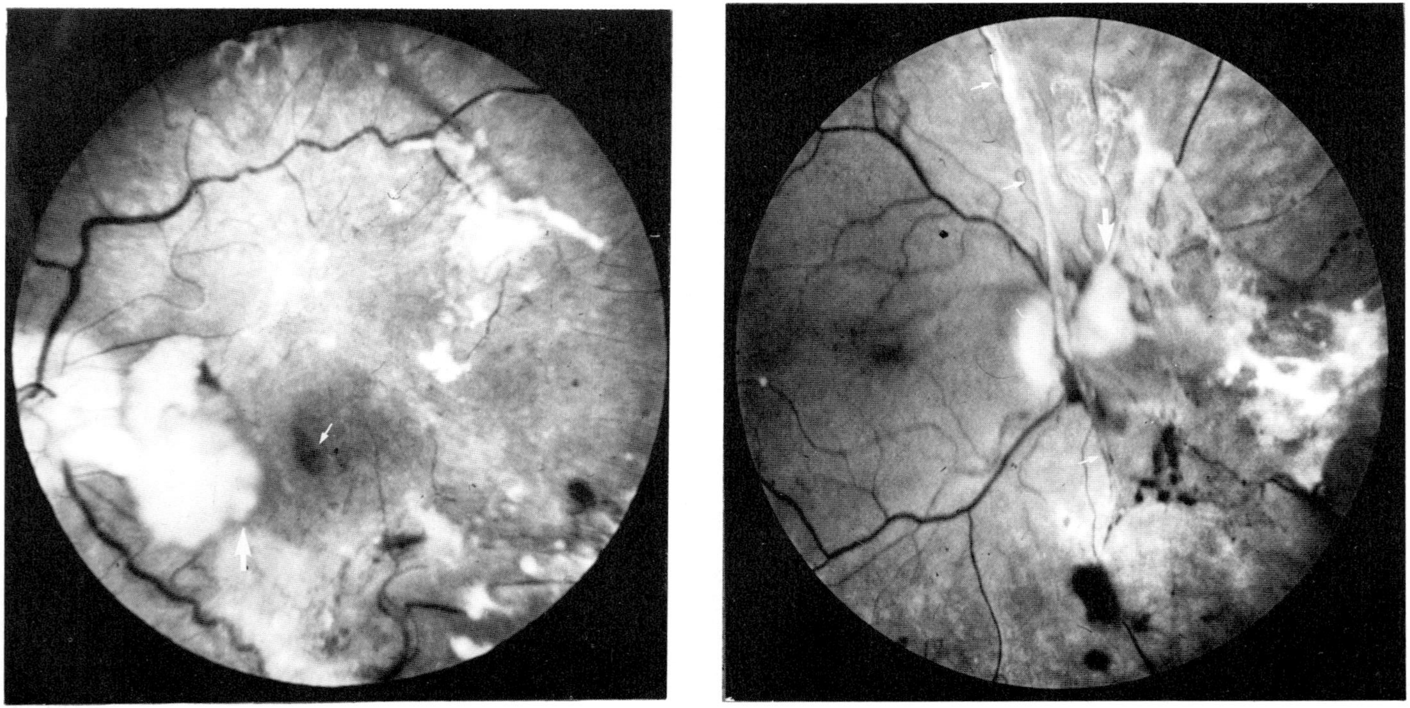

(a) (b)

*Figure 13.7* Fundus photographs after vitrectomy. (*a*) Circumcised diathermized stalk (large arrow) tethering to disc; epimacular fibrocellular membrane and pseudomacular hole (small arrow), as revealed at surgery (acuity 6/24). (*b*) Circumcised diathermized stalk (large arrow) from disc; an extensive fibrocellular epiretinal membrane covering posterior pole, was revealed at surgery, that portion over the macula being peeled up to cut edge (small arrows) (acuity 6/18)

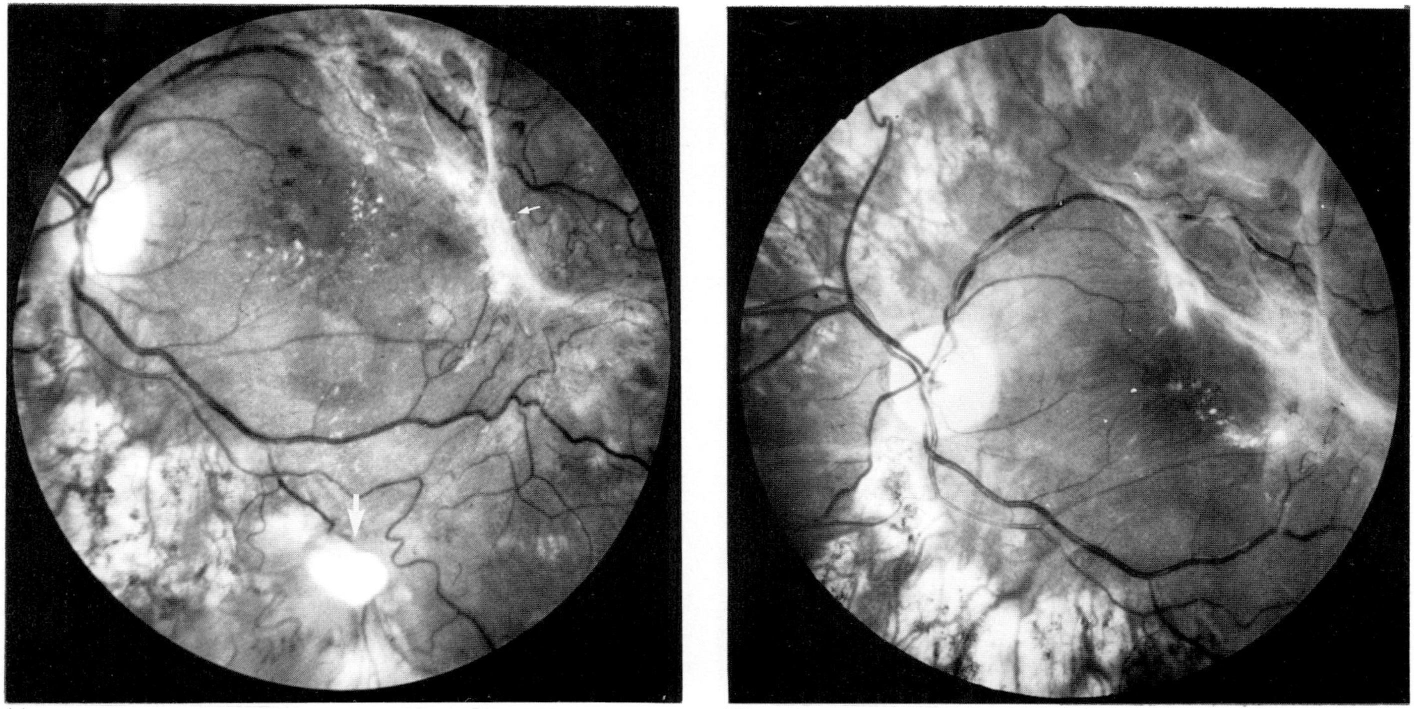

(c) (d)

*Figure 13.7* (*c*) Circumcised diathermized stalk inferiorly (large arrow); early reparative fibrosis superotemporal to fovea (small arrow) after over-enthusiastic peeling of fibrovascular epiretinal membranes (acuity 6/24). (*d*) Same eye 1 month later; progressive proliferation and contraction of reparative fibrocellular membranes (acuity 6/24). (*a*), (*b*) and (*c*) from McLeod, Leaver and Feretis, 1980, courtesy of the Editor and Publishers, *Transactions of the Ophthalmological Societies of the United Kingdom*)

iris (Charles, 1981). The retrolental gel central to Weiger's ligament should, however, be carefully removed so as to avoid blood staining and opacification of this axial gel postoperatively (*see Figure 13.1d*).

## Epiretinal surgery

Fibrovascular membranes proliferating on the retinal surface are dissected in order to relieve tangential traction on the underlying retina and to mobilize retinal breaks. Retinal reapposition to the pigmented epithelium may thus be achieved, and such dissection may also reduce the tendency to rebleeding postoperatively. Dissection may be accomplished by 'scissors-segmentation' using vertically orientated 80° vitreous scissors which are insinuated between the membrane and retina between points of fibrovascular outgrowth (Charles, 1980). Beginning centrally and proceeding outwards, each outgrowth in an extensive membrane can be isolated (*Figures 13.8 and 13.9*). Alternatively, the membrane can be detached from the retina by 'scissors-delamination' using 70° horizontally orientated scissors (Sutherland scissors) whereby the edge of the membrane is progressively peeled centrally and points of origin of fibrovascular outgrowth are sectioned (*Figure 13.8*). The membrane is thus removed *in toto* (Charles, 1981). The latter method is thought to reduce the risk of iatrogenic breaks and damage to the retinal surface which might thereafter lead to reparative, non-vascular proliferation and fibrosis (*see Figures 13.7c and d*); however, this has yet to be substantiated. Whichever method is used, vessels in the membrane, or the 'stem' outgrowths, should be precoagulated by bimanual bipolar diathermy before cutting (Charles *et al.*, 1976). If haemorrhage nevertheless occurs, the bleeding point should be immediately coagulated in order to avoid formation of a fibrin clot which obscures and adheres to the underlying surgical field. Non-vascularized membranes should be removed by peeling, delamination or segmentation if they are causing significant macular distortion (*see Figure 13.7b*).

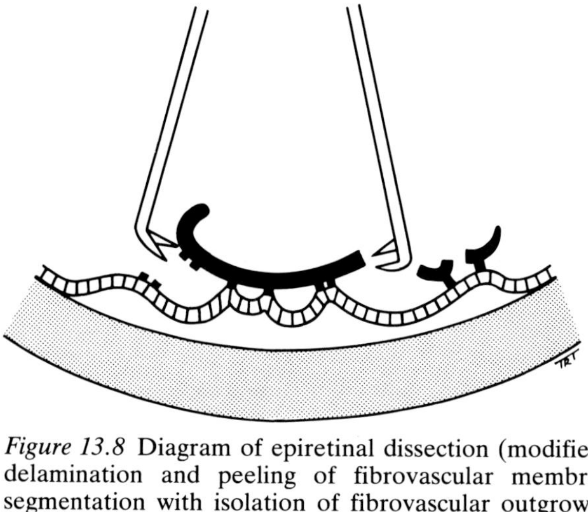

*Figure 13.8* Diagram of epiretinal dissection (modified from Charles). Outside-in scissors-delamination and peeling of fibrovascular membrane (*left*), and inside-out scissors-segmentation with isolation of fibrovascular outgrowths (*right*); angular apices of retinal detachment 'rounded off' as traction is relieved

Such dissection may be difficult to complete in areas of high-density fibrovascular outgrowth, where the retina is very atrophic or if (as is unusual) extensive membranes are present equatorially. Particular problems arise in dissection of peripapillary membranes which are tightly adherent to the retina and contract to cause a 'closed triangle' or tubular configuration of detachment in front of the disc.

## Internal fluid transfer

Eyes with combined rhegmatogenous and traction detachments, and those in which retinal breaks are created during epiretinal dissection, should have the subretinal compartment emptied of fluid by internal drainage using either a flute needle or, preferably, the Charles linear suction system (Charles, 1981). If the open end of the suction implement is placed in the immediate vicinity of a tear, the break tends to stretch (a beneficial variant of 'fish-mouthing'!), and a column of syrup-like fluid, denser and more viscous than infusion fluid, is aspirated. This manoeuvre is readily accomplished if the break is located posteriorly, but is more difficult if the tear is equatorial. Thereafter, the vitreal infusion fluid is exchanged for air or an SF6/air mixture which is injected through the infusion terminal while fluid over the disc is aspirated or vented to the atmosphere in a simultaneous fluid/gas exchange. Internal drainage is continued and completed as residual subretinal fluid (SRF) is displaced posteriorly during the exchange; where necessary, the end of the needle is passed through the retinal break. The exchange is readily visualized through the operating microscope if the eye is aphakic, but in phakic eyes the indirect ophthalmoscope or a biconcave contact lens must be used. Since the entire vitreous cavity is to be filled with gas, the concentration of SF6 should be no higher than 20% in order to prevent postoperative expansion of the bubble and elevation of intraocular pressure. The purpose of using SF6 is to double the duration of the bubble postoperatively, not to exert an expansive force on the retina. Internal gas closure is the most efficient way of sealing a break while postcoagulative adhesion develops during the postoperative period. Nothing is achieved by such an exchange in the absence of a retinal break, other than exposure of the eye to the risk of complications such as cataract and glaucoma. Admittedly, if subretinal fluid is plentiful, its distribution is influenced by the position of the eye and the buoyancy of the enclosed bubble, but its absorption is not accelerated.

Exchange of fluid for liquid silicone has been used in some eyes with multiple breaks and in eyes thought likely to develop reparative fibrosis. The rationale was to achieve a permanent tamponade and inhibit postoperative surface proliferation (Lean *et al.*, 1982). The results, however, proved disappointing since secondary cellular proliferation, contraction, and reopening of breaks did not appear to be favourably influenced by liquid silicone in most cases.

## Tissue coagulation

Bimanual bipolar diathermy is used to ensure haemostasis in severed fibrovascular tissue. Trans-scleral cryopexy or xenon arc endophotocoagulation may be used to promote adherence of the retina around any retinal breaks or to reduce vasopro-

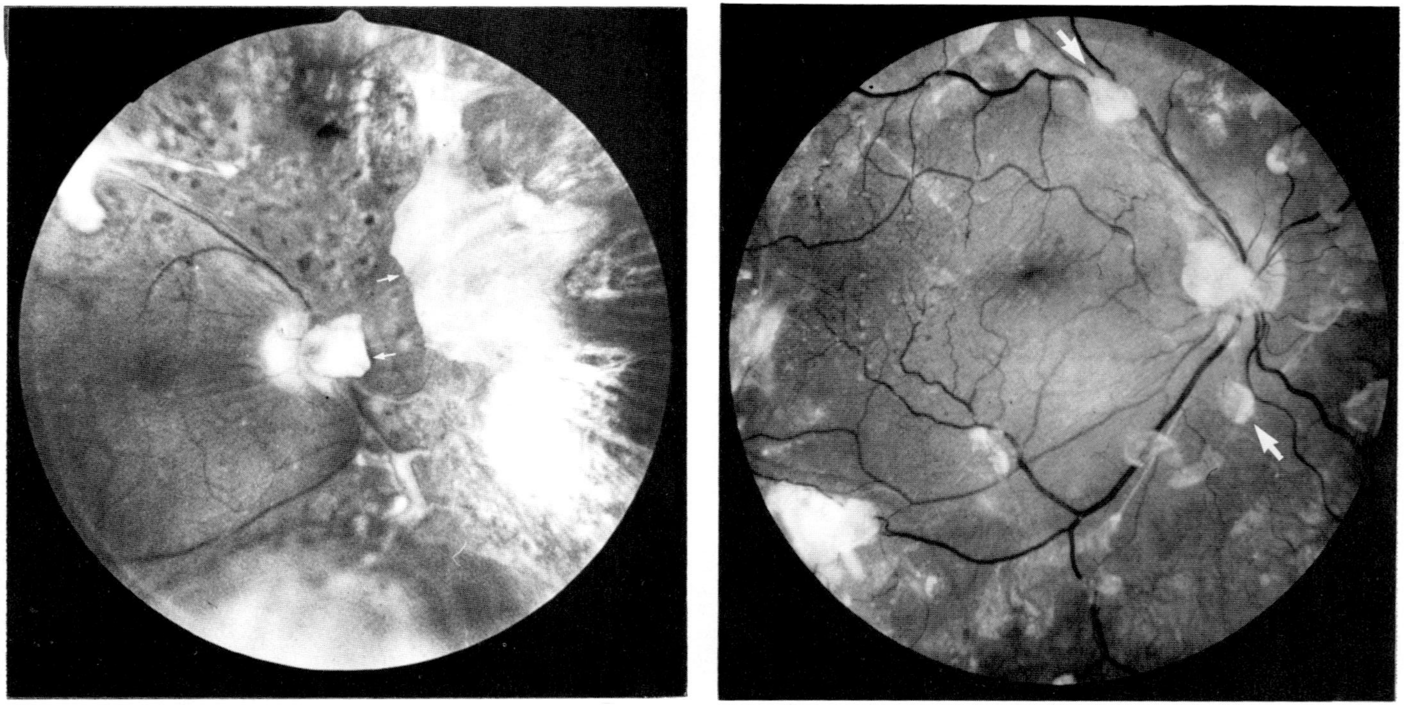

(a) (b)

*Figure 13.9* Fundus photographs (*a*) Vertical scissors-segmentation of thick fibrovascular membrane nasal to disc showing separation of cut edges (small arrows) after relief of traction; rounded elevation from radial buckle below, and chorioretinal scarring from laser and cryocoagulation (acuity 6/6). (*b*) Photographic field showing 18 isolated fibrovascular outgrowths (2 arrowed) after vitrectomy for traction detachment including macula (acuity 6/6)

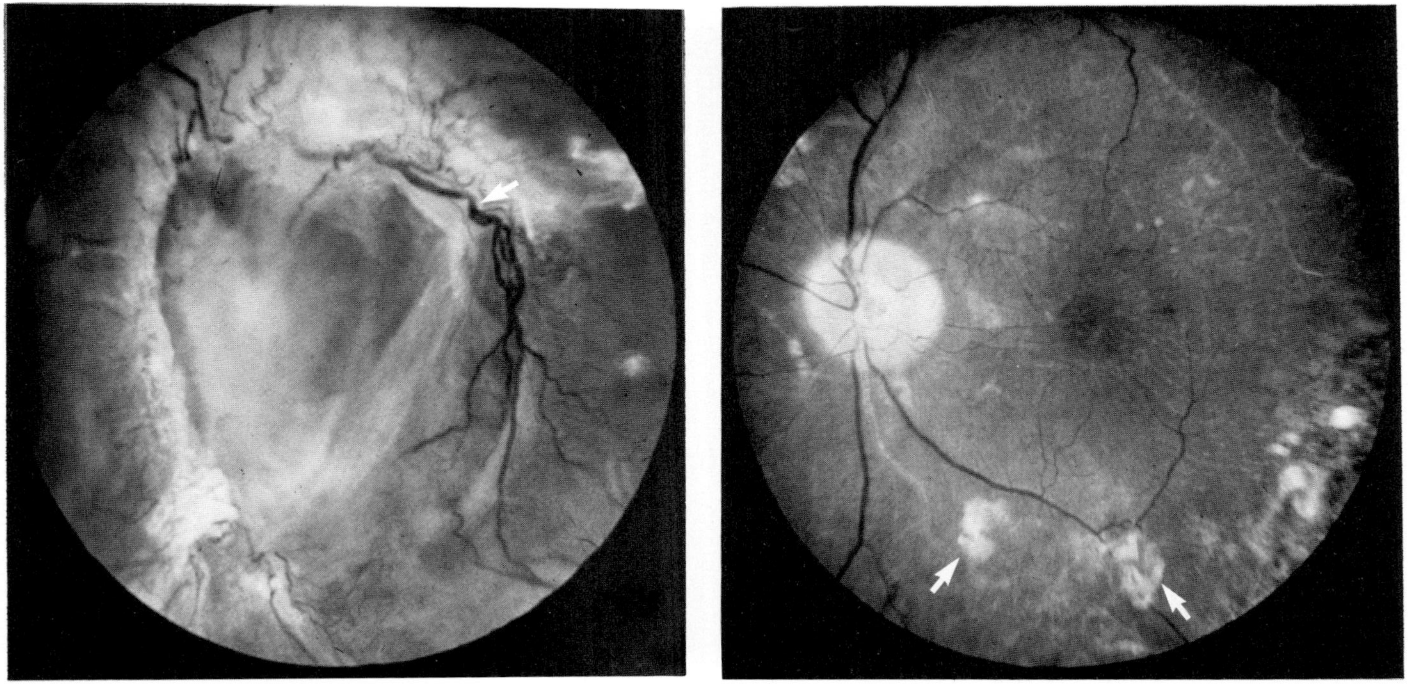

(c) (d)

*Figure 13.9* (*c*) Coalescent fibrovascular membranes with large neovascular channels (arrow) causing traction detachment throughout posterior pole (acuity 2/60). (*d*) Same eye and photographic field as in (*c*) after vitrectomy and retinal reattachment; residual segmented tissue in centre of disc and inferiorly (arrows); attenuated intraretinal vasculature (acuity 6/18). (*b*), (*c*) and (*d*) from Barrie *et al.*, 1982, courtesy of the Editor and Publishers, *British Journal of Ophthalmology*)

liferative activity. Unfortunately, panretinal endophotocoagulation is laborious with current instrumentation and can only be used to treat attached retina. The fibreoptic bundle of the instrument is destroyed if fired in air, so tears are difficult to treat. Panablation is particularly indicated, however, in eyes which are to be left phakic and those with signs of rubeosis or active capillary budding.

Trans-scleral cryopexy is the usual method employed for treating breaks, but transvitreal cryotherapy should not be used. Cryopexy is best carried out after internal SRF drainage and fluid/gas exchange. Because of the internal thermal insulation provided by gas, the retinal ice ball develops more rapidly and persists longer than is usually the case, so it is essential to use an apparatus with a rapid thawing capability. Panretinal cryocoagulation external to the major temporal vascular arcades is indicated in some eyes being treated for extensive detachment.

Some surgeons perform 360° cryotherapy across the posterior border of the vitreous base (usually beneath an encircling strap) in order to seal any undiscovered tears and as part of the overall ablation. Monitored postoral cryopexy in the region of the entry sites should certainly be performed, since some degree of basal gel incarceration is inevitable and may occasionally be complicated by oral disinsertion or tearing along the posterior border of the vitreous base.

Diabetic eyes have a remarkable capacity to withstand the combined effects on tissues of cold, heat and electrocution! To what extent tissue coagulation increases the risk of reparative fibrosis is unknown. Complications of each manoeuvre are nevertheless apparent, for example, choroidal detachment and forward shift of the lens–iris diaphragm from panretinal endophotocoagulation, pigment fall-out from cryotherapy, and diathermy damage to the surface of the retina.

## Scleral buckling and resection

Prophylactic encirclement in the region of the posterior border of the vitreous base is suggested by some surgeons because of the possible development of tears at this site during vitrectomy and to guard against unrecognized entry site complications. The value of this has not been clearly demonstrated, however. The strap may be supplemented by a local tyre where serious entry site complications are recognized or to cover equatorial breaks. More posteriorly located breaks simply require internal closure and cryopexy provided associated traction can be satisfactorily relieved and good postoperative posturing is assured. Radially orientated explants are indicated if a posterior tear cannot be fully mobilized by epiretinal dissection. Tears located between the inferior macular arcade and the equator from the 4 o'clock to 8 o'clock meridians should be indented if there is any doubt regarding posturing or tear-mobilization (*see Figure 13.9a*). If tangential traction persists over a wide area, defying dissection, scleral resection may be indicated (Hanscom and Machemer, 1980).

## Postoperative care

Internal closure of breaks is assured by careful posturing for a few days postoperatively. Other than atropine, no drops are necessary unless specifically indicated by infection or inflammation. Spontaneous lysis can usually be awaited in eyes containing fibrin, for example forming a pupillary membrane; resort to systemic corticosteroid therapy should be resisted, as there is no evidence that it accelerates fibrinolysis. Careful follow-up is essential for early recognition and treatment of complications such as rubeosis and open-angle glaucoma.

## Postoperative complications

Diabetic eyes are, of course, subject to all the postoperative complications that might befall any vitrectomized eye, for example cataract from lens–instrument touch or prolonged contact with a gas bubble, and erythroclastic glaucoma from retained blood. Remarkably, perhaps, postoperative bacterial endophthalmitis is very rare. Certain vitrectomy complications are more likely because diabetes has a deleterious effect on all ocular structures. Problems with corneal epithelial healing, more specifically attachment of the epithelium to the underlying stroma rather than epithelial mitosis and spread, are frequent, especially if the epithelium is removed, or spontaneously erodes, during surgery (Foulks *et al.*, 1979). There is also some evidence to suggest that the endothelium of the cornea is more susceptible to damage than in normal eyes, so prolonged irrigation, adverse effects of ultrasound or endothelium–gas contact should be guarded against. Drugs toxic to the cornea, for example genticin and phenylephrine, should be avoided. Early posterior subcapsular cataracts appear to be more prone to progression postoperatively, and there is more fibrinous exudate owing to generalized vessel disease. However, severe uveitis is unusual except in association with rubeosis; erythrocytes, erythroclasts, lens-laden macrophages and pigment cells may all be mistaken for inflammatory cells. There is also an exaggerated tendency to chronic aphakic open-angle glaucoma, possibly related to trabecular clogging by the various types of cell noted above.

In addition, there are a variety of serious complications which are especially liable to occur after diabetic vitrectomy.

### Rebleeding

If one listens carefully to diabetic patients during prolonged follow-up, it is clear that most vitrectomized eyes undergo some form of rebleeding. This is a problem particularly with phakic eyes – rapid clearing of haemorrhage via the trabecular meshwork is usual in aphakes. Bleeding may arise from residual epiretinal and disc new vessels, from fibrovascular ingrowth at entry sites or from new vessels on the iris. During surgery, bipolar diathermy may reduce the tendency to rebleeding, as may full segmentation of vascularized membranes (Machemer and Blankenship, 1981). The small sclerotomies of common-gauge microsurgery are probably less prone to fibrovascular ingrowth than the large entry sites required for full-function probes. Panretinal photocoagulation, whether intraoperative or postoperative, appears to reduce the risk of haemorrhage substantially (though it is uncertain whether all potential sites of bleeding are similarly favourably affected). Spontaneous clearing can be awaited unless there are other associated complications such as rubeosis or retinal detachment that demand immediate reoperation. Otherwise, the period of delay before washout (and possible lens extraction) is determined by the patient's visual needs.

## Rubeosis iridis

Increased access of vasoproliferative factor to the anterior segment is believed to be responsible for the development (or increase in) of rubeosis iridis following diabetic vitrectomy. Between 10% and 30% of otherwise successful operations are followed by this complication. Rubeosis is much less likely to occur if the eye remains phakic (with an intact anterior hyaloid) or if the retina has undergone panretinal photocoagulation. It develops most frequently if the eye has active neovascularization preoperatively and if the retina becomes, or remains, detached postoperatively (*Table 13.1*). Indeed, rubeosis invariably complicates extensive

*Table 13.1* Diabetic rubeosis

| *Pros* | *Cons* |
|---|---|
| Ischaemic retinopathy | Panretinal photocoagulation |
| Vasoproliferative factor | ? Vitreous inhibitory factor |
| Retinal detachment | Attached retina |
| Vitrectomy | ? Liquid silicone injection |
| Aphakia | Lens and anterior hyaloid intact |

retinal detachment in an aphakic vitrectomized diabetic eye (Michels, 1978); there may be a transient phase of elevated intraocular pressure (often accompanied by haemophthalmos and corneal decompensation), but the ultimate result is phthisis bulbi (*Figure 13.10*). Treatment consists of photocoagulation of attached retina or reattachment of detached retina. These measures are usually successful in reversing early neovascularization and may at least prevent progression of more established rubeosis.

Thus, while removal of a clear lens facilitates certain aspects of surgery and reduces the risk of persistent postoperative haemorrhage, these advantages are only gained at the cost of a high incidence of rubeosis, and, as such, lensectomy should be avoided if possible.

## Retinal detachment and reparative epiretinal fibrosis

Most postoperative detachments have a rhegmatogenous component. Although it is sometimes claimed that certain types of break do not give rise to retinal detachment provided all local traction is eliminated, many would agree that this happy circumstance only obtains in other surgeons' practice! In addition to 'missed breaks', tears may be induced in a variety of ways, for example entry-site dialysis

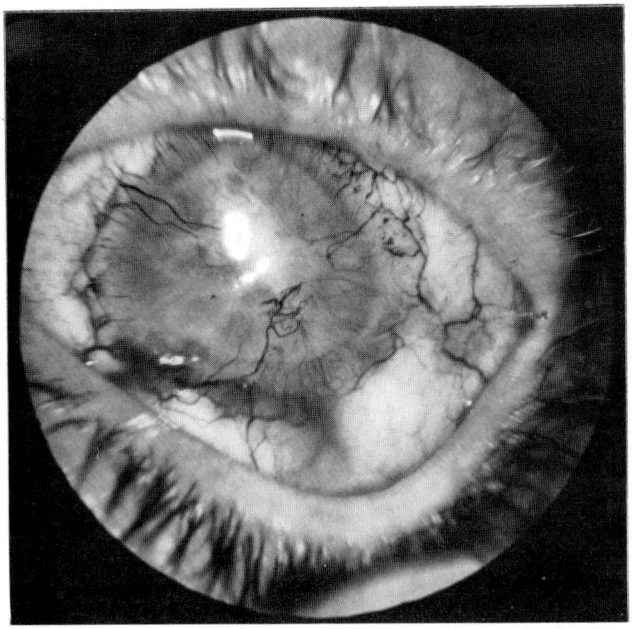

*Figure 13.10* Rubeotic phthisis bulbi and corneal neovascularization after unsuccessful lensectomy/vitrectomy for diabetic traction detachment

from repeated introduction of scissors, breaks at the posterior border of the vitreous base from inefficient suction cutting or vitreous incarceration in entry sites, or tearing/cutting of the retina during epiretinal dissection. The risk of break formation is probably increased in diabetic eyes because the retina is ischaemic and atrophic. Provided such breaks can be recognized, treatment by scleral buckling or internal closure is relatively straightforward. Unfortunately, many postoperative detachments arise from reopening of previously sealed breaks owing to reparative fibrosis; such detachments are less readily repaired. The other major sight-threatening complication of reparative fibrosis is macular pucker (*see Figures 13.7c and d*).

Once an extensive retinal detachment develops in an aphakic vitrectomized eye, rubeosis iridis develops in a matter of days. Immediate reoperation is therefore indicated even if the macula is still attached.

## Results

The degree of visual improvement after technically successful surgery depends essentially on the extent of intrinsic macular damage. In the absence of damage, normal visual acuity is frequently attainable, and remarkable visual improvement may be seen in eyes which have suffered a macular detachment for a relatively short period. Overall results depend, of course, on patient selection, surgical experience and access to available microsurgical technology. At this time, significant visual improvement is an achievable goal in 50–80% of haemorrhage cases (Peyman *et al.*, 1976; Michels, 1978; McLeod, Leaver and Feretis, 1980; Machemer and Blankenship, 1981), and in a similar proportion of detachment cases (Aaberg, 1979, 1981; Charles, 1980, 1981; Barrie *et al.*, 1982), even if surgery is undertaken in many eyes with a guarded prognosis. Visual acuity of 6/60 or more has been obtained in 50–60% of eyes in various series. It is reassuring to note that in successful cases improved visual function can often be maintained for a protracted period (Rice and Michels, 1980; Aaberg, 1981; Blankenship, 1981).

## FUTURE DEVELOPMENTS

At some time in the future, we can look forward to the incidence of PDR being substantially reduced, if not eradicated, by more physiological means of treating diabetes and/or the possible development of a pharmacological inhibitor of vasoproliferative substance. In the meantime, better ophthalmic surveillance of diabetics should lead to earlier recognition of PDR and identification of patients at risk, allowing earlier and more successful treatment by photocoagulation. Identification of the mechanism by which photocoagulation and other measures (such as pituitary ablation) favourably influence PDR may suggest new methods of treatment. It remains to be seen whether there will ever be a widely accepted place for any form of prophylactic vitrectomy in diabetes, and the value of inducing complete posterior vitreous detachment (Scott, 1969), thereby precluding epiretinal vasoproliferation and traction, has yet to be explored.

Assuming, however, that established complications of PDR continue to present to the vitreoretinal surgeon in the foreseeable future, what other developments are likely? Introduction of effective non-mechanical means of removing vitreous gel and dissecting epiretinal membranes, for example by laser disintegration and coagulation, is imminent (Karlin *et al.*, 1979; Fankhauser *et al.*, 1981). Hopefully, the incidence of reparative fibrosis and iatrogenic breaks will diminish substantially. More refined techniques for intraoperative panretinal photocoagulation, for example using laser photocoagulation through the operating microscope or laser endophocoagulation (Fleischman, Swartz and Dixon, 1981; Peyman, Salzano and Green, 1981) should soon be widely available. In addition, some form of glue for instantaneous intraoperative sealing of retinal breaks would be most welcome! One can also look to pharmacological methods of inhibiting reparative fibrosis.

With such developments, relatively early vitrectomy for patients with recurrent transient haemorrhages could be approached with more confidence. More severe types of pathology will also become operable and a better prognosis will be achieved for all patients undergoing surgery.

### Acknowledgements

Particular thanks are due to Mrs Penny Lovelock for preparing the manuscript, and Messrs K. Sehmi and T. R. Tarrant for the illustrations. This work was generously supported by Data Recall Ltd (Diamond Wordprocessors), Dorking.

## References

Aaberg, T. M. (1979) Clinical results in vitrectomy for diabetic traction retinal detachment. *American Journal of Ophthalmology*, **88,** 246–253

Aaberg, T. M. (1981) Pars plana vitrectomy for diabetic traction retinal detachment. *Ophthalmology,* **88,** 639–642

Barrie, T., Feretis, E., Leaver, P. K. and McLeod, D. (1982) Closed microsurgery for diabetic traction macular detachment. *British Journal of Ophthalmology*, **66,** 754–758

Blankenship, G. W. (1981) Stability of pars plana vitrectomy results for diabetic retinopathy complications. *Archives of Ophthalmology*, **99,** 1009–1012

Charles, S. (1980) Vitrectomy for retinal detachment. *Transactions of the Ophthalmological Society of the United Kingdom*, **100,** 542–549

Charles, S. (1981) *Vitreous Microsurgery*. Baltimore/London: Williams and Wilkins

Charles, S. and Flinn, C. E. (1981) The natural history of diabetic extramacular traction retinal detachment. *Archives of Ophthalmology*, **99,** 66–68

Charles, S.,White, J., Dennison, C. and Eichenbaum, D. (1976) Bimanual, bipolar intraocular diathermy. *American Journal of Ophthalmology*, **81,** 101–102

Cohen, H. B., McMeel, J. W. and Franks, E. P. (1979) Diabetic traction detachment. *Archives of Ophthalmology*, **97,** 1268–1272

Davis, M. D. (1965) Vitreous contraction in proliferative diabetic retinopathy. *Archives of Ophthalmology*, **74,** 741–751

Fankhauser, F., Roussel, P., Steffen, J., Van Der Zypen, E. and Chrenkova, A. (1981) Clinical studies on the efficiency of high power laser radiation upon some structures of the anterior segment of the eye. *International Ophthalmology*, **3,** 129–139

Fleischmann, J. A., Swartz, M. and Dixon, J. A. (1981) Argon laser endophotocoagulation – an intraoperative trans-pars plana technique. *Archives of Ophthalmology*, **99,** 1610–1612

Foos, R. Y. (1974) Vitreoretinal juncture: changes in diabetes mellitus. *Concilium Ophthalmologicum 22 (Paris)*, **1,** 373–380

Forrester, J. V., Grierson, I. and Lee, W. R. (1978) Comparative studies of erythrophagocytosis in the rabbit and human vitreous. *von Graefes Archiv für Ophthalmologie*, **208,** 143–158

Foulks, G. N., Thoft, R. A., Perry, H. D. and Tolentino, F. I. (1979) Factors related to corneal epithelial complications after closed vitrectomy in diabetics. *Archives of Ophthalmology*, **97,** 1076–1078

Gragoudas, E. S. and McMeel, J. W. (1976) Treatment of rhegmatogenous retinal detachment secondary to proliferative diabetic retinopathy. *American Journal of Ophthalmology*, **81,** 810–819

Hanscom, T. and Machemer, R. (1980) Scleral resection in combination with vitrectomy. *International Ophthalmology*, **2,** 23–26

Karlin, D. B., Patel, C. K. N., Wood, O. R. and Llovera, I. (1979) $CO_2$ laser in vitreoretinal surgery. *Ophthalmology*, **86,** 290–298

Lean, J., Cooling, R. J., Leaver, P. K. and McLeod, D. (1982) Management of complex retinal detachments by vitrectomy and liquid silicone exchange. *Transactions of the Ophthalmological Societies of the United Kingdom*, **102,** 203–205

Lee, P. F. (1968) Clinical and histological findings in diabetic retinopathy. *American Journal of Ophthalmology*, **65,** 688–695

Machemer, R. (1974) A new concept for vitreous surgery: 7. Two instrument techniques in pars plana vitrectomy. *Archives of Ophthalmology*, **92,** 407–412

Machemer, R. (1978) Pathogenesis of proliferative neovascular retinopathies and the role of vitrectomy: a hypothesis. *International Ophthalmology*, **1,** 1–3

Machemer, R. and Blankenship, G. (1981) Vitrectomy for proliferative diabetic retinopathy associated with vitreous haemorrhage. *Ophthalmology*, **88,** 643–646

McLeod, D., Leaver, P. K. and Feretis, E. (1980) Vitrectomy for severe diabetic eye disease. *Transactions of the Ophthalmological Societies of the United Kingdom*, **100,** 291–298

McLeod, D., Marshall, J. and Grierson, I. (1981) Epimacular membrane peeling. *Transactions of the Ophthalmological Societies of the United Kingdom*, **101,** 170–180

McLeod, D. and Restori, M. (1979). Ultrasonic examination in severe diabetic eye disease. *British Journal of Ophthalmology*, **63,** 533–538

McLeod, D. and Restori, M. (1981) Rapid B-scanning in diabetic eye disease. In *Ultrasonography in Ophthalmology. Documenta Ophthalmologica Proceedings Series*, **29,** 21–31. The Hague: Dr W. Junk Publishers

McMeel, J. W. (1971) Diabetic retinopathy: fibrotic proliferation and retinal detachment. *Transactions of the American Ophthalmological Society*, **69,** 440–493

Michels, R. G. (1978) Vitrectomy for complications of diabetic retinopathy. *Archives of Ophthalmology*, **96,** 237–246

Peyman, G. A., Raichand, M., Huamonte, F. U., Nagpal, K. C., Goldberg, M. F. and Sanders, D. R. (1976) Vitrectomy in 125 eyes with diabetic vitreous haemorrhage. *British Journal of Ophthalmology*, **60,** 752–755

Peyman, G. A., Salzano, T. C. and Green, J. L. (1981) Argon endolaser. *Archives of Ophthalmology*, **99,** 2037–2038

Rice, T. A. and Michels, R. G. (1980) Long-term anatomic and functional results of vitrectomy for diabetic retinopathy. *American Journal of Ophthalmology*, **90,** 297–303

Scott, J. D. (1969) Surgery of advanced diabetic retinopathy. In *Modern Problems in Ophthalmology*, **8,** 505–510. Basel: S. Karger

Shilling, J. S., McLeod, D. and Restori, M. (1979) Control of preretinal neovascularisation. In *Proceedings of the 23rd International Congress of Ophthalmology (Kyoto)*, **1,** 822–825. Amsterdam: Excerpta Medica

Shimizu, K., Kobayashi, Y. and Muraoka, K. (1981) Midperipheral fundus involvement in diabetic retinopathy. *Ophthalmology*, **88,** 601–612

Smith, R. S., Van Heuven, W. A. J. and Streeten, B. (1976) Vitreous membranes: a light and electron microscopical study. *Archives of Ophthalmology*, **94,** 1556–1560

Tardiff, Y. M. and Schepens, C. L. (1977) Closed vitreous surgery. 15. Fibrovascular ingrowth from pars plana sclerotomy. *Archives of Ophthalmology*, **95,** 235–239

Tasman, W. (1972) Retinal detachment secondary to proliferative diabetic retinopathy. *Archives of Ophthalmology*, **87,** 286–289

Trempe, C. L., Takahashi, M. and Topilow, H. W. (1981) Vitreous changes in retinal branch vein occlusion. *Ophthalmology*, **88,** 681–687

Wallow, I. H. L., Greaser, M. L. and Stevens, T. S. (1981) Actin filaments in diabetic fibrovascular preretinal membrane. *Archives of Ophthalmology*, **99,** 2175–2181

# 14
# Current management of giant retinal breaks with an inverted retinal flap

H. MacKenzie Freeman

## INTRODUCTION

Giant retinal breaks have been defined as retinal breaks extending over 90° or more over the circumference of the fundus (Freeman, 1968). They occur in approximately one in 2000000 people per year and in about 1 in 200 rhegmatogenous retinal detachments (Freeman, 1978). In my experience in operating approximately 650 giant retinal breaks according to this definition, I have found a significant variation in their severity and therefore a similar variation in the technique best suited for each case. Results in the management of giant retinal breaks continue to improve as a result of prone positioning of the patient as initiated by Schepens and Freeman (1967), air injection to tamponade the tear as advocated by Norton *et al.* (1969), pars plana vitrectomy pioneered by Machemer and Allen (1976), suturing of the posterior retinal flap utilizing an open sky approach reported by Hirose, Schepens and Lopansri (1981), and transcleral suturing described by Usui *et al.* (1979) and Federman, Shakin and Lanning (1982). I believe there is a role for all of these techniques in our armamentarium in the management of giant tears. What we must continue to do is to put each technique to its optimum use while minimizing the risks in these cases which are often monocular.

## PREOPERATIVE MANAGEMENT

### Preoperative ophthalmoscopic examination

A detailed large drawing is made of the fundus of both eyes with the patient in the supine position. Preoperative examination with the patient in the prone position is important in order to determine the extent to which an inverted flap is capable of unfolding. In addition, examination in the prone position is helpful in identifying where the posterior retinal flap may not unfold completely because of fixed radial or fixed circumferential retinal folds. In order to unfold the posterior retinal flap of a superior giant retinal break, the head is placed in the prone position and the neck

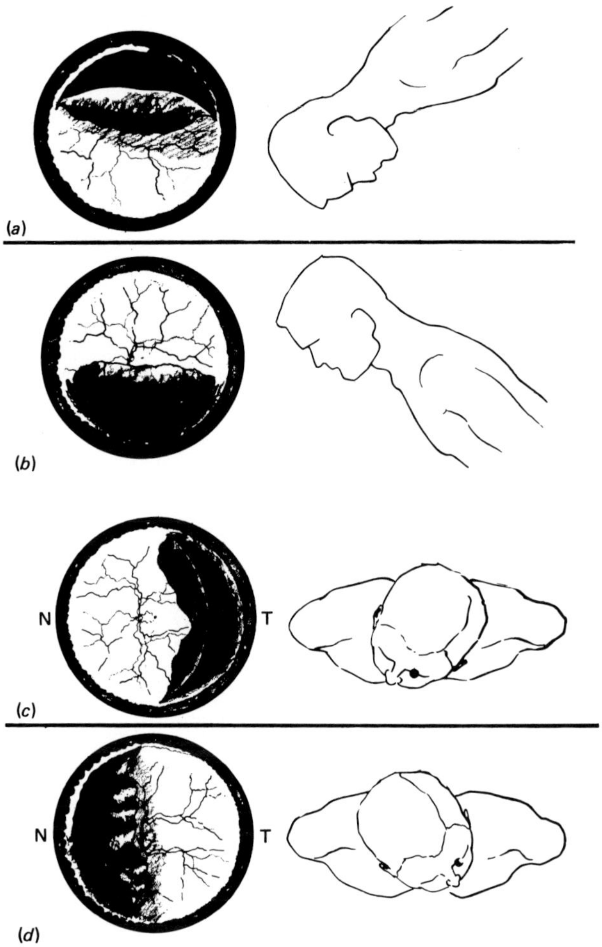

*Figure 14.1* Preoperative positions in order to unfold inverted flaps of variously located giant retinal tears: (*a*) when giant break is superior; (*b*) when break is inferior; (*c*) when break is temporal; (*d*) when break is nasal

is flexed. With inferior giant retinal breaks the neck is hyperextended. The head is rotated toward the shoulder opposite the affected eye with temporally located breaks and rotated toward the shoulder of the affected eye with nasal giant breaks (Freeman, 1969) (*Figure 14.1*). A drawing is made with the patient in the prone position which best unfolds the retinal flap.

## Unfolding the retinal flap with head exercises or forced duction

In some cases, the retinal flap cannot be unfolded by prone positioning but it may be made to unfold with certain head exercises (Freeman, 1968). These head exercises consist of a fast component in the direction the flap is folded, a pause for the count of three followed by a slow return movement. In the case of a superior giant break with an inverted retinal flap, the fast movement of the head consists of a rapid flexion of the neck (*Figure 14.2*). Head exercises are contraindicated in eyes where the giant tear extends in a radial direction (*Figure 14.3*). In such cases these exercises can cause the tear to extend further posteriorly.

A notation is made of the position of the head which results in optimum unfolding of the flap. This information is helpful during surgery to determine the angle to which the giant tear operating table should be rotated in order to unfold the retinal flap prior to the air fluid exchange. The patient's head is secured to the

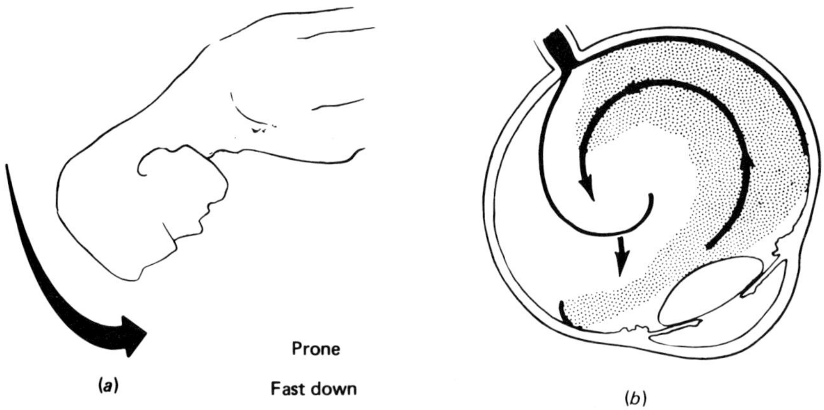


*Figure 14.2* (*a*) Head exercises for a superior giant tear. The arrow indicates the direction of the fast component. (*b*) Movements of fluid vitreous within the eye at the end of the fast component

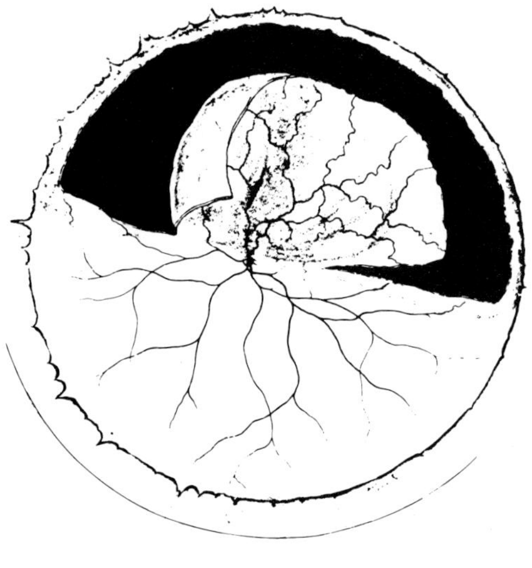

*Figure 14.3* Giant retinal break with the tear extending in a radial direction posteriorly. Head exercises or forced ductions are contraindicated because they may cause the tear to extend further posteriorly

table during surgery so that head exercises cannot be performed, therefore if the flap does not unfold well, forced ductions of the globe are done with the fast component made in the same direction as the fast component of the head exercises.

### Preoperative biomicroscopic examination

Detailed biomicroscopy of the vitreous cavity is performed on both eyes using the Goldmann three-mirror lens, and the findings are recorded on the Tolentino vitreous chart. It is important to record the location of vitreous membranes or vitreous gel which might impede the unfolding of the retinal flap. In the majority of eyes a membrane is attached to the anterior margin of the giant break producing a detachment of the pars plana.

### Preoperative medical consultation

A preoperative medical consultation should be obtained because part of the surgery will be performed in the prone position which can stress the cardiovascular system.

## CURRENT INDICATIONS FOR VARIOUS SURGICAL TECHNIQUES

### Scleral buckling, pars plana vitrectomy, lensectomy

For giant retinal tears extending from 90 to 135° with only a partial inversion of the posterior scleral flap, vitrectomy, lensectomy, air fluid exchange and a 360° scleral buckling is advocated. Retinal suturing is not used in such cases because of the increased risk of choroidal hemorrhage.

### Scleral buckling, pars plana vitrectomy, lensectomy, iridectomy, air fluid exchange and retinal suturing

The author is currently performing a clinical trial of the use of trans-scleral suturing of giant retinal tears over 150° with an inverted flap that unfolds well and is uncomplicated by preretinal organization.

### Open sky vitrectomy and retinal suturing

Open sky retinal suturing is indicated in eyes in which the posterior retinal flap unfolds poorly or becomes immobilized by preretinal organization which causes the posterior edge of the tear to become rolled like a scroll or wrinkled or shortened in a pursestring fashion.

## OPERATIVE MANAGEMENT

### Anesthesia

General anesthesia is preferred because the duration of surgery may exceed 5 hours and part of the surgery is performed with the patient in the prone position. After endotracheal intubation, the nose and pharynx are packed with gauze to absorb nasal and pharyngeal secretions and prevent them from contaminating the operative field when the patient is in the prone position. Extra-long tubes connecting the patient to the anesthesia machine are used to allow the patient to be rotated through 360° on the giant tear operating table. In addition, a reinforced endotracheal tube is used which is less likely to narrow or collapse with undue movements of the head or neck during rotation into the prone position.

### Pars plana vitrectomy

#### Rationale for vitrectomy

Air is used to unfold and tamponade the posterior flap of the giant break (Freeman, Schepens and Couvillion, 1970; Machemer, Aaberg and Norton, 1969). The larger the bubble of air that can be injected, the greater the unfolding of the flap, therefore the aim is to inject as large a bubble as possible. Removal of the lens and most of the vitreous gel makes possible the injection of a large bubble of air.

In addition, removal of the anterior vitreous gel which is often condensed into a vitreous membrane interrupts vitreous traction from this membrane which can result in the formation postoperatively of additional retinal breaks or an extension of the giant retinal tear.

#### Location of the sclerotomy site

The sclerotomy for vitrectomy is placed in the meridian, which allows the greatest freedom of movement of the vitrectomy instrument to make possible the complete removal of the lens via the pars plana route. A temporal sclerotomy site just below the horizontal meridian is generally chosen.

#### Extent of the vitrectomy in the region of the giant break

In order that vitreous gel overlying the bare choroid will not interfere with unfolding of the retinal flap, an attempt is made to remove as much of it as possible. The vitrectomy is extended into the region of the vitreous base along the anterior edge of the giant break in order to remove gel that might prevent the flap from unfolding as far anteriorly as possible.

### Limit of the vitrectomy opposite the giant break

When extending the vitrectomy peripherally one should bear in mind that the vitreous base is strongly attached to the underlying retina. Therefore, in order to avoid causing a circumferential extension of the giant break or retinal tears, one should avoid extending the vitrectomy anterior to the equator beyond the limits of the giant break.

## Lensectomy iridectomy and sphincterotomy

Ultrasonic fragmentation is used to remove a lens having a sclerotic nucleus. A basal iridectomy and inferior sphincterotomy are performed to permit optimal visualization during surgery and to facilitate photocoagulation which is often applied postoperatively.

It is important to examine the fundus periphery with scleral depression following vitrectomy to determine if the giant retinal break has extended circumferentially or to detect new retinal breaks that have been produced during vitrectomy. The sclerotomy is inspected for tight closure and examined ophthalmoscopically for incarceration of vitreous gel. If necessary, additional interrupted sutures are added so that the sclerotomy will not leak and withstand the stress of scleral buckling and air fluid exchange.

## Scleral buckling

I strongly recommend a 360° scleral buckling in all giant breaks with an inverted retinal flap. Postoperative condensation of the vitreous base often causes an elevation of the ends of the giant break with an accumulation of subretinal fluid anteriorly. This fluid can leak posteriorly around the end of a scleral buckle that does not extend around the circumference of the globe.

A 360° scleral buckling is prepared, making the buckle wide on the side of the giant tear. If the eye is of normal size, a lamellar scleral undermining is made approximately 12–13 mm in width. In highly myopic eyes, the globe is usually large, and the undermining may be as wide as 15 mm. In order to preserve the vortex veins on the side of the globe opposite the giant retinal break the buckle is made narrow and placed in the region of the equator (*Figure 14.4*).

Mersiline mattress sutures (4-0) are inserted every 30° through the scleral flaps. A solid, grooved silicone rubber implant, trimmed so that it is 2 mm narrower than the lamellar scleral bed, is placed around the globe under an encircling silicone rubber band. It is desirable to produce a wide low scleral buckle. A high buckling effect tends to shorten the circumference of the globe, producing meridional retinal folds which may leak posteriorly causing a postoperative retinal detachment. By preparing the buckle before the air fluid exchange there are less manipulations of the globe which can cause the unfolded retinal flap to slip posteriorly.

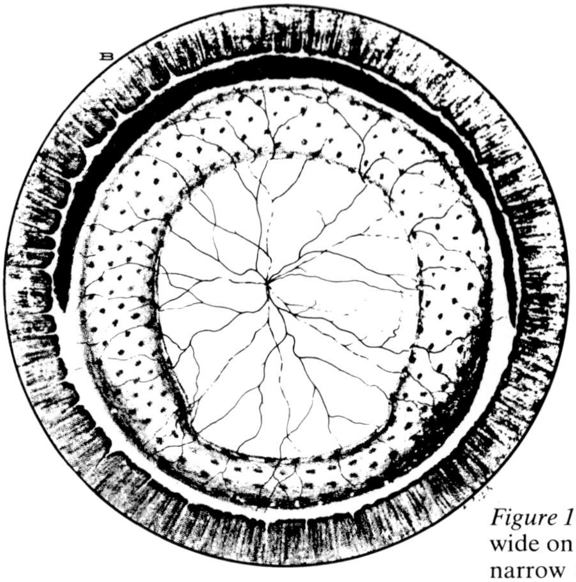

*Figure 14.4* A 360° scleral buckle: this is made wide on the side of the giant retinal break and narrow and more anterior opposite the giant tear in order to avoid encroaching on the vortex veins on that side

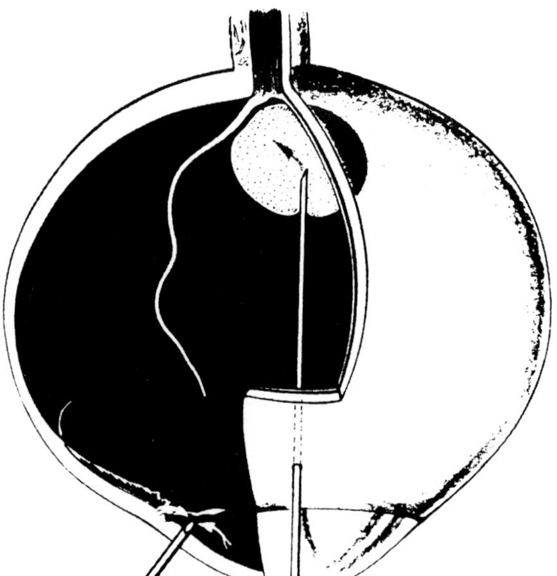

*Figure 14.5* Air fluid exchange: with the patient in the prone position, air is injected under indirect ophthalmoscopic control with the tip of the needle in front of the optic disc

## Air fluid exchange

After the scleral buckle has been prepared, the patient is rotated to the prone position in order to unfold the posterior retinal flap. Ophthalmoscopy is performed to verify that the flap is optimally unfolded. If the flap is not adequately unfolded, forced ductions of the globe are performed by grasping the bridle suture under the muscle nearest the center of the giant retinal break. The ductions consist of a fast component in the direction the flap is folded, followed by a pause then a slow return movement in the opposite direction. These ductions are carried out two or three times, ophthalmoscopy is performed and the ductions are repeated if indicated.

With his elbows supported by a Mayo stand, the surgeon introduces the tip of a 30-gauge needle through the pars plana to the anterior portion of the vitreous cavity. The assistant inserts a short 23-gauge needle through the limbus into the anterior chamber. Then the tip of the 30-gauge needle is directed under indirect ophthalmoscopic control over the optic disc (*Figure 14.5*). Air is slowly injected by the second assistant as fluid drains from the needle in the anterior chamber (Michels, 1981). In the case of a superior giant retinal break, the operating table is rotated upward so that the air bubble moves superiorly over the flap and the inferior edge of the air bubble may become visible in the pupil. To avoid loss of air through the needle in the anterior chamber, the tip of that needle is directed away from the inferior edge of the bubble so that additional fluid can be drained from the globe in order to achieve a near total air fluid exchange.

Indirect ophthalmoscopy is performed to determine whether the posterior flap is unfolded smoothly over the scleral buckle. If the air bubble has caused the retinal flap to slip posteriorly, producing a gaping of the giant tear, then the air is replaced with saline, the patient is rotated to the prone position and the air fluid exchange is repeated. The patient is rotated to the supine position, the intraocular tension is measured and the ophthalmic artery is checked for patency. It is desirable to have the intraocular pressure no higher than 20 mmHg. If the intraocular pressure is elevated above that level, air is aspirated into a syringe through a 30-gauge needle inserted through the pars plana.

## Retinal suturing

Suturing the retina to the choroid or sclera makes it possible to anchor the retinal flap at the time of surgery. Retinal suturing tends to fixate the retinal flap against the pigment epithelium during the formation of the chorioretinal adhesion (Federman, Shakin and Lanning, 1982; Hirose, Schepens and Lopansri, 1981; Usui *et al.*, 1979). In addition, the sutures counteract the tendency for the retinal flap to peel off the scleral buckle as the tamponading effect of the air bubble lessens as the air becomes absorbed.

Sutures can be placed trans-sclerally, using an external approach, tying the knot on the scleral surface or utilizing an open sky approach, tying the knot on the surface of the retina. Providing the retinal flap is mobile so that it unfolds well anteriorly, trans-scleral suturing is preferable because it is technically easier and is associated with less morbidity than open sky suturing which entails the removal of a corneal button, the lens and vitreous. Open sky retinal suturing is preferable in cases in which the posterior retinal flap unfolds poorly or becomes immobilized by preretinal organization which causes the posterior edge of the tear to become rolled like a scroll or wrinkled or shortened in a pursestring contraction. In such cases the wide exposure of the open sky approach makes it possible to peel the extensive preretinal membranes, then handle the retina directly using a spatula to unwrinkle, unfold, then suture it to the choroid that has been treated with diathermy to prevent bleeding.

### Intrascleral retinal suturing

Following the air fluid exchange, meridians for retinal suturing are localized approximately 30° apart and one disc diameter posterior to the edge of the posterior retinal flap. Care is taken to minimize indentation of the sclera that can result in slippage posteriorly of the retinal flap. A hand-held transilluminator is used to identify large choroidal vessels in order to avoid perforating them with the needle of the retinal suture (Freeman *et al.*, 1982; Freeman and Schepens, 1974). The transilluminator is placed on the cornea. The transilluminating beam is directed toward the area localized for suturing. Using a blunt conical electrode a diathermy mark is made in an area devoid of large choroidal blood vessels. An 8-0 monofilament nylon suture with a tapered 5/8 circle curved needle is used to suture the retina. Using a straight-tipped microsurgical needle holder, the needle is passed in and out of the sclera using a rotary motion, then tied with the triple knot on the scleral surface. Additional sutures are placed approximately every 30–45° along the giant retinal break depending on the size of the globe.

## POSTOPERATIVE MANAGEMENT

### Prone positioning

In order that the air bubble will tamponade the flap of the giant tear, the patient is kept on bedrest in the prone position for 3 days. After 3 days, the patient is allowed to adopt a sitting position with the head resting on a pillow on the overbed table. Once the air bubble is less than one-half its original size, prone positioning is discontinued and the patient is allowed to ambulate. As the air bubble decreases in size it may interfere with ophthalmoscopy of the flap of the giant tear. By examining the patient in the prone, supine, and sitting positions with the head tilted in various directions, the air bubble can be moved out of the observation axis of the indirect ophthalmoscope.

## Postoperative photocoagulation

I have found postoperative photocoagulation to be extremely valuable in preventing leakage of thc subretinal fluid posteriorly over the scleral buckle. Using argon photocoagulation applications 500 μ in diameter, three or more rows of burns are applied in areas where the chorioretinal reaction appears too light, or along the edge of the posterior retinal flap that is beginning to become elevated from the buckle. It is important to apply the photocoagulation as soon as possible after surgery.

## OPEN SKY RETINAL SUTURING

The technique of open sky retinal suturing was developed by Hirose and Schepens (Hirose, Schepens and Lopansri, 1981). After corneal trephining, iridotomies, and lens extraction, dense vitreous and preretinal membranes are removed. Solid vitreous gel near the ora serrata, in the area of the giant tear, is carefully grasped with forceps and cut with deWecker microscissors. The quadrant that contains the giant tear is placed in a dependent position so that the retinal flap tends to unfold as a result of gravity. This movement may be helped by a gentle pull of smooth forceps that hold the edge of the retinal flap which floats in vitreous fluid. Sites for retinochoroidal suturing are selected 2–3 mm posterior to the edge of the posterior retinal flap.

Once the location of suturing is determined, the giant tear flap is pushed away temporarily and the pigment epithelium exposed. Underwater diathermy is applied to the bare pigment epithelium, and the latter is removed by scraping. All visible choroidal blood vessels are coagulated in the area where the suture is to be passed. The giant tear flap is then unfolded over the bare choroid. Fluid vitreous is removed by gentle suction. Using a cotton-tipped applicator in one hand, the sclera is indented to form a mound covered by the retinal flap. The other hand is used to pass a fine needle with monofilament nylon through the indented retinal flap and the treated choroid. The tip of the needle passes through the retinal flap from the vitreous side, through the treated choroid, and back through the retina and into the vitreous cavity in one stroke. The suture is tied over the retina. At least one suture is placed in each quadrant that contains the tear. A 13–15 μ monofilament nylon suture is used. The vitreous cavity is washed with balanced saline solution, then as much fluid as possible is removed from the cavity which is filled with hyaluronic acid. The viscous hyaluronic acid pushes the retina against the pigment epithelium and drives subretinal fluid out through the giant tear into the vitreous cavity where it accumulates on top of the hyaluronic acid. This subretinal fluid is removed by gentle suction and additional hyaluronic acid is injected. The iridotomies are closed with 10-0 nylon and the corneal button is sutured as well. A scleral buckling is performed 2–3 weeks after retinal surgery.

## MANAGEMENT OF FELLOW EYES OF NONTRAUMATIC GIANT RETINAL BREAKS

### Incidence of retinal breaks in the fellow eye of giant breaks

In spite of advances in surgical techniques, a considerable number of eyes with giant retinal breaks continue to be lost. In addition, there is a high incidence of retinal breaks and retinal detachment in the fellow eyes of nontraumatic giant breaks. For these reasons, the management of fellow eyes of giant retinal tears is important.

The author has observed retinal breaks to develop in 51 per cent of fellow eyes of nontraumatic giant retinal breaks that have been followed over the past 19 years (Freeman, 1978). The incidence of giant breaks developing in fellow eyes was 13 per cent, retinal tears without detachment developed in 12 per cent of eyes, retinal holes without detachment in 10 per cent, and retinal dialysis without retinal detachment in 0.4 per cent of cases. Retinal detachment caused by either retinal tears, holes or dialyses occurred in 16 per cent of eyes.

### Frequency of followup examination

Even though the fellow eye of a nontraumatic giant retinal break may appear normal at the initial examination, regular and thorough examinations of the retina and vitreous are mandatory. In 17 per cent of fellow eyes which appeared normal there subsequently developed retinal breaks, including one giant retinal break that could not be reattached. The average latent period from the diagnosis of a giant retinal break to the development of giant break in the fellow eyes was 3½ years; for retinal holes the latent period was 1½ years and 3½ years for retinal tears.

These findings indicate that the 5-year period following the development of a giant break in one eye is a critical period for retinal break formation in the fellow eye. It seems prudent that during the 5-year period following a giant retinal break in one eye, the fellow eye should be examined at least every 6 months with subsequent examinations at intervals of 1 year for an additional 5 years.

### Ophthalmoscopic and biomicroscopic findings preceding the development of a giant retinal break

The follow-up of fellow eyes that developed a giant retinal break during the period of observation sheds light on the pathogenesis of nontraumatic giant retinal breaks. The majority of these eyes were highly myopic, i.e. over 10 diopters, they developed increasing vitreous base condensation and increasing areas of white with pressure.

Follow-up of these eyes showed that the earliest change was syneresis and liquefaction of the vitreous gel, so that the posterior and central portions of the vitreous body were converted into a large lacuna while the anterior gel became condensed (*Figure 14.6*). The anterior wall of the lacuna condensed to form a membrane extending across the equatorial region separating the anterior gel from the liquefied vitreous (*Figure 14.7*). This membrane seemed rigid and did not

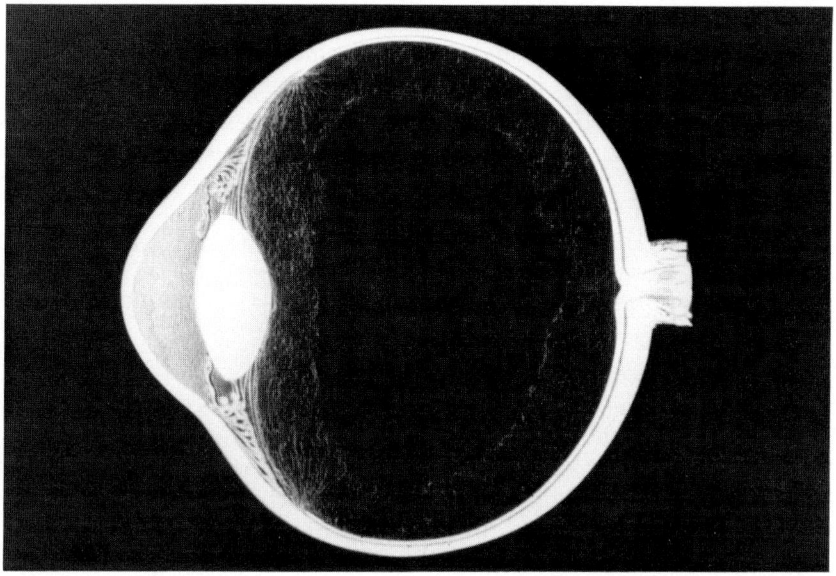

*Figure 14.6* Vitreous changes preceding giant retinal break formation: formation of a giant retinal break is preceded by liquefaction of the central vitreous gel

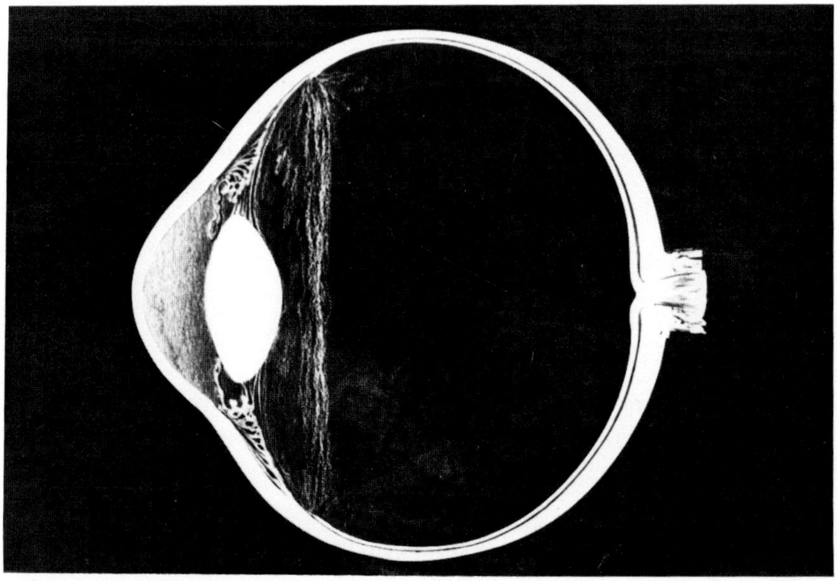

*Figure 14.7* Vitreous changes preceding giant retinal break formation: following liquefaction, anterior vitreous gel becomes condensed forming an equatorial vitreous membrane which originates in the posterior vitreous base

oscillate with ocular movements, suggesting it was under traction between its points of attachment to the vitreous base and areas of white with pressure. Severe contraction of this membrane may be responsible for tearing the retina along the posterior vitreous base (*Figure 14.8*). The posterior retinal flap then easily becomes inverted into the liquefied vitreous (*Figure 14.9*). A similar tense membrane attached to the anterior edge of the giant break is not infrequently encountered during vitrectomy in a giant retinal break operation.

The white with pressure that increases in extent and density may be a result of increasing vitreous base condensation. These findings indicate that areas of white with pressure should be carefully studied in order to determine whether they are increasing in size and density.

The use of a semi-transparent acetate overlay over the initial large fundus drawing has proved especially useful in recognizing subtle changes in white with pressure. Recording not only the extent but the density of the white with pressure is helpful for comparison at future examinations. The density of white with pressure may be graded + to ++++ depending on the degree of opacification of the retina. When increasing white with pressure with increasing vitreous base condensation in a highly myopic eye can be documented, then scleral buckling is performed to relieve vitreous traction.

## CURRENT INDICATIONS FOR PROPHYLACTIC TREATMENT OF THE FELLOW EYE

### Retinal holes

When retinal holes are present in a fellow eye of a giant retinal break, then prophylactic treatment with cryo is indicated.

### Retinal tears

The author treats all symptomatic and asymptomatic retinal tears in fellow eyes of giant retinal breaks. In order to relieve vitreous traction to the tear and lessen the formation of additional retinal tears, a scleral buckling is performed. In order to achieve a more permanent buckling effect, a circling band is placed around the greater circle of the globe.

### Lattice degeneration and retinal breaks

The prognosis of retinal detachment and especially giant retinal breaks in eyes with lattice degeneration is poor. For that reason I treat lattice degeneration with retinal breaks with a scleral buckling.

### High myopia, increasing white with pressure, increasing condensation of the vitreous base

The high incidence of giant retinal breaks which develop in eyes in which there is a combination of myopia in excess of 10 diopters, increasing white with pressure, and

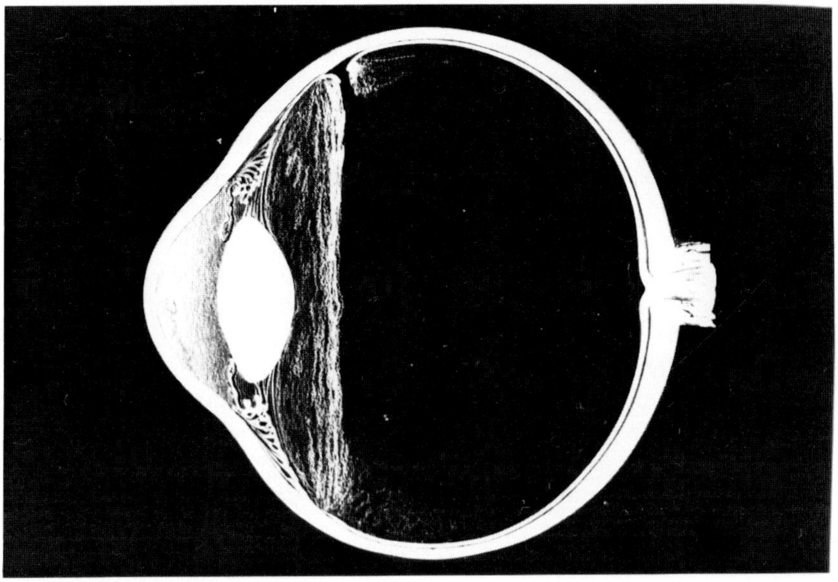

*Figure 14.8* Vitreous changes preceding giant retinal break formation: as a result of contraction of equatorial vitreous membrane, a retinal tear forms where membrane attaches to the peripheral retinal superiorly

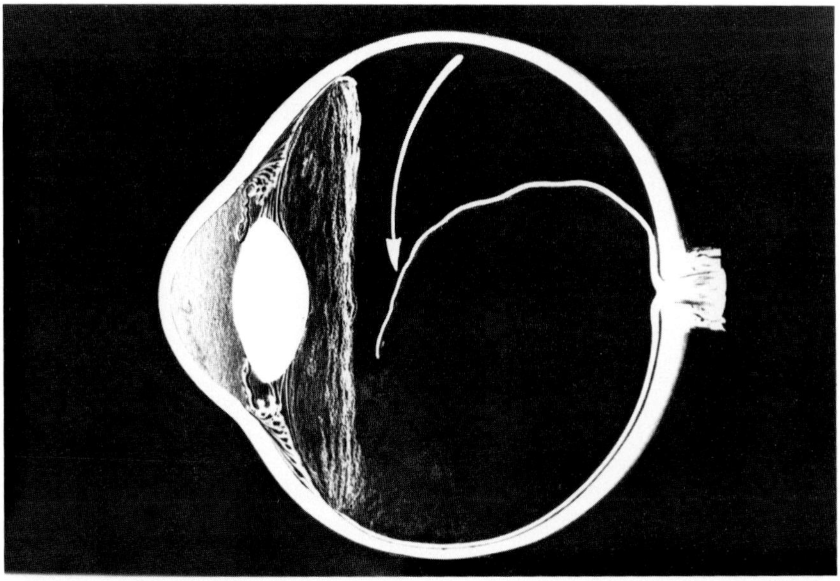

*Figure 14.9* Giant retinal break formation: as retinal tear increases in circumference to become a giant retinal break, the posterior retinal flap easily inverts into the liquefied vitreous gel

increasing condensation of the vitreous base, have prompted prophylactic treatment of such eyes with a scleral buckling and an encircling element. Results thus far in 24 treated eyes are encouraging in that only two eyes have developed retinal breaks while there has been a 100 per cent incidence of giant retinal breaks in a similar group of untreated eyes.

An osmotic agent and a carbonic anhydrase inhibitor are used to lower the intraocular pressure during surgery, therefore a Foley catheter is inserted into the bladder. A very light diathermy mark is made to localize the posterior edge of areas of white with pressure selected for buckling. In eyes where the sclera is of normal thickness, an 8 mm lamellar scleral undermining is performed in an attempt to buckle approximately 180–240° of the globe, selecting an arc which encompasses the most vitreoretinal pathology. Using a blunt conical electrode and low intensity current, diathermy applications are placed 2 mm apart in the scleral bed. In order to avoid damaging the long posterior ciliary arteries or nerves, their location is determined by transillumination of the sclera. To obtain a uniform and light diathermy reaction on the fundus, applications should be frequently monitored with indirect ophthalmoscopy. The relatively wide spacing of the diathermy is designed to decrease the amount of scleral shrinkage which tends to elevate intraocular pressure and to minimize the area of chorioretinal reaction. Postoperatively, properly spaced diathermy produces a leopardskin appearance with a substantial area of intact choroid and retina between the pigmented scars. This is important in the event of reoperation. Three or four mattress sutures per quadrant are placed through the scleral flaps. A grooved silicone rubber impant 6 mm wide and 2 mm thick is placed in the lamellar scleral bed. In order to provide a permanent buckling effect, a circling band is inserted in the groove of the implant and around the globe. The mattress sutures are gently tightened and tied in a slip-knot while the intraocular pressure and patency of the ophthalmic artery are carefully monitored. If the combination of carbonic anhydrase inhibitor and osmotic agent have failed to lower the intraocular pressure sufficiently, then it can be lowered with repeated paracentesis. Syneresis fluid which percolates into the anterior chamber is removed from the eye to produce the moderate buckling effect desired. The encircling band and sutures are also adjusted so that the closing intraocular pressure does not exceed 25 mmHg. An anchoring suture is placed over the encircling band near the middle of the untreated quadrant of the globe.

In eyes with thin sclera, two rows of extremely light cryocoagulation are applied over the arc previously described and external buckling is performed with a grooved silicone implant and encircling element.

## SUMMARY

### Incidence of giant retinal breaks

Giant retinal breaks occur in approximately 1 in 2 million people per year and in approximately 1 in 200 rhegmatogenous retinal detachments.

## Preoperative workup

In order to determine the extent to which the posterior retinal flap is capable of unfolding, a large fundus drawing should be made with the patient in both supine and prone positions. In addition, preoperative biomicroscopy of the vitreous is important to identify vitreous membranes or vitreous gel that may interfere with the unfolding of the posterior retinal flap.

## Indications for various techniques

(1) For giant retinal tears extending from 90 to 135° with only a partial inversion of the retinal flap, the author advocates vitrectomy, lensectomy, air fluid exchange and a 360° scleral buckling.
(2) For giant retinal tears extending over 150° with an inverted retinal flap that unfolds well, the author is currently using trans-scleral retinal suturing in combination with pars plana vitrectomy, lensectomy, iridectomy and air fluid exchange.
(3) Open sky retinal suturing is indicated in eyes in which the posterior retinal flap unfolds poorly or becomes immobilized by preretinal organization which causes the posterior edge of the tear to become rolled like a scroll or wrinkled in a pursestring fashion.

## Pars plana vitrectomy

Removal of most of the vitreous gel makes possible the injection of a large bubble of air which will promote optimal unfolding of the flap.

## Scleral buckling

A scleral buckle which extends 360° around the globe is indicated in all giant retinal breaks with an inverted retinal flap.

## Air fluid exchange

It is mandatory to perform an air fluid exchange with the patient in the prone position.

## Intrascleral retinal suturing

Transillumination of the choroidal vasculature is helpful to detect large choroidal blood vessels in order to avoid perforating them during the placement of intrascleral retinal sutures.

## Followup of fellow eyes of giant retinal breaks

Retinal breaks were observed to develop in 51 per cent of fellow eyes of nontraumatic giant retinal breaks. Retinal holes without detachment were treated with cryo; retinal tears and lattice degeneration associated with retinal breaks were treated with a scleral buckling procedure.

## Management of high-risk eyes

The high incidence of giant retinal breaks that develop in eyes having a combination of myopia over 10 diopters, increasing vitreous base traction and increasing white with pressure has prompted the author to treat such eyes with a prophylactic scleral buckling.

## References

Federman, J. L., Shakin, J. L. and Lanning, R. C. (1982) The microsurgical management of giant retinal tears with trans-scleral retinal sutures. *Ophthalmology*, **89**, 832–838

Freeman, H. M. (1968) The treatment of giant retinal tears. In *New and Controversial Aspects of Retinal Detachment*, edited by A. McPherson, 391–399. New York: Hoeber Medical Division, Harper & Row

Freeman, H. M. (1969) Current management of giant retinal breaks. In *Symposium of Retina and Retinal Surgery, New Orleans Academy of Ophthalmology, Chapter 11*, 171–183. St Louis: C. V. Mosby

Freeman, H. M. (1978) Fellow eyes of giant retinal breaks. *Transactions of the American Ophthalmological Society*, **76**, 343–382

Freeman, H. M., Federman, J. L., Shakin, J. L. and Lanning, R. C. (1982) Discussion of microsurgical management of giant retinal tears with trans-scleral retinal sutures. *Ophthalmology*, **89**, 838–839

Freeman, H. M. and Schepens, C. L. (1974) Innovations in the technique for drainage of subretinal fluid: transillumination and choroidal diathermy. *Transactions of the American Academy of Ophthalmology and Otolaryngology*, **78**, 829–836

Freeman, H. M., Schepens, C. L. and Couvillion, G. C. (1970) Current management of giant retinal breaks. Part II. *Transactions of the American Academy of Ophthalmology and Otolaryngology*, **74**, 59–74

Hirose, T., Schepens, C. L. and Lopansri, C. (1981) Subtotal open sky vitrectomy for severe retinal detachment occurring as a late complication of ocular trauma. *Ophthalmology*, **88**, 1–9

Machemer, R. and Allen, A. (1976) Retinal tears 180° and greater. Management with vitrectomy and intravitreal gas. *Archives of Ophthalmology (Chicago)*, **94**, 1340–1346

Machemer, R., Aaberg, T. and Norton, E. W. D. (1969) Giant retinal tears. II. Experimental production and management with intravitreal air. *American Journal of Ophthalmology*, **68**, 1022–1029

Michels, R. G. (1981) *Vitreous Surgery*, 250–255. St Louis: C. V. Mosby

Norton, E. W. D., Aaberg, T. M., Fung, W. *et al. (1969)* Giant retinal tears. I. Clinical management with intravitreal air. *American Journal of Ophthalmology*, **68**, 1101–1021

Schepens, C. L. and Freeman, H. M. (1967) Current management of giant retinal breaks. *Transactions of the American Academy of Ophthalmology and Otolaryngology*, **71**, 474–487

Usui, M., Hamazaki, S., Takano, S. and Matsuo, H. (1979) A new surgical technique for the treatment of giant tear: transvitreoretinal fixation. *Japanese Journal of Ophthalmology*, **23**, 206–215

# 15
# Surgery of periretinal membranes

Jay L. Federman, Miriam E. Ridley and Jeffrey L. Shakin

## INTRODUCTION

Periretinal membranes can be discussed in several different ways. We have elected to use an anatomical approach to describe their clinical appearance, pathology and management. We shall consider membranes involving the vitreoretinal interface and retinal surface (epiretinal membranes), as well as subretinal membranes. These membranes can also be divided into vascular and avascular types. Vascular membranes occurring in proliferative retinopathies and choroidal neovascularization in degenerative macular disorders are discussed elsewhere. We shall therefore confine our discussion to avascular membranes, which proliferate perhaps in order to repair a defect in the continuity of a smooth surface.

Periretinal membranes may cause interference of visual function by blocking light, or by causing distortion or detachment of the retina. Attempts at medical treatment have been unrewarding, and early surgical attempts were not promising (Wise, 1975). However, with the recent development of automated microsurgical instruments and newer concepts of closed intraocular microsurgery, successful surgical approaches are now possible (Machemer, 1974, 1976; Shea, 1980; Charles, 1981; Michels, 1981).

## MEMBRANES INVOLVING THE VITREORETINAL INTERFACE

Early in life the vitreoretinal interface extends from the base of the vitreous to the edge of the optic disc. The vitreous adheres to the edge of the optic disc, is less adherent to the surface of the retina, and is permanently attached to the tissue that straddles the ora serrata. Here the collagen meshwork of the vitreous base interdigitates with Müller's cells and attaches to the basement membranes of the unpigmented epithelium of the pars plana and Müller's cells of the retina (Hogan, Alvarado and Weddell, 1971). The collagen meshwork is more firmly adherent along the major vessels, which are superficial in the retina; collagen fibrils from the vitreous intermesh with the basal lamina of these larger vessels. Pockets of liquefaction form and coalesce as the vitreous deteriorates with age, and the collagen mesh collapses forward to be suspended by its firm attachment at the vitreous base. As this process takes place, the vitreoretinal interface begins to

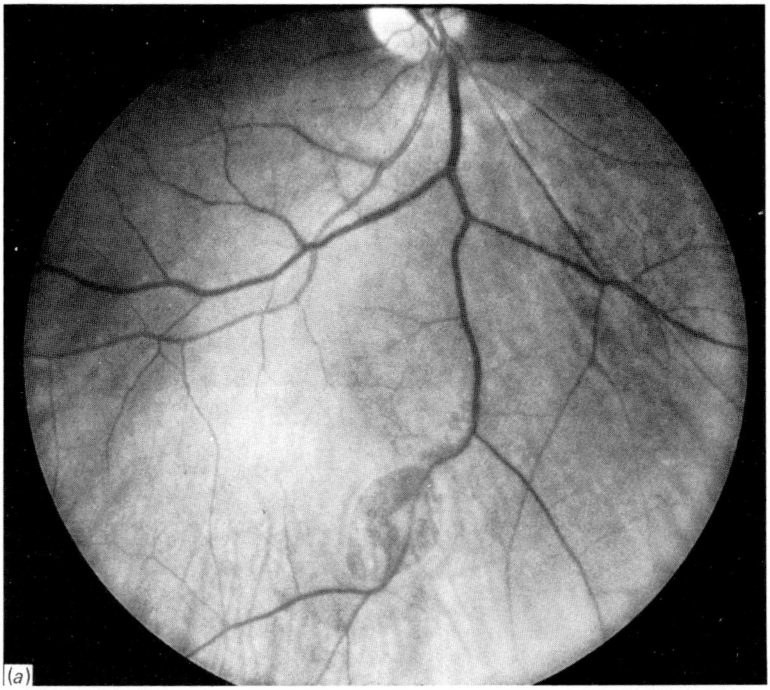


*Figure 15.1a* Vitreoretinal traction causing avulsion of a large retinal vein with a full-thickness retinal tear and surrounding subretinal fluid

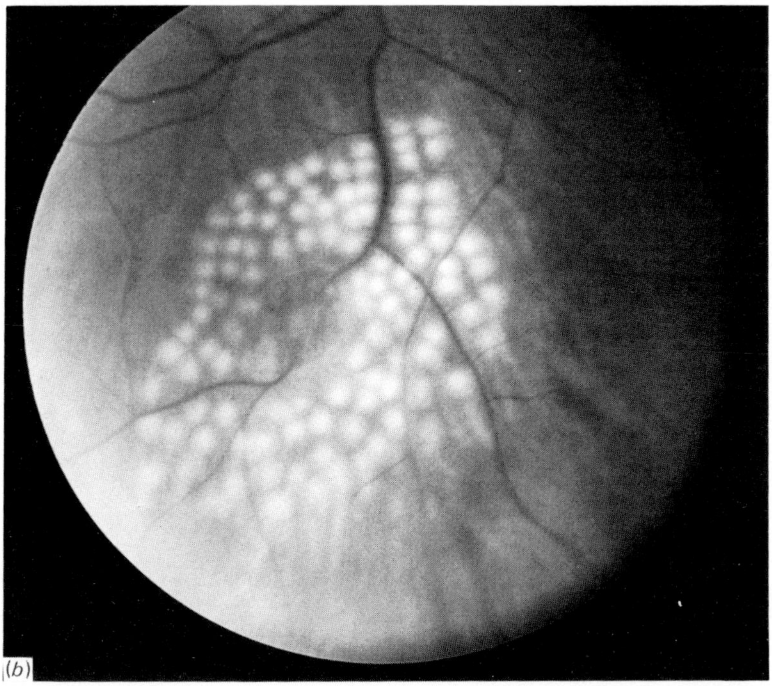


*Figure 15.1b* Argon laser photocoagulation burns surround the retinal tear

separate, and at sites of exaggerated adherence between the vitreous and the surface of the retina focal tractional complications may develop.

The first approach to a small focal traction detachment may be to surround the area with photocoagulation (*Figure 15.1a and b*). However, this may be dangerous if light energy is absorbed by the vitreous, causing further contraction and traction. The adherence caused by photocoagulation may be insufficient to counteract the increasing traction and, in fact, may contribute to the formation of multiple small retinal holes. When vitreoretinal traction continues to increase and threatens the macula, surgery becomes necessary. Although scleral shortening procedures have been employed in the past, an internal closed surgical approach to remove the vitreous and thus relieve the vitreoretinal traction directly has the highest chance of success. If there is a retinal tear and internal temporary gas tamponade is not technically feasible, external scleral buckling may be necessary.

In some eyes with incomplete posterior vitreous detachment, a strand of vitreous may remain attached to the macula and cause traction and cystoid degeneration within the macula, which may progress to a full-thickness macular hole (*Figure 15.2*). Rarely does the ophthalmologist or the pathologist have the opportunity to see the attachment of the cortical vitreous to the surface of the retina in the macular zone during this process, but we have seen sufficient examples of persistent foveal traction to accept it as a factor contributing to cystoid macular degeneration and macular hole formation. Although so far vitrectomy surgeons have had only limited experience in managing this problem, the removal of persistent traction before irreversible changes occur may be a logical approach.

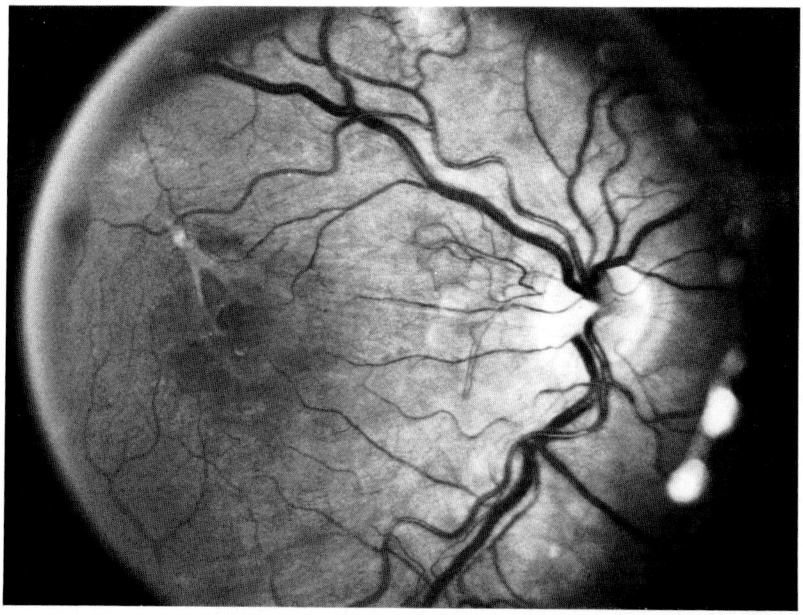

*Figure 15.2* Incomplete posterior vitreous detachment with persistent foveal traction causing cystoid degeneration of the fovea and a full-thickness retinal hole

## EPIRETINAL MEMBRANES

### Cellophane maculopathy

Focal avascular epiretinal membrane formation may be seen in elderly patients in the form of so-called cellophane maculopathy. Numerous authors have shown the membranes to be composed of monolayers, usually of glial cells that have migrated through a break in the internal limiting membrane (ILM) (Roth and Foos, 1971; Bellhorn *et al.*, 1975; Laqua and Machemer, 1975; Clarkson, Green and Massof, 1977). The subsequent contraction of the cells causes wrinkling of the underlying ILM and occasionally of the inner nerve fiber layer. A glinting surface reflex, often with distortion of the small macular vessels, is seen in the posterior fundus (*Figure 15.3a and 15.4a*). In most cases there is neither leakage of fluorescein (*Figure 15.3b*) nor retinal edema, and most patients remain asymptomatic. However, in those with symptoms, leakage of fluorescein is usually seen from the distorted retinal vessels (*Figure 15.4b*). In a small number of patients thickening of the membrane with more distortion leads to a significant decrease in visual acuity.

### Macular pucker

Macular pucker is, in our opinion, a more complex disorder, seen usually after blunt, penetrating or surgical trauma. It may also occur secondary to ocular inflammation. Here the membrane is composed of several layers of cells. As in cellophane maculopathy, these are frequently derived from glial cells in the retina, but have an additional complement of fibrocytes, macrophages and cells derived from pigment epithelium, which may or may not contain pigment. These membranes contain collagen (Clarkson, Green and Massof, 1977; Kampik *et al.*, 1980, 1981). Clinically, the membrane is easily recognized because of its opaque white appearance and the more pronounced distortion of the retina (*Figure 15.5a*). Visual acuity in eyes with macular pucker is markedly reduced, in contrast to that of cellophane maculopathy. In recent years we have found surgical intervention to be the most successful form of treatment for patients with macular pucker (*Figure 15.5b*).

The surgical management of eyes with severe cellophane maculopathy and macular pucker is most efficiently carried out through a pars plana approach with closed intraocular microsurgical techniques. A three-incision technique is preferred, with an infusion cannula fixed in place through the third incision. Because some of the membranes are transparent, internal illumination allows the surgeon to visualize the membrane more clearly. Oblique and retroillumination also help to delineate its edges and thickness more accurately.

First the vitreous is cleared in the area of the membrane, ensuring that no attachments of the vitreous to the membrane persist. The membrane is then dissected, using a 22-gauge disposable needle bent toward the bevel. A disposable needle is used because the edges and the tip of the needle are extremely sharp and can be used for horizontal delamination. An infusion line is then attached, taking

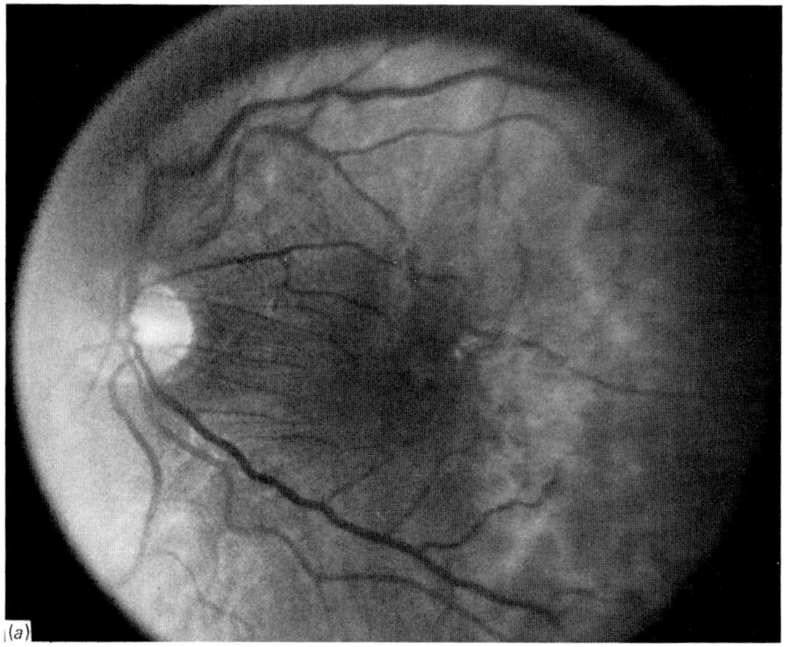

*Figure 15.3a* Clinical appearance of cellophane maculopathy in the left eye of an asymptomatic female aged 62 years. Note the retinal vessels which are pulled toward the membrane

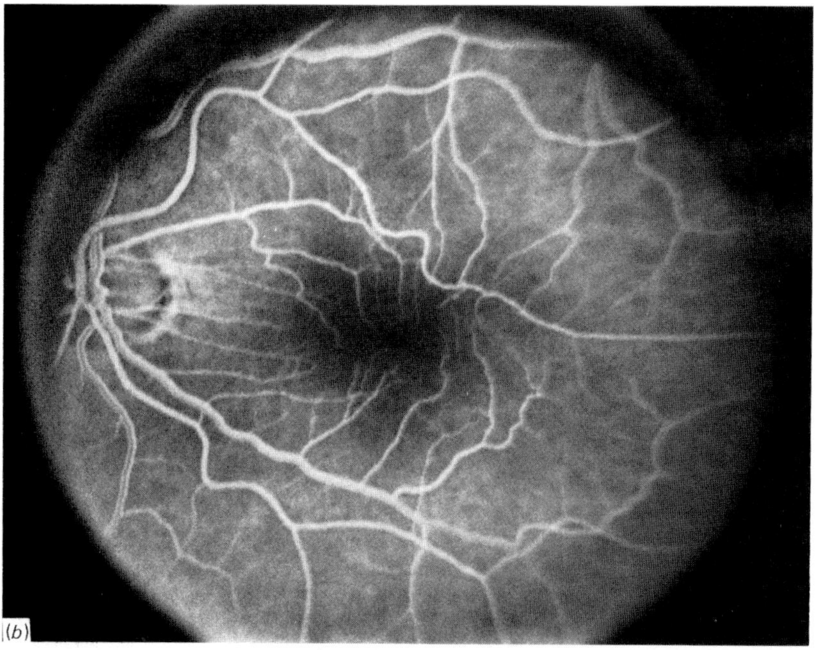

*Figure 15.3b* Same patient as in *Figure 15.3a*. Fluorescein angiogram showing more vivid distortion of the retinal vessels but no leakage of dye

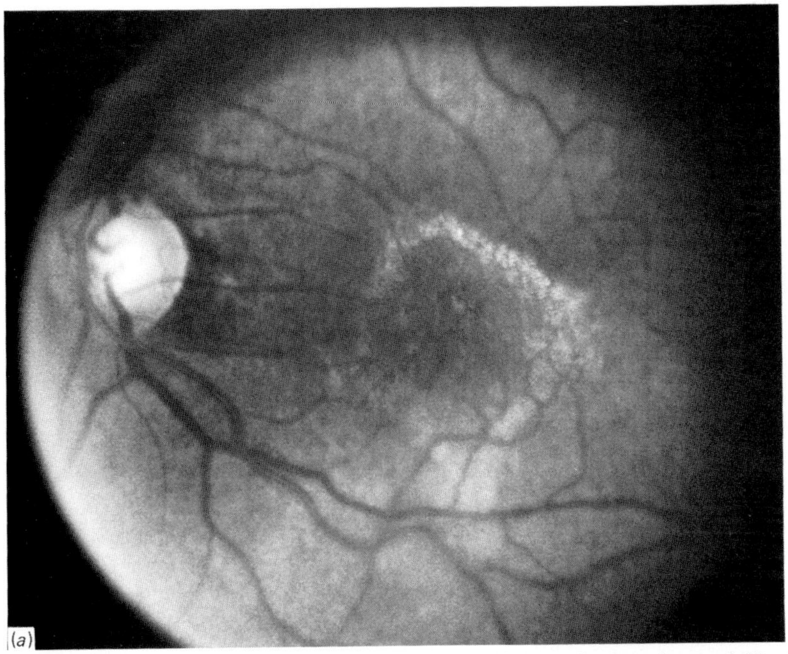

*Figure 15.4a* Cellophane maculopathy in the left eye of a female aged 68 with a visual acuity of 20/80. Note the abnormal reflex off the surface of the membrane with distortion of the retinal vessels

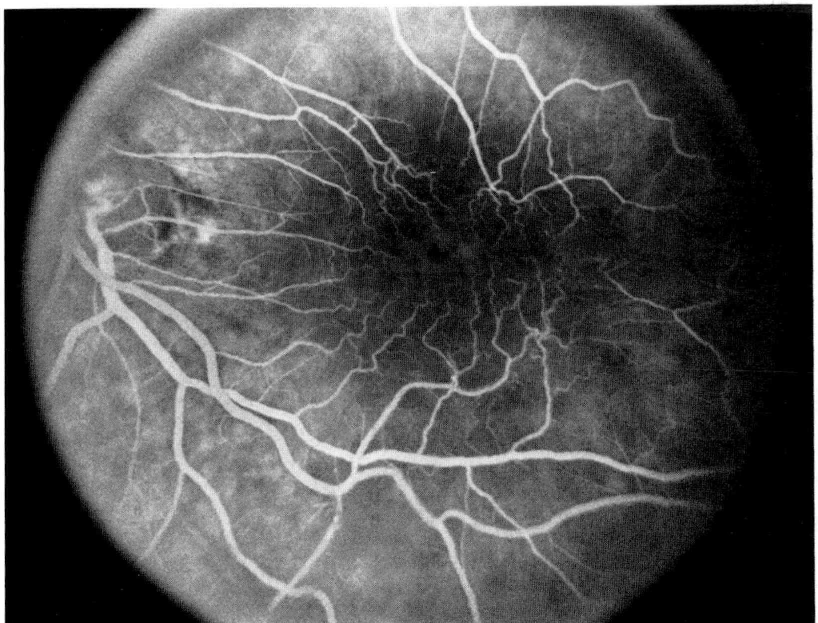

*Figure 15.4b* Fluorescein angiogram of the same area as in *Figure 15.4a* showing the tortuosity and distortion of the vessels, with leakage of fluorescein into the fovea

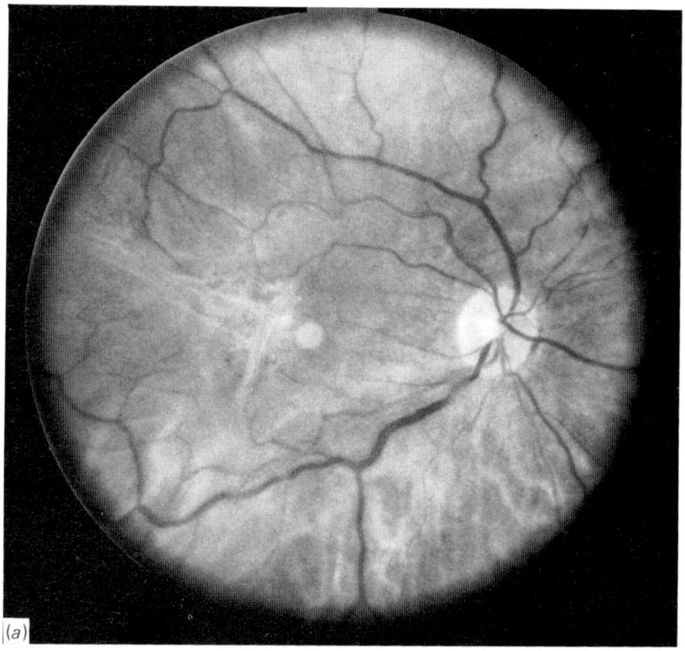

(a)

*Figure 15.5a* Preoperative clinical appearance of a macular pucker, in a male patient aged 54 years, which developed 8 weeks after retinal detachment surgery. The abnormal reflex on the surface of the epiretinal macular membrane and the distortion of the retinal vessels are more prominent than in cellophane maculopathy. Visual acuity is 20/200

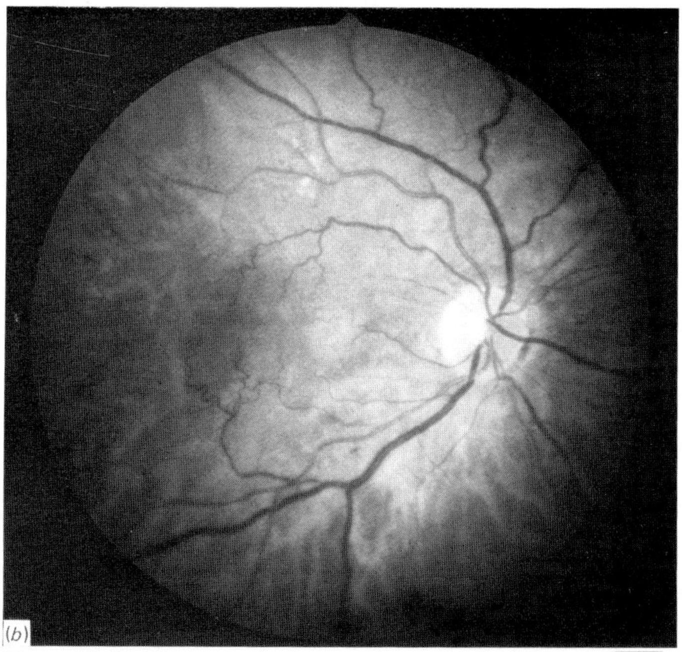

(b)

*Figure 15.5b* Postoperative appearance of the same eye as in *Figure 15.5a* 6 weeks after epiretinal membrane peeling. Visual acuity is now 20/30

care that the flow of infusion fluid is directed across the tip of the needle. This is sometimes advantageous during the dissection of the membrane. An edge to the membrane is identified and the membrane is lifted *en bloc* from the surface of the retina (*Figure 15.6*). The frequently less transparent appearance of the retina immediately beneath the membrane must not be mistaken for residual membrane.

The SITE end cutter can be used to remove scattered remnants of membrane from the retinal surface. Alternatively, the released membrane can be grasped with straight intraocular forceps (Sutherland) and removed *en bloc*. Postoperatively it may take a few days before the retina returns to its normal anatomical position.

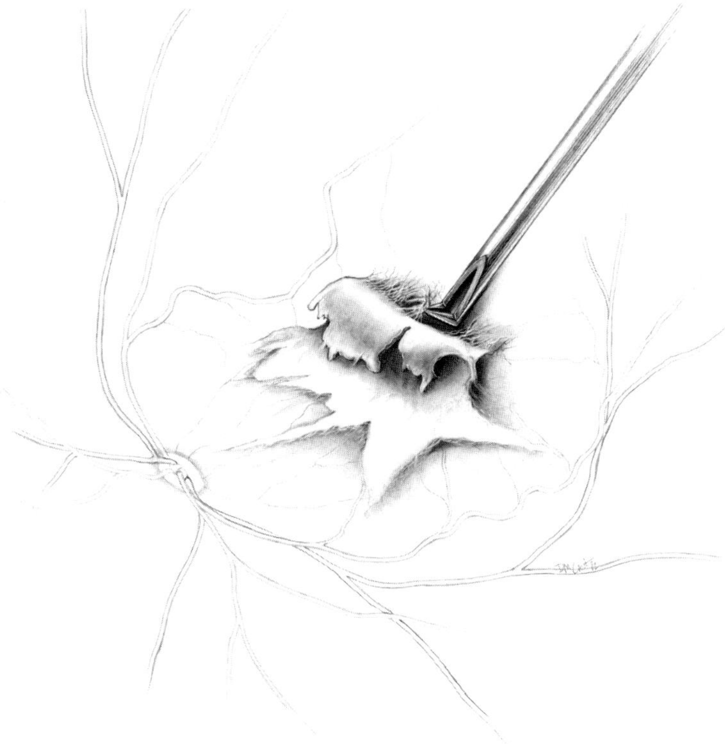

*Figure 15.6* Diagram of a 22-gauge bent needle being used to dissect an epiretinal membrane in an eye with macular pucker. The membrane is dissected in one block or in one mass

Most patients experience an improvement in vision (*see Figure 15.5b*), which in some may be as good as 20/20 (Michels, 1981; Federman, unpublished observation). In our experience restoration of good acuity is less likely in long-standing cases with established cystoid macular degeneration. Like other authors, we have found that inadvertent creation of macular or peripheral holes is the most common surgical complication (Charles, 1981; Michels, 1981). These retinal breaks can be successfuly managed by endophotocoagulation or cryopexy and, if necessary, gas tamponade. Macular pucker recurs in up to 4 per cent of patients (Charles, 1981; Michels, 1981).

## Massive periretinal proliferation

Diffuse avascular preretinal membrane formation is seen in eyes with massive periretinal proliferation (MPP). Recent histological studies have confirmed the presence of pigment epithelial cells, glial cells, fibroblasts, myofibroblasts and macrophages in membranes from eyes with MPP (Van Horn *et al.*, 1977; Kampik *et al.*, 1981; Newsome, Rodrigues and Machemer, 1981). The sources have been presumed to be the retina, the pigment epithelium, and blood (Machemer *et al.*, 1978; Kampik *et al.*, 1981). The cellular migration and growth may be considered as a repair mechanism that is particularly active in the young. Preretinal cells grow in sheets along the ILM and may involve the entire retinal surface. Subsequent contraction of cells produces 'star folds' and 'fixed folds' in the retina (*Figures 15.7 and 15.8*).

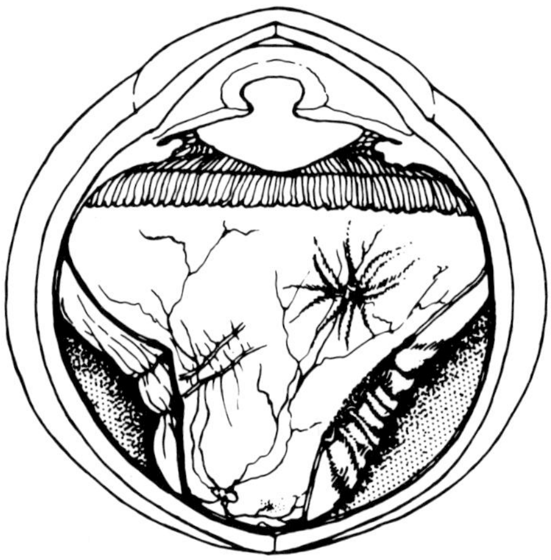

*Figure 15.7* Drawing of an eye with massive periretinal proliferation showing fixed folds radiating from the disc and a focal star-fold in the superotemporal quadrant. These folds are due predominantly to epiretinal membrane formation. A subretinal band extends from 2 o'clock to 6 o'clock in the temporal mid-periphery, causing pleats in the overlying retina

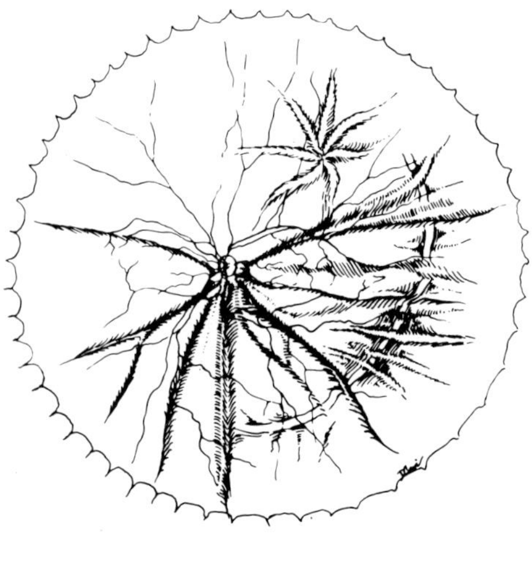

*Figure 15.8* Diagrammatic cross-section of an eye with massive periretinal proliferation. The star fixed-folds from the epiretinal membranes on the temporal side are caused by contraction of sheets of preretinal cells. On the nasal side, the subretinal bands elevate and cause folding of the overlying retina

The clinical presentation of MPP varies widely, ranging from one or two foci of star folds to diffuse fixed folds involving the entire fundus with or without subretinal bands (*Figures 15.7 and 15.8*). In its extreme form, MPP causes a tight funnel retinal detachment that obscures the disc (*Figure 15.9*). These various clinical manifestations have to be managed in different ways. Eyes with just one or two areas of fixed folds can be managed successfully with encircling buckling

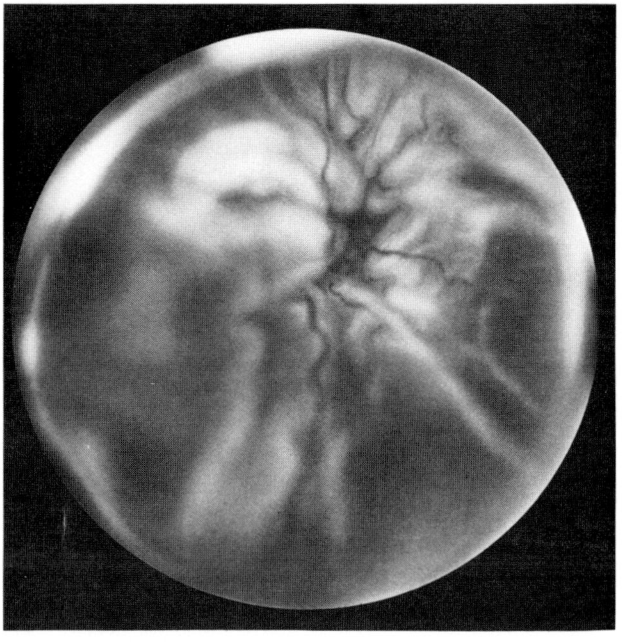

*Figure 15.9* Appearance of extreme massive periretinal proliferation. The disc is obscured by a funnel of retinal folds

procedures alone (Machemer, 1978). However, for more massive diffuse periretinal proliferation involving both surfaces of the retina, closed intraocular microsurgical procedures in conjunction with external buckles are indicated. We usually have to remove the lens in order to achieve adequate excision of the anterior vitreous, which exerts traction on the anterior retina.

It is unnecessary, and probably also unwise, to attempt to remove the entire epiretinal membrane. Membranes bridging fixed retinal folds should be lifted or divided as atraumatically as possible using a bent 22-gauge disposable needle or automated microsurgical scissors. Once the retina has been mobilized, a total air–gas fluid exchange is performed by draining fluid through the SITE end cutter or tapered extrusion needle and simultaneously injecting a 20 per cent SF6/air mixture through the infusion cannula (*Figure 15.10*). Trans-scleral cryopexy is then applied to all retinal breaks. If there is residual retinal traction, the retina is supported with a 360 degree buckle.

It is difficult to supply meaningful statistics of successful reattachment because of the wide spectrum of the disease (Machemer, 1977). Certainly, even the most advanced funnel-shaped detachments with subretinal components can be attached successfully with these techniques. In many cases of extensive MPP, however, the cellular proliferation continues postoperatively despite reattachment of the retina

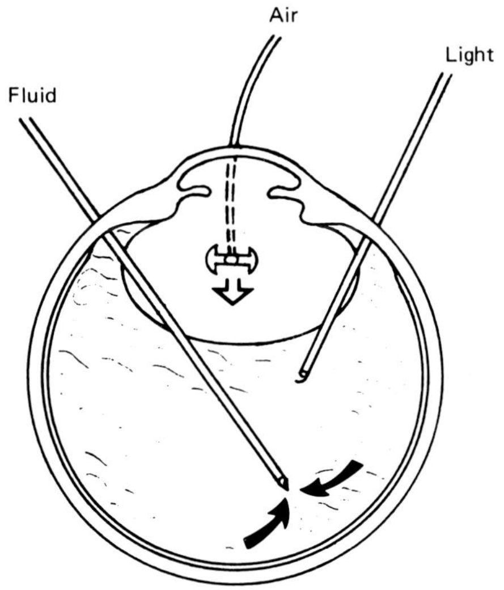


*Figure 15.10* A three-incision closed system showing the technique of air–gas fluid exchange. Air is injected through the cannula superiorly while fluid is drained inferiorly

at the time of surgery, and subsequent contracture causes redetachment. Corticosteroids and other drugs have been employed in an attempt to prevent further proliferation after the retina has been reattached (Tano, Chandler and Machemer, 1980; Tano *et al.*, 1980), but their value is only speculative at present. In certain cases in which multiple procedures have failed to reattach the retina, injection of silicone oil into the vitreous may be successful (Kanski and Daniel, 1973; Scott, 1973; Cairns, J. and Charles, S., personal communication).

## SUBRETINAL MEMBRANES

Cells may also proliferate in the subretinal space, particularly in eyes with long-standing detachments (Wallyn and Hilton, 1979). The subretinal components have been investigated in monkeys by Machemer and have been found to be derived from glial and pigment epithelial cells (Laqua and Machemer, 1975; Machemer and Laqua, 1975). In contrast to preretinal cells, which grow in sheets, cells in the subretinal space grow in strands or tubules (*Figure 15.11*). These subretinal bands bridge foci of presumed outer retina and pigment epithelial injury, and otherwise are suspended through the subretinal space (Laqua and Machemer, 1975). As these tubular membranes contract, the overlying retina is thrown into folds (*see Figures 15.7 and 15.8*).

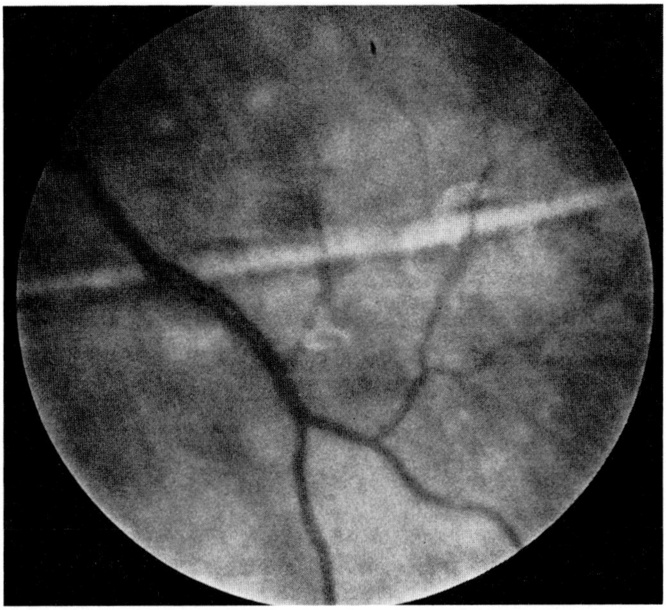

*Figure 15.11* Clinical appearance of a subretinal band. There is an overlying retinal detachment and the retinal vessels are slightly distorted

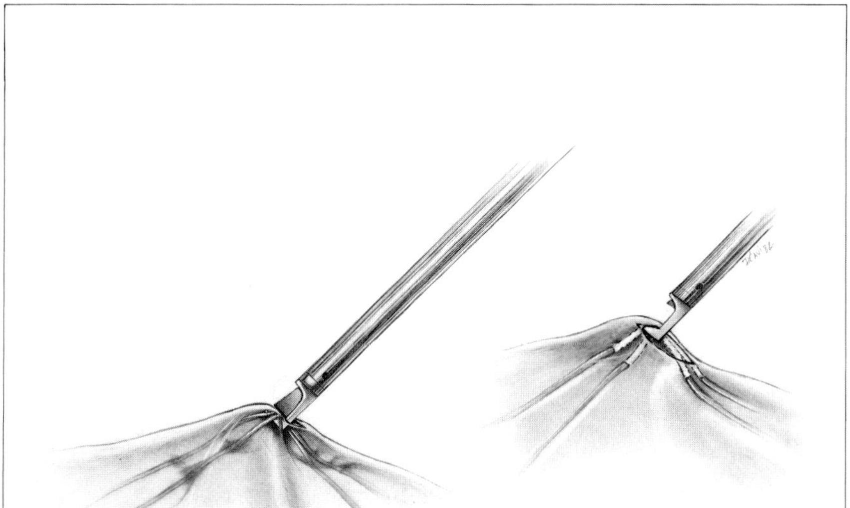

*Figure 15.12* Section of subretinal bands. Automated microsurgical scissors are placed through a retinotomy and under the subretinal bands (*left*). The scissors are then activated and the bands are cut (*right*). The divided bands retract into the subretinal space

If subretinal bands prevent reattachment of the retina it may be necessary to support the involved area with a scleral buckle. Machemer has described techniques by which these subretinal strands can be cut either through the sclera and choroid or internally via a peripheral retinal tear (Machemer, 1980). We have successfully divided subretinal bands directly through the retina (*Figure 15.12*). The retinotomies are then closed with transvitreal or trans-scleral cryopexy. In several of our patients in whom more conventional methods had failed, this technique has allowed reattachment of the retina.

## SUMMARY

Periretinal proliferation is manifest as either preretinal or subretinal avascular or vascular membrane formation. We have concentrated only on the avascular membranes, which are most effectively managed by closed intraocular microsurgical techniques. Increasing technological advances, such as the development of the YAG laser, may enable us in the future to disrupt these membranes by non-invasive techniques. Medical management may play a role in preventing membrane formation or reformation, but this has not yet been established.

## References

Bellhorn, M. B., Friedman, A. H., Wise, G. N. and Henkind, P. (1975). Ultrastructure and clinicopathologic correlation of idiopathic preretinal macular fibrosis. *American Journal of Ophthalmology*, **79**, 366–373

Charles, S. (1981). *Vitreous Microsurgery*, 1st edition, 131–133. Baltimore: Williams and Wilkins

Clarkson, J. G., Green, W. R. and Massof, D. (1977). A histopathologic review of 168 cases of preretinal membrane. *American Journal of Ophthalmology*, **84**, 1–17

Hogan, M. J., Alvarado, J. A. and Weddell, J. E. (1971). *Histology of the Human Eye*, 1st edition, 488–490, 607–657. Philadelphia: W. B. Saunders

Kampik, A., Green, W. R., Michels, R. G. and Nase, P. K. (1980). Ultrastructural features of progressive idiopathic epiretinal membrane removed by vitreous surgery. *American Journal of Ophthalmology*, **90**, 797–809

Kampik, A., Kenyon, K. R., Michels, R. G., Green, W. R. and De La Cruz, Z. C. (1981). Epiretinal and vitreous membranes. Comparative study of 56 cases. *Archives of Ophthalmology*, **99**, 1445–1454

Kanski, J. J. and Daniel, R. (1973). Intravitreal silicone injection in retinal detachment. *British Journal of Ophthalmology*, **51**, 542–545

Laqua, H. and Machemer, R. (1975). Glial cell proliferation in retinal detachment. *American Journal of Ophthalmology*, **80**, 602–618

Machemer, R. (1974). A new concept for vitreous surgery. Two instrument techniques in pars plana vitrectomy. *Archives of Ophthalmology,* **92**, 407–412

Machemer, R. (1976). Removal of preretinal membranes. *Transactions of the American Academy of Ophthalmology and Otolaryngology*, **81**, 420–425

Machemer, R. (1977). Massive periretinal proliferation: a logical approach to therapy. *Transactions of the American Ophthalmic Society*, **75**, 556–586

Machemer, R. (1978). Pathogenesis and classification of massive periretinal proliferation. *British Journal of Ophthalmology*, **62**, 737–747

Machemer, R. (1980). Surgical approaches to subretinal strands. *American Journal of Ophthalmology*, **90**, 81–85

Machemer, R. and Laqua, H. (1975). Pigment epithelial proliferation in retinal detachment. *American Journal of Ophthalmology*, **80**, 1–23

Machemer, R., Van Horn, D. and Aaberg, T. M. (1978). Pigment epithelial proliferation in human retinal detachment with massive periretinal proliferation. *American Journal of Ophthalmology*, **85**, 181–191

Michels, R. G. (1981). Vitreous surgery for macular pucker. *American Journal of Ophthalmology*, **92**, 628–639

Newsome, D. A., Rodrigues, M. M. and Machemer, R. (1981). Human massive periretinal proliferation. *In vitro* characteristics of cellular components. *Archives of Ophthalmology*, **99**, 873–880

Roth, A. M. and Foos, R. Y. (1971). Surface wrinkling retinopathy in eyes enucleated at autopsy. *Transactions of the American Academy of Ophthalmology and Otolaryngology*, **75**, 1047–1058

Scott, J. D. (1973). The treatment of massive vitreous retraction. *Transactions of the Ophthalmological Society of the UK*, **93**, 417–423

Shea, M. (1980). The surgical management of macular pucker in rhegmatogenous retinal detachment. *Ophthalmology*, **87**, 70–74

Tano, Y., Chandler, D. and Machemer, R. (1980). Treatment of intraocular proliferation with intravitreal injection of triamcinolone acetonide. *American Journal of Ophthalmology*, **90**, 810–816

Tano, Y., Sugita, G., Abrams, G. and Machemer, R. (1980). Inhibition of intraocular proliferation with intravitreal corticosteroids. *American Journal of Ophthalmology*, **89**, 131–136

Van Horn, D., Aaberg, T. M., Machemer, R. and Fenzl, R. (1977). Glial cell proliferation in human retinal detachment with massive periretinal proliferation. *American Journal of Ophthalmology*, **84**, 383–393

Wallyn, R. H. and Hilton, G. F. (1979). Subretinal fibrosis in retinal detachment. *Archives of Ophthalmology*, **97**, 2128–2129

Wise, G. N. (1975). Clinical features of idiopathic preretinal macular fibrosis. *American Journal of Ophthalmology*, **79**, 349–357

# 16
# Closed intraocular microsurgical techniques in the anterior segment

M. Madison Slusher, Jay L. Federman and Jack J. Kanski

## INTRODUCTION

The term 'closed intraocular microsurgery' (CIOM) refers to the removal of intraocular tissue through small incisions with automated suction-cutting devices while maintaining the intraocular pressure at a normal or slightly elevated level. This chapter will deal with CIOM of the anterior segment in terms of broad principles and techniques.

## INDICATIONS AND TECHNIQUES

### Vitreous touch syndrome

A frequent indication for anterior vitrectomy either via a limbal or pars plana approach is corneal contact by the anterior hyaloid face leading to endothelial decompensation and corneal oedema (Michels, Machemer and Mueller-Jensen, 1974, *Figure 16.1*). Pre-existing endothelial disease such as Fuchs' dystrophy may predispose to this complication. Early intervention is necessary if the patient is to be spared a keratoplasty, as there is a strong relationship between the chronicity of corneal oedema and visual results (Taylor, Michels and Stark, 1979; Wilkinson and Rowsey, 1980; Leibowitz *et al.*, 1981).

### Aphakic pupil-block glaucoma

Anterior vitrectomy is also a satisfactory procedure in the management of aphakic pupil-block glaucoma (*Figure 16.1*). An adequate amount of vitreous should be removed and air introduced into the anterior chamber. This is aimed at relieving the pupil-block, opening the angle, and normalizing intraocular pressure. The air should be introduced into the anterior chamber before the cutter is withdrawn in order to prevent 'formed' vitreous following the instrument out of the eye and becoming incarcerated in the wound. This technique is also very useful in the

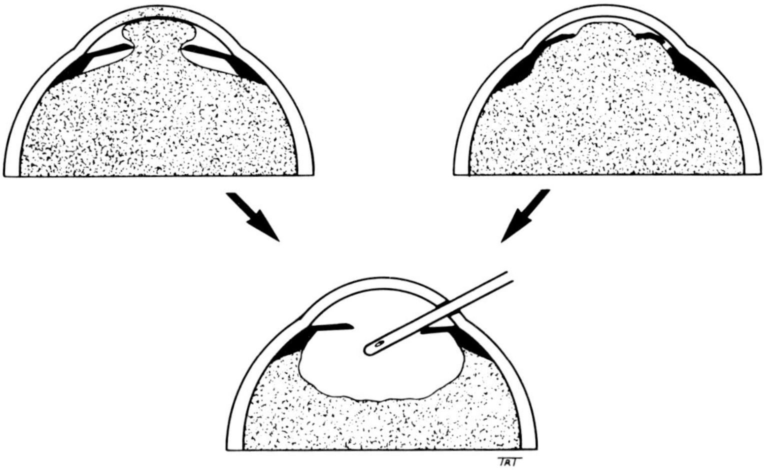

*Figure 16.1* Corneal oedema due to vitreous touch (*top left*) and aphakic pupil-block glaucoma (*top right*) can be managed by anterior vitrectomy (*bottom*)

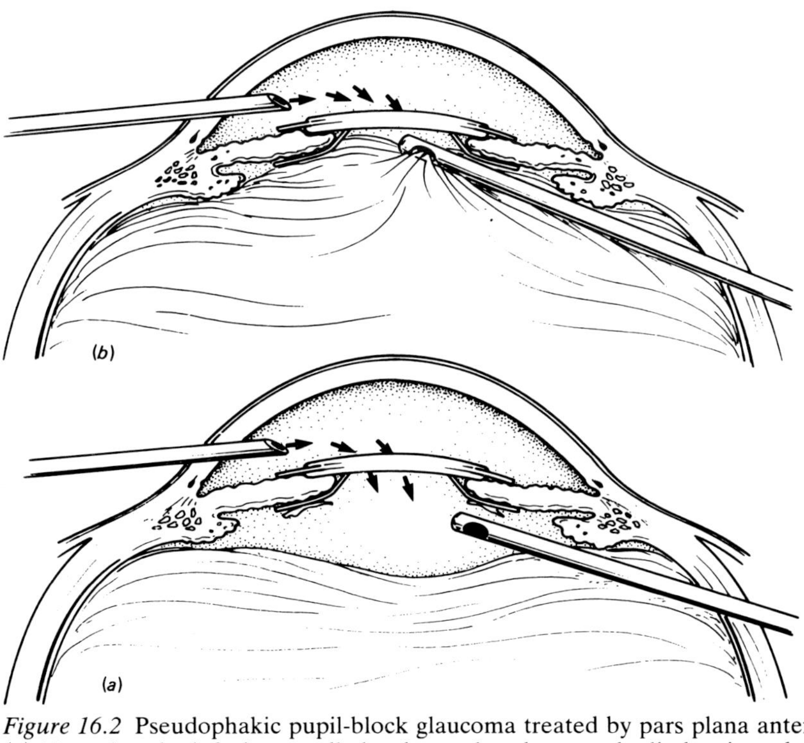


*Figure 16.2* Pseudophakic pupil-block glaucoma treated by pars plana anterior vitrectomy. (*a*) Note that the infusion needle has been placed across the limbus in order to prevent the intraocular lens from damaging the corneal endothelium. (*b*) Free passage of perfusion fluid is possible once anterior vitreous has been excised. The same technique can be used to provide laminar flow between a retropseudophakic membrane and an intraocular lens, allowing the cutter to engage the membrane without displacing the intraocular lens

management of pseudophakic glaucoma due to adhesion of vitreous to the entire posterior surface of an intraocular lens and iris, with obstruction of the peripheral iridectomies (*Figure 16.2*). When treating the 'aqueous misdirection syndromes' a larger amount of vitreous should be removed from the mid-vitreous cavity so that aqueous can percolate freely (Taylor, Michels and Stark, 1979).

## Vitreous wick syndrome

This is a rare complication of cataract extraction in which vitreous gel protrudes either through an oversized limbal suture track or a small dehiscence in the wound. Treatment is by excision of incarcerated vitreous, anterior vitrectomy and repair of the defect (Rice and Michels, 1978).

## Filtration surgery in aphakia

It has long been recognized that the results of filtration surgery in aphakic eyes with vitreous gel in the anterior chamber are inferior to similar procedures in phakic eyes. Herschler (1981) has reported that anterior vitrectomy enhances the pressure-lowering effects of filtration procedures in aphakic eyes. Vitrectomy can be performed as a separate procedure, preceding glaucoma surgery (usually trabeculectomy), or the vitreous can be removed at the time of filtration surgery. Some authors remove vitreous through the trabeculectomy incision, whilst others prefer a pars plana approach. Since the actual mechanism of surgical success is frequently unclear, some advocate a 'total' posterior vitrectomy, whilst others stress the importance of removing that portion of the vitreous likely to find its way to the filtration site (Taylor, Michels and Stark, 1979; Herschler, 1981).

## Irvine–Gass syndrome

Although most cases of cystoid macular oedema following cataract extraction (Irvine–Gass syndrome) are transient, occasionally prolonged oedema may cause a significant impairment of central vision. Several recent studies have reported not only lessening of the cystoid macular oedema and improvement of vision but also a significant decrease in pain and irritability of these eyes following vitrectomy (Aaberg, 1977; Taylor, Michels and Stark, 1979; Federman *et al*., 1980; Fung, 1980).

Although at present case selection for vitrectomy is still controversial, eyes with vitritis associated with adhesion of anteriorly herniated vitreous to the wound and iris distortion in which cystoid macular oedema is both clinically and angiographically significant should be considered for surgical intervention. Patients in whom a course of systemic or periocular injections of steroids has led to an improvement of vitreous inflammation, which then regresses when therapy is discontinued, are thought to be particularly good candidates.

## Epithelial ingrowth

This rare but devastating complication of cataract extraction frequently leads to intractable glaucoma. The source of the ingrowth is the conjunctival epithelium. Predisposing factors include implantation of epithelial cells by instruments, delayed wound closure, incarceration of vitreous or iris in the wound, and 'through-and-through' suturing of the section. In 1978 Stark *et al.* described a method by which this condition could be treated successfully. The extent of iris involvement is first

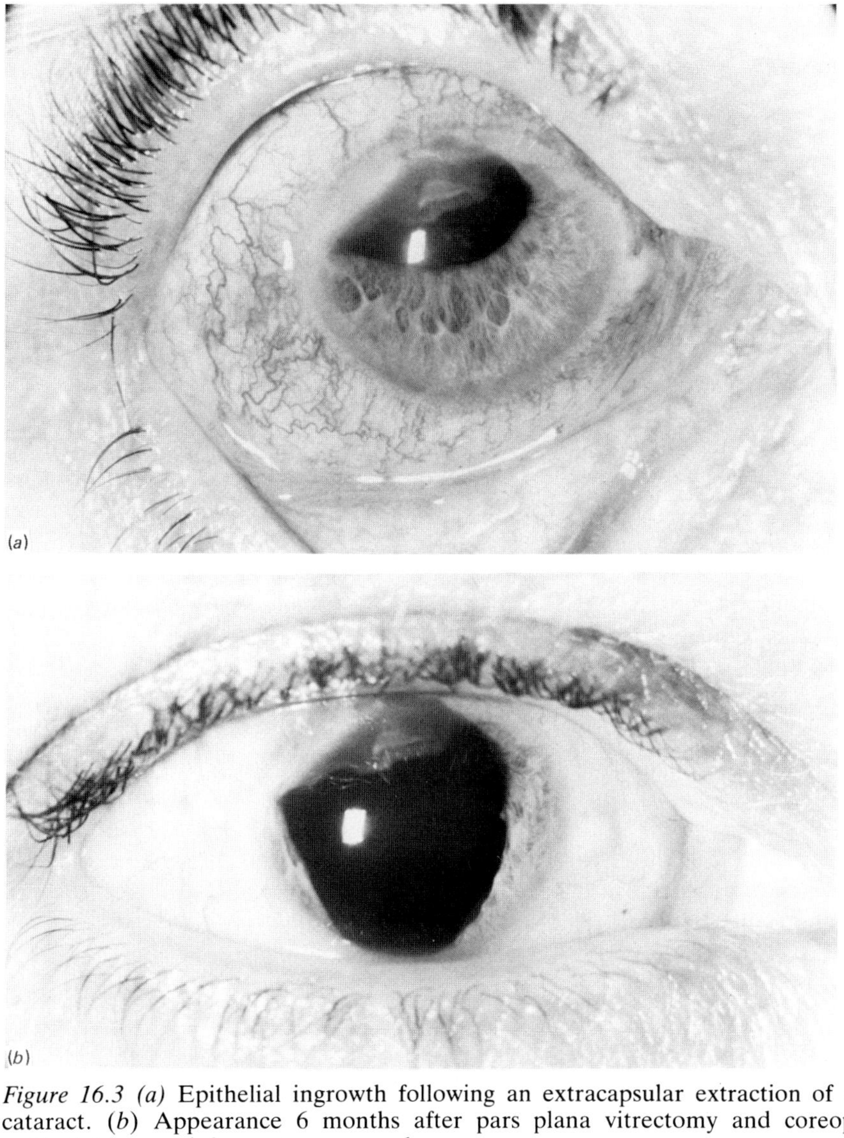

*Figure 16.3 (a)* Epithelial ingrowth following an extracapsular extraction of a traumatic cataract. (*b*) Appearance 6 months after pars plana vitrectomy and coreoplasty. The epithelial ingrowth has not progressed

identified by applying argon laser photocoagulation to suspicious areas. The fistula is then identified and closed, and the involved iris tissue and vitreous are excised with a vitreous cutter. The anterior chamber is then filled with air to insulate the effects of cryotherapy, which is applied to the angle, cornea and ciliary body in order to destroy the epithelial cells. *Figure 16.3* shows the pre- and postoperative appearance of a successfully treated case. Giant epithelial cysts in the anterior chamber can be treated in a similar manner.

## Angle neovascularization and spontaneous hyphaema

Thin inflammatory pupillary membranes and recurrent vitritis or blood-tinged vitreous adhesions to the corneal endothelium with secondary stromal oedema may occur in association with angle neovascularization and spontaneous hyphaema following uncomplicated extracapsular cataract extraction. Anterior vitrectomy through a limbal incision, combined with bipolar diathermy to the angle vessels, has been shown to be effective in preventing further bleeding, reversing the corneal oedema and correcting the iris distortion secondary to the inflamed, blood-tinged vitreous (Michels and Rice, 1977).

## Pupillary membranes

Probably no other area of anterior segment surgery has been so revolutionized by the advent of CIOM techniques as the management of pupillary membranes (Kanski and Crick, 1977a; Treister and Machemer, 1978; Kanski and Ramsay, 1980; Van Oldenborgh, 1980; Diddie *et al.*, 1982). In the past many of these cases had numerous procedures, which frequently resulted in failure. Even now, with CIOM techniques, the excision of tough fibrous and non-malleable membranes may pose significant difficulties unless accessory instruments capable of creating a 'ribbon' or edge to the membrane are used (*Figure 16.4*). Automated intraocular scissors primarily designed for cutting and segmentation of epiretinal membranes are very suitable for this purpose.

Inflammatory membranes in eyes with intraocular lenses offer their own set of challenges, as both the anterior and posterior surface of the implant may be involved. In certain cases a bimanual approach utilizing an infusion needle introduced through the limbus and a vitreous cutter via the pars plana may be successful in scraping or polishing both surfaces of the implant, and at the same time maintaining the depth of the anterior chamber and preventing damage to the corneal endothelium by the lens.

## Posteriorly dislocated intraocular lenses

CIOM techniques are useful in the management of posteriorly dislocated intraocular lenses that cannot be repositioned by posture and miotics (Mackool, 1981).

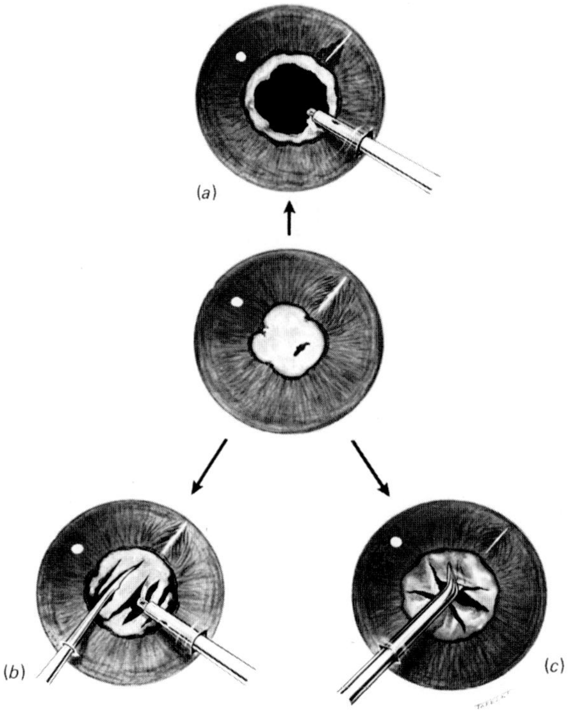


*Figure 16.4* Excision of pupillary membranes. (*a*) Soft and pliable membranes can be removed with the cutter alone. Tough fibrous and non-malleable membranes have to be sectioned first so as to create tissue edges that can be aspirated by the cutting port. This can be achieved by using either a Ziegler's knife (*b*) or intraocular scissors (*c*)

First a subtotal pars plana vitrectomy is performed and then the lens is grasped with intraocular foreign body forceps. Using the fibreoptic endoilluminator for support the lens is then repositioned in the plane of the iris and refixated with a McCannel suture. If complete removal of the intraocular lens is required, the implant can be held in position with foreign body forceps with one hand while the second hand prepares a limbal incision through which the psuedophakos can be extracted.

## Persistent hyperplastic primary vitreous (PHPV)

Because of its unique features, PHPV should be approached with caution. Preoperative B-scan ultrasonography must be performed in order to evaluate the thickness and vascularity of the retrolental membrane, as well as to detect the presence of tractional retinal detachment. Because in eyes with PHPV the retina frequently inserts anteriorly directly into the pars plicata, the incision should be placed 1–2 mm behind the limbus in order to avoid retinal damage (Federman *et al.*, 1982). However, this approach may also present potential problems since branches of the anterior ciliary vessels as well as the major arterial circle vessels in the iris may be encountered. The lens and the retrolental membrane should be excised first. Vitreous should then be removed from around the fibrovascular 'stalk', which may extend all the way from the retrolental membrane to the optic nerve head and which contains remnants of the hyaloid artery system. In order to prevent bleeding, intraocular cautery should be applied distal to the point at which the stalk is sectioned.

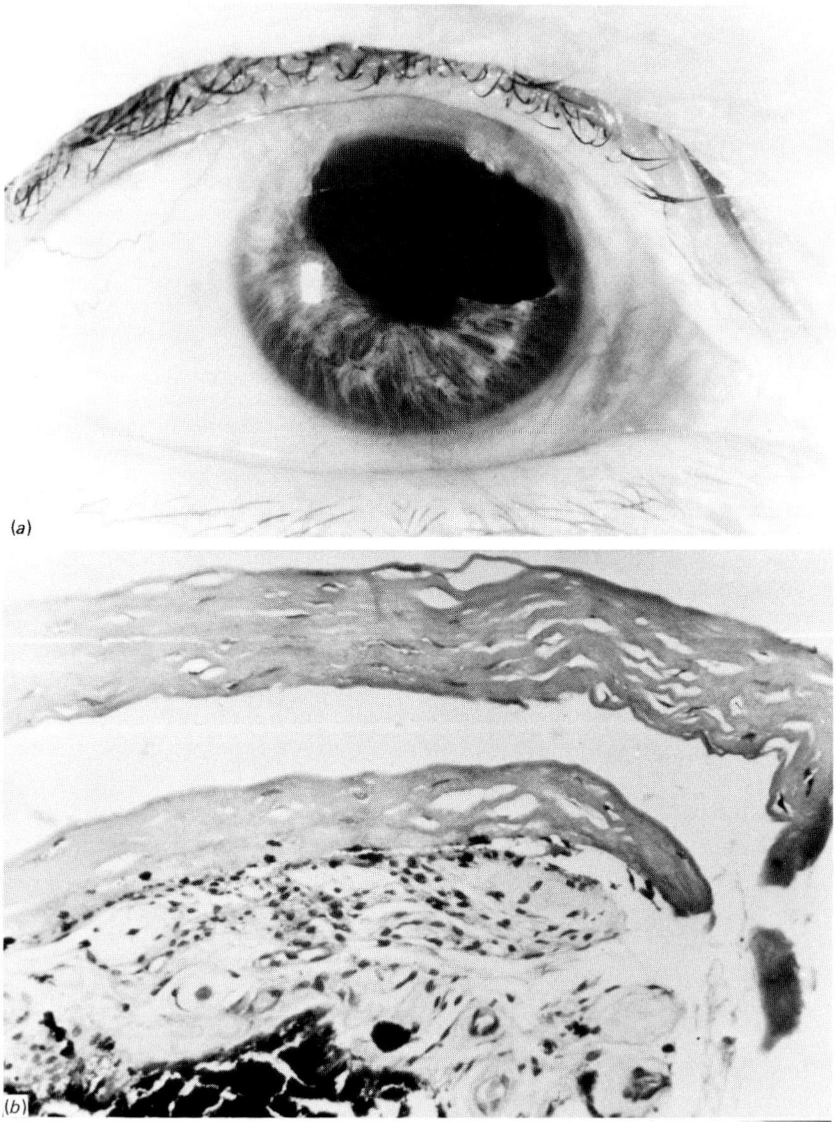

*Figure 16.5* (*a*) Postoperative appearance following *en bloc* removal of a dense pupillary membrane and section of iris to provide tissue for microscopical study. (*b*) Photomicrograph of membrane-iris tissue shows a rare stromalization process involving the anterior chamber (PAS ×16)

## Anterior segment biopsy

Although the value of posterior segment biopsy is well recognized (Michels *et al.*, 1975), only recently has an *en bloc* excision and examination of anterior segment tissue been reported using CIOM techniques (Slusher, 1981; *Figure 16.5*).

## Removal of cortical lens material

Technical improvements in the linear suction apparatus for cortical stripping in adult extracapsular extraction have popularized the use of vitreous cutters for this purpose. The advantage of vitreous cutters over other irrigation–aspiration devices is that a cutting potential is instantly available should it be required in the event of rupture of the posterior capsule, vitreous loss, or the dislodgement of lens material into the vitreous cavity. Vitreous cutters whose aspiration ports can be aligned while only suction is activated are most suitable. Technically, probes with end ports, as opposed to side ports, are also preferred, since cortical lens material may be more readily engaged and stripped from the capsular recess with an end-cutting probe.

## Lensectomy

Lensectomy (*Figure 16.6*) is an operation in which the lens is removed using a vitreous cutter. It can be performed either through a limbal incision or through the pars plana. The choice of a limbal versus a pars plana approach is determined mainly by the desirability of leaving the posterior capsule *in situ*. For example, in young patients certain cataracts may be removed without resorting to ultrasonic fragmentation. In these cases the lens cortex and nucleus are first hydrated and then simply aspirated with the probe without activating the cutting mode. The posterior capsule can then be 'polished' if necessary.

In the treatment of congenital cataract the posterior capsule is usually excised in order to enable the surgeon to obtain a good view of the fundus and also to perform an accurate refraction against the clear red reflex. Several studies have suggested that lensectomy is probably a superior procedure than older techniques such as discission, linear extraction, and aspiration in the treatment of congenital cataracts (Harcourt, 1980; Taylor, 1981; Peyman *et al.*, 1981). The main disadvantage of lensectomy at present is the lack of long-term results, particularly regarding the incidence of retinal detachment.

Lensectomy has revolutionized the management of cataracts secondary to chronic anterior uveitis (Kanski and Crick, 1977b; Diamond and Kaplan, 1978, 1979). These eyes frequently have extensive posterior synechiae and small pupils, making access to the lens difficult. Using the vitreous cutter, the pupil can be enlarged, making access to the lens much easier. It is essential to excise the posterior capsule together with a generous amount of anterior vitreous in order to eliminate the 'scaffold' along which postoperative inflammatory membranes can

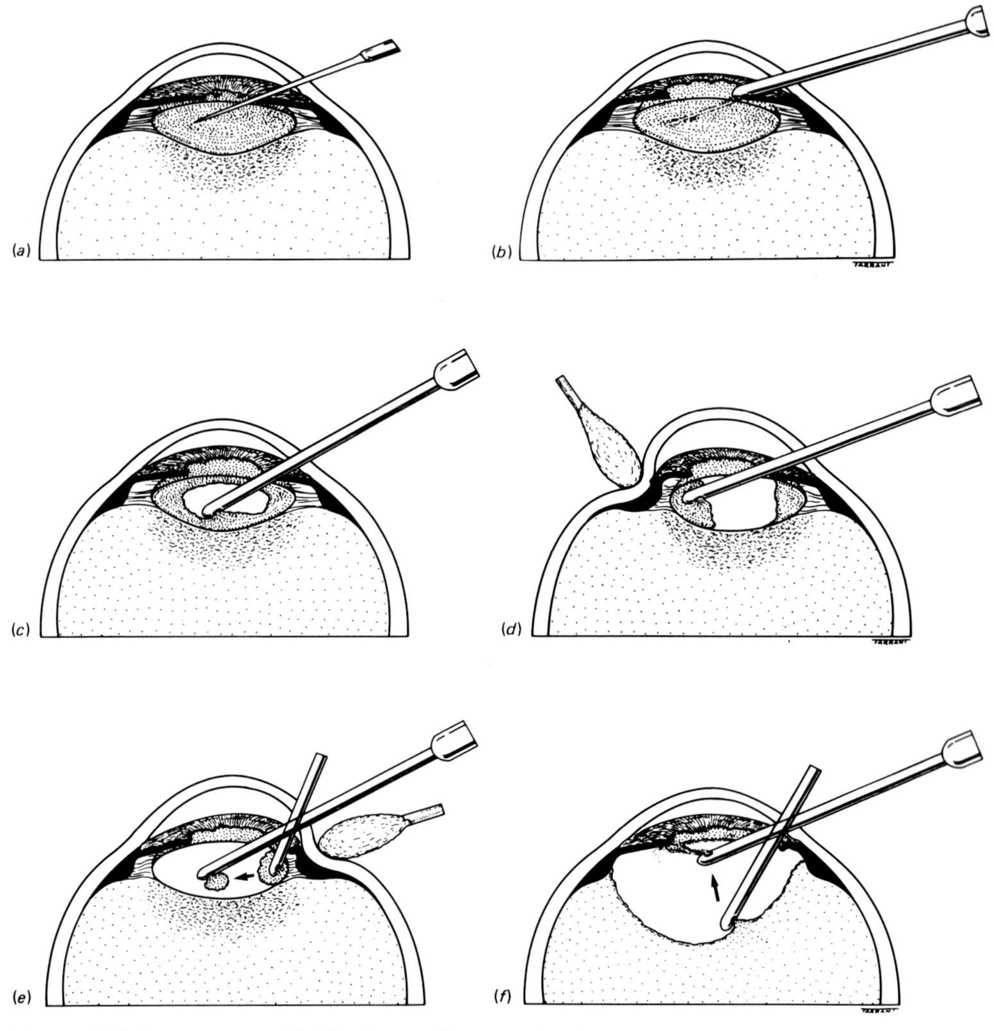


*Figure 16.6* Lensectomy. (*a*) Hardness of lens nucleus is tested with a knife. (*b*) If necessary, pupil is enlarged. (*c*) Nuclear and cortical material is removed while working within the 'capsular bag'. (*d*) The limbus is indented to remove cortical lens material from under the iris. (*e*) Lens material adjacent to site of incision is removed. (*f*) Posterior capsule together with a variable amount of anterior vitreous is excised. The anterior capsule is removed last

proliferate. It has been suggested by some that operation should not be undertaken in the presence of active ocular inflammation (Praeger *et al.*, 1976). Although this is an ideal objective it is very difficult to achieve in practice. As lensectomy is a relatively atraumatic procedure compared with older techniques, eyes with active uveitis seem to tolerate the operation well without any significant exacerbation of inflammation, provided a subconjunctival injection of corticosteroids is given after the completion of surgery and topical steroids are administered at frequent intervals during the immediate postoperative period.

## Anterior segment trauma

The ability to excise injured tissue or blood by CIOM techniques has radically altered the basic approach to a variety of traumatic anterior segment disorders. For example, non-resolving organized blood clots in the anterior chamber can be evacuated without endangering the lens or iris (McCuen and Fung, 1979; Stern and Mondal, 1979) and traumatically subluxated lenses can be removed (Kanski, 1978; Peyman *et al.*, 1979). In the management of subluxated lenses, a bimanual technique utilizing a vitreous cutter and a fibreoptic endoilluminator via the pars plana enables the surgeon to 'feed' the lens into the aspiration port of the cutter by using the sharp-tipped endoilluminator for fixation. The endoilluminator may also be necessary should lens fragments become displaced posteriorly.

The greatest applicability of CIOM techniques has been in the management of trauma to the lens and anterior vitreous, which may or may not be associated with laceration to the cornea or sclera. Although in these cases the degree of lens disruption and the extent of lens–vitreous–blood admixture posteriorly shows great variability, the first priority is to restore normal ocular contours and to normalize intraocular pressure by meticulous closure of all wounds. Non-viable tissue prolapsing through any laceration should also be carefully excised. Once this has been achieved the extent of posterior segment involvement should be assessed by B-scan ultrasonography.

Several reports have pointed out that selected penetrating injuries involving the posterior segment may be most satisfactorily approached after an interval of 10–14 days, during which the posterior vitreous has detached. This ostensibly reduces the risk of causing vitreoretinal traction and retinal tear formation during vitrectomy.

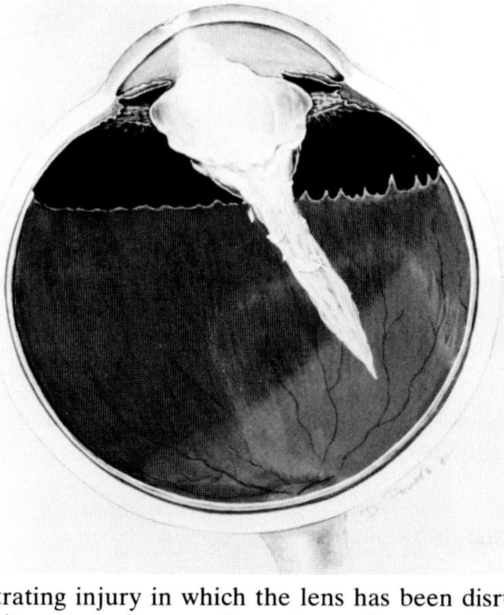

*Figure 16.7* Penetrating injury in which the lens has been disrupted and lens material has tracked into the vitreous cavity, creating a lens–vitreous admixture which also frequently contains blood

However, because of the marked inflammatory response and potential corneal endothelial decompensation in eyes with corneoscleral lacerations associated with massive lens rupture and lens–vitreous–blood admixture (*Figure 16.7*), few surgeons would advocate such a long delay in the removal of damaged intraocular tissue once primary repair has been carried out. The rationale for a meticulous removal of all traumatized tissue via a pars plana approach is to eliminate the matrix for infection, vitreous surface cell proliferation, and the potential for phakogenic uveitis. The most feared long-term complication of such a massive inflammatory reaction is tractional retinal detachment.

Because of the difficulties in performing and interpreting B-scan ultrasonography of the peripheral globe, it is extremely important for the surgeon to examine the peripheral retina using the fibreoptic endoilluminator at the end of vitrectomy in order to detect and repair any occult shallow retinal detachment, which is not uncommon in these cases. Recent emphasis on the simultaneous microscopical management of retinal detachment and anterior segment disorders imposes added measures of responsibility on the surgeon (Bonnet, 1980; Slusher, 1982). He must not only be capable of assessing accurately the extent of ocular damage but also of judging the feasibility of performing a successful one-stage surgical repair.

## COMPLICATIONS

### Corneal complications

Recent studies have shown that corneal endothelial cell counts decrease with any CIOM procedure, regardless of the presence or absence of the lens (Buettner and Bourne, 1982). Since this is partly due to the effect of the infusion fluid on the endothelial cells, it is important to reduce both the volume and the turbulence of the perfusate to a minimum. Two ways in which this can be achieved are to use watertight incisions which do not allow leakage of fluid from the eye and also to separate the infusion system from the cutting probe.

Corneal oedema can also be due to the 'dissection' of infusion fluid into the corneal stromal lamellae. This complication can be avoided by not placing the limbal incision too anteriorly and also by ensuring that the infusion fluid is not running until the irrigating sleeve or needle is in the anterior chamber. An excessive elevation of intraocular pressure due to hanging the infusion bottle too high above the patient's eye can also cause corneal oedema. Striate keratopathy is particularly common following anterior segment CIOM procedures in eyes with traumatically ruptured lenses in which lens material and vitreous is contiguous with the corneal endothelium. Another important cause of endothelial damage is careless manoeuvring of the cutting probe in the anterior chamber.

### Wound-related complications

It is possible for vitreous or lens capsule to 'follow' the tip of the probe out of the eye and become incarcerated in the wound. If the tissue is still attached to the vitreous base, secondary traction may lead to retinal break formation. External use of the cutter at the wound lips can generally cut such strands of vitreous or capsule satisfactorily and allow them to retract into the eye. However, herniation of tissue can usually be prevented by allowing the eye to become slightly hypotonous by closing off the infusion and evacuating a small amount of fluid before withdrawing the probe.

## Lens-related complications

Lensectomy should be performed thoroughly in every instance, since retained lens material may act as a source of inflammation, leading to secondary glaucoma as well as obstructing the pupil (*Figure 16.8*). It is extremely time-consuming and dangerous to try to remove hard nuclear material with a vitreous cutter, as this will inevitably lead to damage to the iris and corneal endothelium. Another serious complication is dislocation of lens material into the vitreous cavity (*Figure 16.9a*). This can be avoided by being very careful not to damage the posterior lens capsule prematurely either with the von Graefe knife or vitreous cutter. Although the eye will usually tolerate the presence of small pieces of soft lens matter in the vitreous, large pieces of hard nucleus should be removed. This involves making two pars plana incisions and then crushing the lens material between the cutter and a

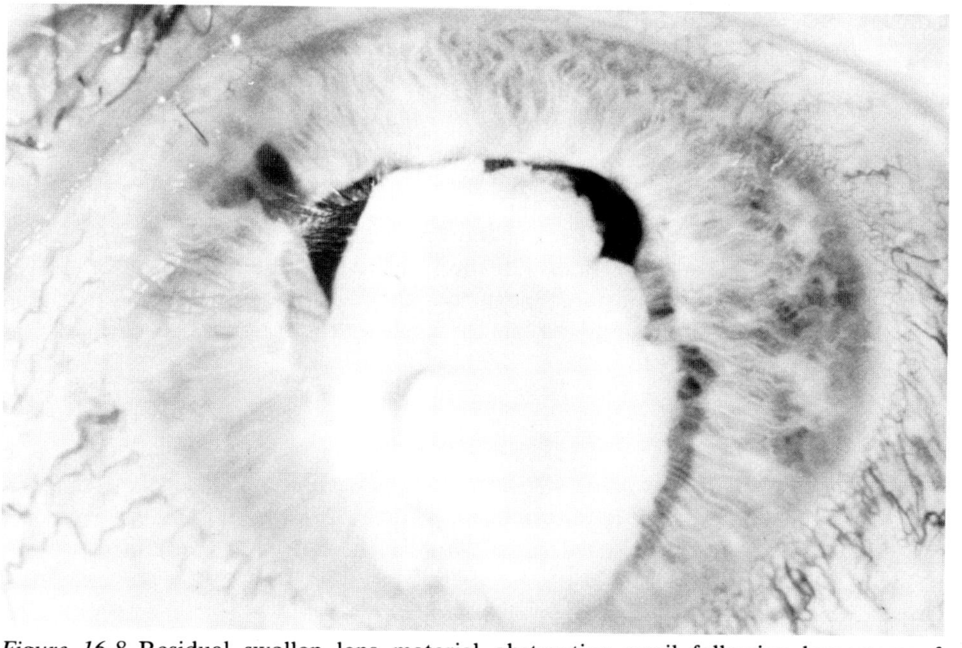

*Figure 16.8* Residual swollen lens material obstructing pupil following lensectomy for complicated cataract. In this instance a limbal incision was used with a full-function probe. In retrospect this was a poor choice, since an inadequate amount of lens material was removed

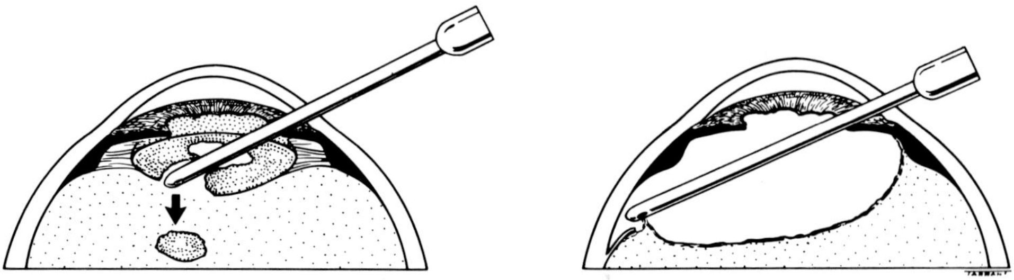

*Figure 16.9* (*Left*) Dislocation of lens material into vitreous cavity is usually caused by a premature rupture of the posterior capsule. (*Right*) The retina can be damaged by working too close to the vitreous base

22-gauge needle and forcing it into the cutting port. This should be performed in the mid-vitreous cavity so as to avoid damage to the retina (Hutton, Snyder and Vaiser, 1978).

## Retinal damage

The most feared complication is retinal detachment. This can be avoided by ensuring that the surgeon is fully aware which way the aspiration port is pointing when he is working behind the iris and not using excessive suction when working in the area of the vitreous base (*Figure 16.9b*). A key preventive measure is maximal pupillary dilatation. Currently the most popular method is to use 0.5 ml of 1:1000 cardiac adrenaline (epinephrine) without preservative* mixed with 500 ml of intraocular infusion fluid.

## Metal shavings

Uniquely related to vitreous cutters is the production of metallic 'shavings' with 'fatiguing' of the metal due to friction of the cutter within the probe's outer sleeve. Although these particles are usually inert, they may very occasionally be associated with a postoperative inflammatory reaction, making their removal desirable.

## References

Aaberg, T. M. (1977). Pars plana vitrectomy for persistent aphakic cystoid macular edema secondary to vitreous incarceration in the cataract wound. In *New and Controversial Aspects of Vitreoretinal Surgery*, edited by A. McPherson, 230–233. St Louis: C. V. Mosby

Bonnet, M. (1980). *Microsurgery of Retinal Detachment* (American adaptation by Alexander J. Brucker), 51–74. New York: Masson Publishing

* To the best of the authors' knowledge, this is available only from Parke-Davis.

Buettner, H. and Bourne, W. M. (1982). Effect of trans pars plana surgery on the corneal endothelium. In *Current Concepts in Diagnosis and Treatment of Vitreoretinal Diseases*, edited by W. Straub. *Developments in Ophthalmology*, **2**, 28–33. Basel, Switzerland: S. Karger

Diamond, J. G. and Kaplan, H. J. (1978). Lensectomy and vitrectomy for complicated cataract secondary to uveitis. *Archives of Ophthalmology*, **96**, 1798–1804

Diamond, J. G. and Kaplan, H. J. (1979). Uveitis: effect of vitrectomy combined with lensectomy. *Ophthalmology*, **86**, 1320–1327

Diddie, K. R., Wallace, D. A., Ober, R. R. and Smith, R. E. (1982). Results of anterior segment surgery with vitrectomy instruments. *American Journal of Ophthalmology*, **93**, 172–185

Federman, J. L., Annesley, W. H. Jr, Sarin, L. K. and Remer, P. (1980). Vitrectomy and cystoid macular edema. *Ophthalmology*, **87**, 622–628

Federman, J. L., Shields, J. A., Altman, B. and Koller, H. (1982). The surgical and nonsurgical management of persistent hyperplastic primary vitreous. *Ophthalmology*, **89**, 20–24

Fung, W. E. (1980). Anterior vitrectomy for chronic cystoid macular edema. *Ophthalmology*, **87**, 189–193

Harcourt, B. (1980). Cataract surgery in childhood. *Transactions of the Ophthalmological Society of the United Kingdom*, **100**, 212–215

Herschler, J. (1981). The effect of total vitrectomy on filtration surgery in the aphakic eye. *Ophthalmology*, **88**, 229–232

Hutton, W. L., Snyder, W. B. and Vaiser, A. (1978). Management of surgically dislocated intravitreal lens fragments by pars plana vitrectomy. *Ophthalmology*, **85**, 176–189

Kanski, J. J. (1978). Closed intraocular microsurgery in ocular trauma. *Transactions of the Ophthalmological Society of the United Kingdom*, **98**, 51–54

Kanski, J. J. and Crick, M. D. P. (1977a). Vitrectomy technique in anterior segment surgery. *British Journal of Ophthalmology*, **61**, 209–215

Kanski, J. J. and Crick, M. D. P. (1977b). Lensectomy. *Transactions of the Ophthalmological Society of the United Kingdom*, **97**, 52–57

Kanski, J. J. and Ramsay, J. H. (1980). Vitrectomy techniques in the management of complications in cataract surgery. *Transactions of the Ophthalmological Society of the United Kingdom*, **100**, 216–218

Leibowitz, H. M., Laing, R. A., Chang, R., Theodore, J. and Oak, S. S. (1981). Corneal edema secondary to vitreocorneal contact. *Archives of Ophthalmology*, **99**, 417–421

Mackool, R. J. (1981). Closed vitrectomy and the intraocular implant. *Ophthalmology*, **88**, 414–423

McCuen, B. W. and Fung, W. E. (1979). The role of vitrectomy instrumentation in the treatment of severe traumatic hyphaema. *American Journal of Ophthalmology*, **88**, 930–934

Michels, R. G., Machemer, R. and Mueller-Jensen, K. (1974). Vitreous surgery: history and current concepts. *Ophthalmic Surgery*, **5**, 13–59

Michels, R. G., Knox, D. L., Erozan, Y. S. and Green, W. R. (1975). Intraocular reticulum cell sarcoma. Diagnosis by pars plana vitrectomy. *Archives of Ophthalmology*, **93**, 1331–1335

Michels, R. G. and Rice, T. A. (1977). Bimanual bipolar diathermy for treatment of bleeding from the anterior chamber angle. *American Journal of Ophthalmology*, **84**, 873–874

Peyman, G. A., Raichand, M., Goldberg, M. F. and Ritacca, D. (1979). Management of subluxated and dislocated lenses with the vitrophage. *British Journal of Ophthalmology*, **63**, 771–778

Peyman, G. A., Raichand, M., Oesterle, C. and Goldberg, M. F. (1981). Pars plicata lensectomy in the management of congenital cataracts. *Ophthalmology*, **88**, 437–439

Praeger, D. L., Schneider, H. A., Sakowski, A. D. and Jacobs, J. C. (1976). Kelman procedure in the treatment of complicated cataract of the uveitis of Still's disease. *Transactions of the Ophthalmological Society of the United Kingdom*, **96**, 168–171

Rice, T. A. and Michels, R. G. (1978). Current surgical management of the vitreous wick syndrome. *American Journal of Ophthalmology*, **85**, 656–661

Slusher, M. M. (1981). Anterior segment biopsy using vitreous surgical instruments. *Ophthalmic Surgery*, **12**, 586–588

Slusher, M. M. (1982). Microsurgical management of pupillary membranes and retinal detachment. *Retina*, **2,** 80–83

Stark, W. J., Michels, R. G., Maumenee, A. E. and Cupples, H. (1978). Surgical management of epithelial ingrowth. *American Journal of Ophthalmology*, **85**, 772–780

Stern, W. H. and Mondal, K. M. (1979). Vitrectomy instrumentation for surgical evacuation of recurrent anterior-chamber hemorrhage. *Ophthalmic Surgery*, **10**, 34–38

Taylor, D. (1981). Choice of surgical technique in the management of congenital cataract. *Transactions of the Ophthalmological Society of the United Kingdom*, **101**, 114–117

Taylor, H. R., Michels, R. G. and Stark, W. J. (1979). Vitrectomy methods in anterior segment surgery. *Ophthalmic Surgery*, **10**, 25–58

Treister, G. and Machemer, R. (1978). Pars plana approach for pupillary membranes. *Archives of Ophthalmology*, **96**, 1014–1016

Van Oldenborgh, H. M. (1980). Correction of late operative complications by means of a suction cutter. *Transactions of the Ophthalmological Society of the United Kingdom*, **100**, 219–221

Wilkinson, C. P. and Rowsey, J. J. (1980). Closed vitrectomy for the vitreous touch syndrome. *American Journal of Ophthalmology*, **90**, 304–308

# 17
# Scleral buckling operations for rhegmatogenous retinal detachment

Peter H. Morse

## INTRODUCTION

Numerous scleral buckling techniques have been devised as treatment for retinal detachment (separation). One, evolved from the encircling polyethylene tube, consists of a soft silicone rubber implant or explant with encircling elements and usually drainage of subretinal fluid, and the other is a modification of the Custodis plombage, often without drainage of subretinal fluid (Schepens, Okamura and Brockhurst, 1957; Schepens *et al.*, 1960; Regan *et al.*, 1962; Lincoff, Baras and McLean, 1965). More recently, some complicated cases have been approached intraocularly by pars plana vitrectomy or injection of silicone oil.

The surgeon's preference as to the use of cryotherapy, diathermy, explant, implant, encircling elements, and drainage or non-drainage of subretinal fluid is usually immaterial as long as certain details in the examination of the patient and operation are meticulously observed. Topics which have no influence on the success or failure of the operation have been omitted from this discussion.

Prior to scleral buckling surgery, both eyes must be carefully examined for retinal breaks and predisposing vitreoretinal degeneration using the indirect opthalmoscope and scleral depressor, and the Goldmann 3-mirror lens and slit-lamp. A careful detailed drawing, not only for reference during surgery but also for case review, is advisable.

## PROPHYLAXIS

Following induction of anesthesia the entire fundus should be re-examined; the cryoprobe can be used as the scleral depressor. All retinal breaks and areas of retinal degeneration, such as lattice (palisade) and vitreoretinal traction sites in both detached and attached retina, are treated under direct ophthalmoscopic observation. Such areas, if not treated, may later lead to another detachment of the retina.

One sometimes encounters cases of subclinical retinal detachment affecting neither the visual acuity nor the visual field, yet with enough underlying subretinal fluid to make one uncertain whether or not prophylactic cryotherapy or photocoagulation will be sufficient to prevent progression (Davis, 1974). Foci of lattice degeneration with round retinal holes and subretinal fluid located inferiorly in the fundus may seem to carry a low risk, yet a certain number of these will later progress to clinical detachment of the retina in spite of prophylactic treatment. On the other hand, a tractional type of retinal break, such as a horseshoe-shaped tear with a significant amount of subretinal fluid, may not settle adequately after prophylaxis because of continuous vitreous traction upon the flap of the tear. In such cases a localized scleral buckling operation is probably the safest type of therapy.

## LOCALIZATION OF BREAKS

At operation, the posterior margin of the retinal break is localized by indenting the sclera while observing the fundus with the indirect ophthalmoscope. If there are a number of breaks at varying distances from the limbus, it is important to localize the posterior margin of the most posteriorly located retinal break. In localizing giant retinal tears one should not only mark the posterior extent but also each extremity. Following accurate localization the sclera must be marked either with diathermy, a marking pencil or a suture. The size of a retinal break can be estimated by comparing it to the ophthalmoscopically visible size of the optic nerve head, which is between 1.5 and 1.85 mm in diameter. When dealing with an isolated retinal break, one may also estimate the facility of its closure without drainage of subretinal fluid at the time of localization. If the retinal pigmented epithelium is easily approximated to the sensory retina with gentle indentation, the outcome of such a limited operation is likely to be favourable.

## SCLERAL BUCKLING

The objective of scleral buckling surgery is to place the entire retinal break on the indentation (buckle). There must be an adequate margin of the buckle of 2 mm or more anteriorly, posteriorly, and on either extremity of the retinal break. The majority of retinal detachments are most effectively treated by using material that is 5 to 7.5 mm in width, which will create an indentation extending from the ora serrata to a point 5 mm posterior to the posteriorly localized margin of the retinal break (*Figure 17.1*). Using buckling material of lesser width is usually inadequate. Whether one uses an explant (material sutured directly to the sclera), or an implant (suturing material beneath dissected lamellar scleral flaps), is unimportant. The width of the bed used to create the buckle should be 2–3 mm wider than the width of the material. The width of the bed may be increased by up to 1 mm if the substance used is quite thick. For example, when using a silicone sponge or tire 7.0–7.5 mm wide, the bed should be 10.5–11.0 mm wide, and when using 5 mm wide buckling material, the bed should be 7–8 mm wide (*Figure 17.2*). The size of the bed can be estimated by measuring the distance from a point 5 mm posterior to

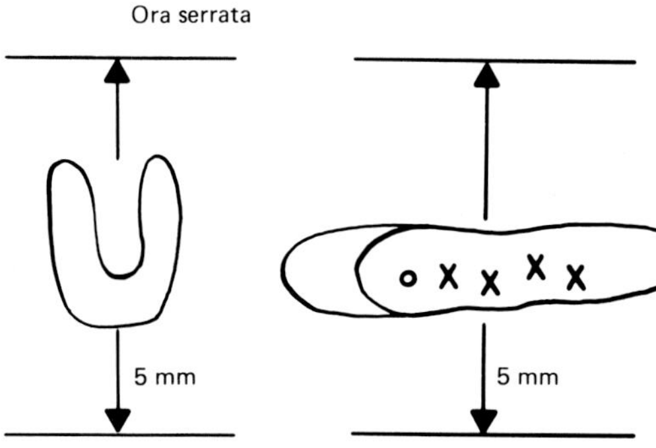


*Figure 17.1* Drawing illustrating the concept of extending the bed of the scleral buckling operation for retinal detachment from the ora serrata to a point 5 mm posterior to the localized posterior margin of a retinal break in either a horseshoe-shaped retinal tear or holes and tears associated with lattice degeneration of the retina

the posterior margin of the retinal break to the ora serrata, which is located roughly at the insertion of the rectus muscles. The bed may be created by lamellar scleral dissection over this width or by the placement of the bites of a scleral mattress suture over the same distance.

The choice of operation is often governed by the type and location of the vitreoretinal disease causing the detachment, as well as the extent of the detachment itself (Schepens, 1971, 1976). Retinal detachments with a break in only one quadrant may be treated by a localized procedure. The orientation of the buckle may be either circumferential or radial. Despite many theoretical advantages, a radial buckle offers no significant practical advantage (Lincoff and Kreissig, 1975). An anteroposterior retinal tear with a longer, thinner flap may be more effectively closed using a radially oriented buckle. A localized radially oriented posterior extension from a circumferential buckle, also known as a meridional implant, may be of use in closing a break more posteriorly than the other retinal breaks closed by the circumferential buckle, which may extend from 45 to 360 degrees.

When deciding upon the circumferential extent of the buckle, one must consider the extent or completeness of posterior vitreous detachment, the circumferential extent of the retinal detachment, the severity and extent of associated

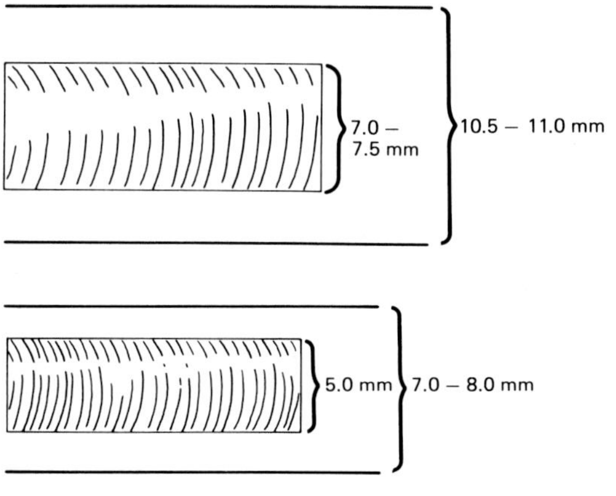


*Figure 17.2* Drawing illustrating the relationship between the size of the implant or explant and the width of the bed. For a 7–7.5 mm wide silicone sponge or tire the bed should be 10.5 –11 mm wide, and for a 5 mm wide silicone sponge the bed should be 7–8 mm wide

vitreoretinal degeneration and the amount of vitreous traction exerted on the retinal breaks. The presence of widespread vitreoretinal degeneration, multiple retinal breaks in different quadrants, as well as severe vitreoretinal traction, are indications for a greater circumferential extent of the scleral buckle. Some aphakic eyes are treated by using a greater circumferential extent of the buckle in order to relieve traction over the vitreous base. When extending the buckle circumferentially for more than 90 degrees, it is usually necessary to drain subretinal fluid in order to obtain an adequate indentation without excessive elevation of the intraocular pressure. The greater extent of the circumferential buckle compensates for the lost intraocular volume following drainage of subretinal fluid, and eliminates hypotony. Localized buckles of 45 to 90 degrees of arc will not be effective in closing retinal breaks after drainage of large volumes of subretinal fluid, as the eye will not have enough internal resistance or force to appose the sensory retina to the retinal pigmented epithelium. If one desires to use a localized buckle in such circumstances, air or other gases may be injected into the vitreous in order to restore normal intraocular pressure. Indications for 360 degree scleral buckling are total detachment without visible breaks, total detachment with breaks in all quadrants, and massive periretinal proliferation (Morse, 1977).

Not all subretinal fluid needs to be evacuated at the time of operation. However, in order to avoid postoperative reaccumulation of fluid, one should ensure that the buckle is accurately positioned to close the retinal breaks and that no large retinal folds connect the break to a significant volume of subretinal fluid posterior to the buckle (Morse, 1978). Postoperatively the position of the patient may have to be adjusted in order to avoid redetachment of the retina due to gravitational shift of the fluid to the location of the retinal breaks and buckle.

## DRAINAGE OF SUBRETINAL FLUID

Drainage of subretinal fluid remains a controversial issue (Scott, 1970; O'Connor, 1973; Freeman and Schepens, 1974; Lincoff, Kreissig and Goldbaum, 1976). Whether or not subretinal fluid is drained is determined by a number of factors and should never be a predetermined decision. One major safety factor is to avoid high intraocular pressure at the time of perforation.

Patients with viscous subretinal fluid, highly elevated (bullous) retinal detachment, posteriorly located retinal breaks, and shifting subretinal fluid are poor candidates for scleral buckling procedures without drainage of subretinal fluid. Those with breaks in the inferior quadrants of the fundus and large amounts of subretinal fluid are also poor candidates because gravity may cause subretinal fluid to keep the retina elevated above the buckle. Patients with preretinal or vitreoretinal membranes which prevent an even settling of the retina are not good candidates for non-drainage procedures and may well be considered for combined scleral buckling and vitrectomy operations. However, because careful drainage of subretinal fluid carries few risks, one should not subject a patient to postoperative bedrest and uncomfortable positioning when this may be avoided by drainage.

It must be remembered that subretinal fluid which is not drained at operation may occasionally take 72 hours or longer to be absorbed. Younger patients tend to resorb fluid more rapidly than elderly patients, but this is not invariable. Patients who have had an operation without drainage of subretinal fluid tend to have fewer folds on the buckle. In non-drainage operations there is also the reassuring knowledge that the retinal break has been successfully closed if resorption of subretinal fluid occurs within 48 hours. Continuous reaccumulation of fluid is an adverse sign.

## ENCIRCLEMENT

The routine use of encircling elements has been advocated for buckles extending over 180 degrees, and to give permanence to the buckle. They are also cited as indicated in patients with large or multiple retinal breaks, retinal detachments with extensive chorioretinal degeneration or vitreous hemorrhage; in aphakic patients with retinal detachment; for vitreous traction on the retina, fixed retinal folds, massive periretinal proliferation and thin sclera; for fellow eyes of patients with previously unsuccessfully operated retinal detachments, and in aged patients to avoid reoperation (Schepens, 1964). The author has obtained long-standing buckles and equally good results without using encircling elements. The technique consists of burying a half-thickness silicone sponge beneath lamellar scleral flaps. The same operation in terms of extent of the buckle, width of the bed, drainage or non-drainage of subretinal fluid is performed, but the encircling element is omitted (Morse, 1975). It has also been shown that permanence of a buckle is not needed for successful surgery in many cases (Dellaporta, 1970).

## INTRAVITREOUS INJECTIONS

Intravitreous injection of air or gas should be considered to counteract hypotony at the end of the operation, especially if the scleral buckle does not restore normal intraocular pressure following drainage of subretinal fluid, if there is fishmouthing of the retinal break, if large retinal folds allow communication of the retinal break with an area of subretinal fluid posterior to the buckle, in some patients with giant retinal tears, if a high buckle is undesirable, and in patients where a longer-lasting intraocular tamponade is desired (Norton, 1973; Lincoff *et al.*, 1980).

## CAUSES OF FAILURE

The only acceptable reason for failure of a scleral buckling operation is the pre- or postoperative presence of massive periretinal proliferation. New retinal breaks or redetachment of the retina may be successfully treated by reoperation. Malpositioning of the buckle or not visualizing retinal holes are faults on the part of the surgeon.

## POSTOPERATIVE MANAGEMENT

Postoperatively patients are allowed essentially full activity although they are cautioned against any activity which may cause sudden forceful or repetitive jerking of the head or body for a period of 3 to 4 weeks. Patients are discharged from hospital 1–3 days after operation, depending on their comfort and the appearance of the fundus.

## Acknowledgement

This work was supported in part by an unrestricted grant from Research to Prevent Blindness, New York.

## References

Davis, M. D. (1974). Natural history of retinal breaks. *Archives of Ophthalmology*, **92**, 183

Dellaporta, A. (1970). Experimental and clinical studies on scleral encircling operations. *Transactions of the American Ophthalmological Society*, **68**, 595

Freeman, H. M. and Schepens, C. L. (1974). Innovations in the technique for drainage of subretinal fluid: transillumination and choroidal diathermy. *Transactions of the American Academy of Ophthalmology and Otolaryngology*, **78**, 829

Lincoff, H. A., Baras, I. and McLean, J. (1965). Modifications to the Custodis procedure for retinal detachment. *Archives of Ophthalmology*, **73**, 160

Lincoff, H. and Kreissig, I. (1975). Advantages of radial buckling. *American Journal of Ophthalmology*, **79**, 955

Lincoff, H., Kreissig, i. and Goldbaum, M. (1976). Selection of patients for non-drainage operations. In *Retina Congress*, edited by R. C. Pruett and C. D. J. Regan, 397–411. New York: Appleton-Century-Crofts

Morse, P. H. (1975). Scleral buckling with soft silicone sponge and lamellar scleral dissection. *Annals of Ophthalmology*, **7**, 731

Morse, P. H. (1977). Encirclement versus 360° buckling and prognostic factors in retinal separation surgery. *Transactions of the Ophthalmological Society of the United Kingdom*, **97**, 36

Morse, P. H. (1978). Selection of type of operation for rhegmatogenous retinal detachment. *Transactions of the Ophthalmological Society of the United Kingdom*, **98**, 147

Norton, E. W. D. (1973). Intraocular gas in the management of selected retinal detachments. *Transactions of the American Academy of Ophthalmology and Otolaryngology*, **77**, 85

O'Connor, P. R. (1973). Absorption of subretinal fluid after external scleral buckling without drainage. *American Journal of Ophthalmology*, **76**, 30

Regan, C. D. J., Schepens, C. L., Okamura, I. D., Brockhurst, R. J. and McMeel, J. W. (1962). Scleral buckling procedures. VI. Further notes on silicone in primary operations. *Archives of Ophthalmology*, **68**, 313

Schepens, C. L. (1964). Scleral buckling with circling element. *Transactions of the American Academy of Ophthalmology and Otolaryngology*, **68**, 959

Schepens, C. L. (1971). Current management of retinal detachment. Progress or chaos? *Annals of Ophthalmology*, **3**, 21

Schepens, C. L. (1976). Rationale of surgical procedures. In *Retina Congress*, edited by R. C. Pruett and C. D. J. Regan, 297. New York: Appleton-Century-Crofts

Schepens, C. L., Okamura, I. D. and Brockhurst, R. J. (1957). The scleral buckling procedures. I. Surgical techniques and management. *Archives of Ophthalmology*, **58**, 797

Schepens, C. L., Okamura, I. D., Brockhurst, R. J. and Regan, C. D. J. (1960). Scleral buckling procedures. V. Synthetic sutures and silicone implants. *Archives of Ophthalmology*, **64**, 868

Scott, J. D. (1970). Retinal detachment surgery without drainage. *Transactions of the Ophthalmological Society of the United Kingdom*, **90**, 57

# Index